Fitness and Exercise
SOURCEBOOK

Volume Twenty

Fitness and Exercise SOURCEBOOK

Basic Information on Fitness and Exercise, Including Fitness Activities for Specific Age Groups, Exercise for People with Specific Medical Conditions, How to Begin a Fitness Program in Running, Walking, Swimming, Cycling, and Other Athletic Activities, and Recent Research in Fitness and Exercise.

Edited by
Dan R. Harris

Edited by Dan R. Harris

Omnigraphics, Inc.

Matthew P. Barbour, *Production Manager*
Laurie Lanzen Harris, *Vice President, Editorial*
Peter E. Ruffner, *Vice President, Administration*
James A. Sellgren, *Vice President, Operations and Finance*
Jane J. Steele, *Marketing Consultant*

Frederick G. Ruffner, Jr., *Publisher*
Copyright © 1996 Omnigraphics, Inc.

Library of Congress Cataloging-in-Publication Data

Fitness & exercise sourcebook / edited by Dan R. Harris.
    p.   cm. — (Health reference series ; v. 20)
    "Basic information on fitness and exercise, including fitness activities for specific age groups, exercise for people with specific medical conditions, how to begin a fitness program in running, walking, swimming, cycling, and other athletic activities, and recent research in fitness and exercise."
    Includes bibliographical references and index.
    ISBN 0-7808-0186-5 (lib. bdg. : alk. paper)
    1. Physical fitness—Handbooks, manuals, etc.   2. Exercise—Handbooks, manuals, etc.   I. Harris, Dan R.   II. Series.
GV436.F53 1997
613.7—dc21   96-54057
                                                                  CIP

∞

This book is printed on acid-free paper meeting the ANSI Z39.48 Standard. The infinity symbol that appears above indicates that the paper in this book meets that standard.

Printed in the United States of America

Contents

v

Part V: Recent Research in Fitness

Preface

About This Book

According to *Healthy People 2000,* released in 1990 by the U.S. Department of Health and Human Services, chronic diseases, such as diabetes, cancer and heart disease, are now the leading cause of death in the United States. Recommendations for improving the general health of the population now consistently include increased physical fitness, due to the fact that research has shown that regular physical activity helps lower blood pressure, reduces risk for diabetes, and decreases the likelihood of obesity. Yet despite these recommendation, less than one fourth of the U.S. population currently engages in light-to-moderate physical activity.

The requirements for achieving the recommended levels of physical fitness are surprisingly modest. Physical fitness is often defined as the ability to perform typical activities and chores, such as raking leaves or cleaning windows, without getting fatigued. Furthermore, the regimen usually prescribed for attaining this level of fitness calls for moderate aerobic activity, such as walking, cycling, swimming or jogging for only 20 to 30 minutes, 3 or 4 days a week.

The material collected in this volume explores the subject of physical fitness and exercise from a wide variety of perspectives. One of the common themes the reader will encounter throughout the book is the discussion of the four basic components of physical fitness: **Cardiorespiratory Endurance, Muscular Strength, Muscular**

Endurance and Flexibility. These components represent the fundamental building blocks for achieving the desired levels of physical fitness, and serve as a touchstone for understanding the various contextual issues presented in this volume.

This book contains numerous publications produced by a wide variety of government agencies, including the President's Council on Physical Fitness and Sports, the National Institutes of Health, and the Food and Drug Administration; private foundations such as The American Academy of Pediatrics, American Association of Retired Persons, American College of Sports Medicine, American Diabetes Association, American Running and Fitness Association, Arthritis Foundation, Johns Hopkins University, and the Maryland Department of Health and Mental Hygiene; consumer magazines including *American Fitness, American Health, Bicycling Magazine, Consumer Digest, Diabetes Self-Management, Fitness Swimmer, Flower & Garden, Men's Health, Parents Magazine, Prevention, Tennis Magazine, and Women's Sports and Fitness,* and various publications from Human Kinetics. The documents chosen present basic information regarding physical fitness and exercise for the interested layperson.

Physical fitness is intrinsically linked to other vital health-related concerns, such as nutrition and diet, as well as the prevention or management of major chronic medical conditions, including diabetes, cancer and heart disease. The reader is therefore encouraged to consult other related volumes in the *Health Reference Series,* including the *Diet and Nutrition Sourcebook, Respiratory Diseases and Disorders Sourcebook, Diabetes Sourcebook, Cardiovascular Diseases and Disorders Sourcebook,* the *New Cancer Sourcebook,* and *Cancer Sourcebook for Women.*

How to Use This Book

This book is organized into parts and chapters. The parts of this volume are arranged in broad topic areas. Individual chapters focus on specific areas of concern. In many cases, chapters contain several sections from a variety of reprinted documents from government and private sources. To help you quickly identify areas of interest, a "Chapter Contents" listing appears at the beginning of each chapter containing more than a single document.

Part I: *General Fitness and Exercise* contains information regarding the fundamentals of physical fitness. The chapters outline the basic definitions of physical fitness and its health benefits, provide methods for assessing fitness levels, offer advice on establishing and maintaining a long-term exercise regimen, and assess the role of physical activity in the control of body weight.

Part II: *Fitness for Specific Age Groups* discusses the role of physical activity in promoting health in children, teens, middle-aged, and older persons. Also included are materials that explore the link between physical fitness and intellectual development, the influence of nutrition on sports performance, safety considerations for youth sports, and advice on assessing local school physical education programs.

Part III: *Exercise and Specific Medical Conditions* provides information regarding the role of physical activity in the management of chronic medical conditions such as arthritis, diabetes and heart disease. Additionally, advice on maintaining physical activity for people with asthma and people with hip replacements is included. Materials are also included that explore the effects of exercise on pregnancy and mental health.

Part IV: *Specific Activities* provides information and advice for a wide variety of sports and activities. Also, qualification criteria for the Presidential Sports Award are included, as well as information regarding footwear, home fitness equipment and health spas.

Part V: *Recent Research in Fitness* comprises a number of research abstracts published by the President's Council on Physical Fitness and Sports, that survey the latest understanding on the role of physical fitness on a broad range of health topics.

Acknowledgements

The editor wishes to thank the organizations that generously provided much of the information included in this volume free of charge: the American Association of Retired Persons, American College of Sports Medicine, American Diabetes Association, *Diabetes Self-Management Magazine, Fitness Swimmer Magazine,* and the Maryland Department of Health and Mental Hygiene. Additionally, the diligent research efforts of Margaret Mary Missar, and valuable assistance from Jeanne Gough in obtaining reprint permissions for the coyrighted material used in this book are gratefully acknowledged.

Bibliographic Note

This volume contains individual publications issued by the President's Council on Physical Fitness and Sports, many of them unnumbered. Numbered publications from this category are OM 85-0053, OM 87-0063, and GPO: 1994-155-072; as well as Series 1 and 2 of the *Physical Activity and Fitness Research Digest* (Feb. 1993-Sept., 1995). Also included are publications from the U.S. Department of Health and Human Services. Numbered publications from this category are NIH Publication No. 93-1677, and DHHS Publication No. (ADM) 84-1364. Material from *FDA Consumer* is also included. Additionally, this volume includes many copyrighted articles and publications from various foundations and consumer magazine publications. These sources are as follows: American Academy of Pediatrics, HE0090; American Association of Retired Persons, PF 3248(1193) D549; American College of Sports Medicine, 6083-86, 6083-87, 6083-88 6083-89 6083-90 6085-42, 6085-43, and additional unnumbered publications; American Diabetes Association, *Diabetes Day-by-Day* series, Nos. 8, 9, *Diabetes Forecast* magazine, Jan. 1990, Jan. 1992; *American Fitness*, Nov./Dec. 1995; *American Health*, August, 1993, March 1994, June, 1995; American Running and Fitness Association, unnumbered; Arthritis Foundation, 9704/6-95; *Bicycling*, Jan. 1996; *Consumers Digest*, Nov./Dec. 1994; *Diabetes Self-Management*, March 1992, May/June 1992; *Fitness Swimmer*, Dec. 1992, March 1993, Dec. 1993; *Flower & Garden*, June/July 1993; *Fitness Cycling*, Human Kinetics; *Johns Hopkins Medical Letter*, Aug. 1995; Maryland Department of Health and Mental Hygiene, GPO: 1993 0-150-565 (QL 3); *Men's Health*, Sept. 1994; *Parents Magazine*, July 1994, Oct. 1994; *Prevention*, Feb. 1996; *Tennis*, May 1992; *Women's Sports and Fitness*, Nov./Dec. 1993. These are used by permission. Every effort has been made to obtain the appropriate permissions to reprint the above copyrighted material. Any omissions will be corrected in subsequent editions.

Note from the Editor

This book is part of Omnigraphics' *Health Reference Series*. The series provides basic information about a broad range of medical concerns. It is not intended to serve as a tool for diagnosing illness, in prescribing treatments, or as a substitute for the physician/patient relationship. All persons concerned about medical symptoms or the possibility of disease are encouraged to seek professional care from an appropriate health care provider.

Because exercise is an important part of managing the symptoms of diabetes, the American Diabetes Association devotes a considerable amount of its resources to providing information regarding physical fitness activities. Much of this material represents some of the best available introductory information for various physical activities. For this reason, the chapters regarding cross-country skiing and weight training are included in this volume, and intended for all readers, even though these chapters contain some information specific to people with diabetes.

Part One

General Fitness and Exercise

Chapter 1

Fitness Fundamentals: Guidelines for Personal Exercise Programs

Making a Commitment

You have taken the important first step on the path to physical fitness by seeking information. The next step is to decide that you are going to be physically fit. This chapter is designed to help you reach that decision and your goal.

The decision to carry out a physical fitness program cannot be taken lightly. It requires a lifelong commitment of time and effort. Exercise must become one of those things that you do without question, like bathing and brushing your teeth. Unless you are convinced of the benefits of fitness and the risks of unfitness. you will not succeed.

Patience is essential. Don't try to do too much too soon and don't quit before you have a chance to experience the rewards of improved fitness. You can't regain in a few days or weeks what you have lost in years of sedentary living, but you can get it back if you persevere. And the prize is worth the price.

In the following pages you will find the basic information you need to begin and maintain a personal physical fitness program. These guidelines are intended for the average healthy adult. It tells you what your goals should be and how often, how long and how hard you must exercise to achieve them. It also includes information that will make your workouts easier, safer and more satisfying. The rest is up to you.

U.S. Government Printing Office: 1990-279-047-814/21139

Checking Your Health

If you're under 35 and in good health, you don't need to see a doctor before beginning an exercise program. But if you are over 35 and have been inactive for several years, you should consult your physician, who may or may not recommend a graded exercise test. Other conditions that indicate a need for medical clearance are:

- High blood pressure

- Heart trouble

- Family history of early stroke or heart attack deaths

- Frequent dizzy spells

- Extreme breathlessness after mild exertion

- Arthritis or other bone problems

- Severe muscular, ligament or tendon problems

- Other known or suspected disease

Vigorous exercise involves minimal health risks for persons in good health or those following a doctor's advice. Far greater risks are presented by habitual inactivity and obesity.

Defining Fitness

Physical fitness is to the human body what fine tuning is to an engine. It enables us to perform up to our potential. Fitness can be described as a condition that helps us look, feel and do our best. More specifically, it is:

> "The ability to perform daily tasks vigorously and alertly, with energy left over for enjoying leisure-time activities and meeting emergency demands. It is the ability to endure, to bear up, to withstand stress, to carry on in circumstances where an unfit person could not continue, and is a major basis for good health and well-being."

Physical fitness involves the performance of the heart and lungs, and the muscles of the body. And, since what we do with our bodies also affects what we can do with our minds, fitness influences to some degree qualities such as mental alertness and emotional stability.

As you undertake your fitness program, it's important to remember that fitness is an individual quality that varies from person to person. It is influenced by age, sex, heredity, personal habits, exercise and eating practices. You can't do anything about the first three factors. However, it is within your power to change and improve the others where needed.

Knowing the Basics

Physical fitness is most easily understood by examining its components, or "parts." There is widespread agreement that these four components are basic:

Cardiorespiratory Endurance—the ability to deliver oxygen and nutrients to tissues, and to remove wastes, over sustained periods of time. Long runs and swims are among the methods employed in measuring this component.

Muscular Strength—the ability of a muscle to exert force for a brief period of time. Upper-body strength, for example, can be measured by various weight-lifting exercises.

Muscular Endurance—the ability of a muscle, or a group of muscles, to sustain repeated contractions or to continue applying force against a fixed object. Pushups are often used to test endurance of arm and shoulder muscles.

Flexibility—the ability to move joints and use muscles through their full range of motion. The sit-and-reach test is a good measure of flexibility of the lower back and backs of the upper legs.

Body Composition is often considered a component of fitness. it refers to the makeup of the body in terms of lean mass (muscle, bone, vital tissue and organs) and fat mass. An optimal ratio of fat to lean mass is an indication of fitness, and the right types of exercises will help you decrease body fat and increase or maintain muscle mass.

A Workout Schedule

How often, how long and how hard you exercise, and what kinds of exercises you do should be determined by what you are trying to accomplish. Your goals, your present fitness level, age, health, skills, interest and convenience are among the factors you should consider. For example, an athlete training for high-level competition would follow a different program than a person whose goals are good health and the ability to meet work and recreational needs.

Your exercise program should include something from each of the four basic fitness components described previously. Each workout should begin with a warmup and end with a cooldown. As a general rule, space your workouts throughout the week and avoid consecutive days of hard exercise.

Here are the amounts of activity necessary for the average, healthy person to maintain a minimum level of overall fitness. Included are some of the popular exercises for each category.

Warmup—5-10 minutes of exercises such as walking, slow jogging, knee lifts, arm circles or trunk rotations. Low intensity movements that simulate movements to be used in the activity can also be included in the warmup.

Muscular Strength—a minimum of two 20-minute sessions per week that include exercises for all the major muscle groups. Lifting weights is the most effective way to increase strength.

Muscular Endurance—at least three 30-minute sessions each week that include exercises such as calisthenics, pushups, situps, pullups, and weight training for all the major muscle groups.

Cardiorespiratory Endurance—at least three 20-minute bouts of continuous aerobic (activity requiring oxygen) rhythmic exercise each week. Popular aerobic conditioning activities include brisk walking, jogging, swimming, cycling, rope-jumping, rowing, cross-country skiing. and some continuous action games like racquetball and handball.

Flexibility—0-12 minutes of daily stretching exercises performed slowly, without a bouncing motion. This can be included after a warmup or during a cooldown.

Cool Down—a minimum of 5-10 minutes of slow walking, low-level exercise, combined with stretching.

A Matter Of Principle

The keys to selecting the right kinds of exercises for developing and maintaining each of the basic components of fitness are found in these principles:

Specificity—pick the right kind of activities to affect each component. Strength training results in specific strength changes. Also, train for the specific activity you're interested in. For example, optimal swimming performance is best achieved when the muscles involved in swimming are trained for the movements required. It does not necessarily follow that a good runner is a good swimmer.

Overload—work hard enough, at levels that are vigorous and long enough to overload your body above its resting level, to bring about improvement.

Regularity—you can't hoard physical fitness. At least three balanced workouts a week are necessary to maintain a desirable level of fitness.

Progression—increase the intensity, frequency and/or duration of activity over periods of time in order to improve.

Some activities can be used to fulfill more than one of your basic exercise requirements. For example, in addition to increasing cardiorespiratory endurance, running builds muscular endurance in the legs, and swimming develops the arm, shoulder and chest muscles. If you select the proper activities, it is possible to fit parts of your muscular endurance workout into your cardiorespiratory workout and save time.

Measuring Your Heart Rate

Heart rate is widely accepted as a good method for measuring intensity during running, swimming, cycling and other aerobic activities. Exercise that doesn't raise your heart rate to a certain level and keep it there for 20 minutes won't contribute significantly to cardiovascular fitness.

The heart rate you should maintain is called your **target heart rate**. There are several ways of arriving at this figure. One of the sim-

7

plest is: **maximum heart rate** (220 - age) x 70%. Thus, the target heart rate for a 40 year-old would be 126.

Some methods for figuring the target rate take individual differences into consideration. Here is one of them:

1. Subtract age from 220 to find **maximum heart rate**.

2. Subtract resting heart rate (see below) from maximum heart rate to determine heart rate reserve.

3. Take 70% of heart rate reserve to determine heart rate raise.

4. Add heart rate raise to resting heart rate to find target rate.

Resting heart rate should be determined by taking your pulse after sitting quietly for five minutes. When checking heart rate during a workout, take your pulse within five seconds after interrupting exercise because it starts to go down once you stop moving. Count pulse for 10 seconds and multiply by six to get the per-minute rate.

Controlling Your Weight

The key to weight control is keeping energy intake (food) and energy output (physical activity) in balance. When you consume only as many calories as your body needs, your weight will usually remain constant. If you take in more calories than your body needs, you will put on excess fat. If you expend more energy than you take in you will burn excess fat.

Exercise plays an important role in weight control by increasing energy output, calling on stored calories for extra fuel. Recent studies show that not only does exercise increase metabolism during a workout, but it causes your metabolism to stay increased for a period of time after exercising, allowing you to burn more calories.

How much exercise is needed to make a difference in your weight depends on the amount and type of activity, and on how much you eat. Aerobic exercise burns body fat. A medium-sized adult would have to walk more than 30 miles to burn up 3,500 calories, the equivalent of one pound of fat. Although that may seem like a lot, you don't have to walk the 30 miles all at once. Walking a mile a day for 30 days will achieve the same result, providing you don't increase your food intake to negate the effects of walking.

If you consume 100 calories a day more than your body needs, you will gain approximately 10 pounds in a year. You could take that weight off, or keep it off, by doing 30 minutes of moderate exercise daily. The combination of exercise and diet offers the most flexible and effective approach to weight control.

Since muscle tissue weighs more than fat tissue, and exercise develops muscle to a certain degree, your bathroom scale won't necessarily tell you whether or not you are "fat." Well-muscled individuals, with relatively little body fat, invariably are "overweight" according to standard weight charts. If you are doing a regular program of strength training, your muscles will increase in weight, and possibly your overall weight will increase. Body composition is a better indicator of your condition than body weight.

Lack of physical activity causes muscles to get soft, and if food intake is not decreased, added body weight is almost always fat. Once-active people, who continue to eat as they always have after settling into sedentary lifestyles, tend to suffer from "creeping obesity."

Clothing

All exercise clothing should be loose-fitting to permit freedom of movement, and should make the wearer feel comfortable and self-assured.

As a general rule, you should wear lighter clothes than temperatures might indicate. Exercise generates great amounts of body heat. Light-colored clothing that reflects the sun's rays is cooler in the summer, and dark clothes are warmer in winter. When the weather is very cold, it's better to wear several layers of light clothing than one or two heavy layers. The extra layers help trap heat, and it's easy to shed one of them if you become too warm.

In cold weather, and in hot, sunny weather, it's a good idea to wear something on your head. Wool watch or ski caps are recommended for winter wear, and some form of tennis or sailor's hat that provides shade and can be soaked in water is good for summer.

Never wear rubberized or plastic clothing. Such garments interfere with the evaporation of perspiration and can cause body temperature to rise to dangerous levels.

The most important item of equipment for the runner is a pair of sturdy, properly-fitting running shoes. Training shoes with heavy, cushioned soles and arch supports are preferable to flimsy sneakers and light racing flats.

When to Exercise

The hour just before the evening meal is a popular time for exercise. The late afternoon workout provides a welcome change of pace at the end of the work day and helps dissolve the day's worries and tensions.

Another popular time to work out is early morning, before the work day begins. Advocates of the early start say it makes them more alert and energetic on the job.

Among the factors you should consider in developing your workout schedule are personal preference, job and family responsibilities, availability of exercise facilities and weather. It's important to schedule your workouts for a time when there is little chance that you will have to cancel or interrupt them because of other demands on your time.

You should not exercise strenuously during extremely hot, humid weather or within two hours after eating. Heat and/or digestion both make heavy demands on the circulatory system, and in combination with exercise can be an overtaxing double load.

Chapter 2

How Fit are You?

By Susan Rees

By now you know that regular exercise is essential to health and well-being. But are you sure your regimen is giving you results? Fitness tests of aerobic endurance, strength, body composition and flexibility can help you zero in on where you're succeeding and where you're falling short.

The latest state-of-the-art evaluations bear little resemblance to those humiliating tests you suffered through in gym class. They range from plunges into tanks of water (to measure your body fat) to simple sit-and-reach flexibility tests.

The question is, is testing necessary? Isn't it enough to do the requisite 20 minutes of aerobic activity three times a week and hope for the best? "Certain fitness glitches tend to crop up during testing," says Stu Mittleman, director of the physiology lab at Equinox Fitness Club in New York City. Some classic examples: the muscle-bound jock who is easily winded, the marathoner who has strong aerobic power but can't touch her toes, or the weekend warrior who logs hours on the stair machine but lacks muscle definition.

"Fitness evaluations let us see which activities are doing the trick and which aren't, so we can restructure a client' s program if necessary," says Mittleman. Essentially, they take the guesswork out of working out. They can also steer a beginner toward a regimen that suits his ability.

American Health, March 1994

Until recently, fitness tests with all the high-tech bells and whistles have been the province of elite athletes, available only at university exercise physiology labs, at pulmonary rehabilitation facilities or in physical therapists' offices. Now a growing number of health clubs are making them available to ordinary exercisers. Equinox, for instance, offers a comprehensive fitness assessment that costs $125 for members and $265 for nonmembers. Among other things you'll get a rating of your VO₂ *max* (the amount of oxygen you consume during exercise) and your resting metabolic rate, which lets you know how many calories you burn while channel surfing from the couch.

Attaching yourself to a machine to gauge your overall fitness is certainly not mandatory, but testing its components—endurance, strength, body composition and flexibility—can help athletes and ordinary exercisers alike. The VO₂ *max* test, for instance, is good for anyone who wants to improve his cardiovascular capacity, such as first-time exercisers and casual athletes with a yen to run a 10K. "VO₂ *max* tells you your true cardiovascular capacity, maximum heart rate and training range," says Dawn James, health fitness director at Wenmat Sports and Fitness in Sacramento, Calif. "It provides a great baseline measurement."

To find your VO₂ *max*, you run on a treadmill or ride a stationary bike while exhaling into a tube connected to a machine that measures expired gases. The average college-aged man, for instance, uses a bit more than 40 milliliters (ml) of oxygen per kilogram (kg) of body weight. By comparison, top distance runners use 75 ml to 80 ml. The higher the number, the better your aerobic fitness. And the fitter you are, the more efficiently your body transports oxygen in the blood to hard-working muscles.

Body composition testing is also gaining popularity among weekend athletes. The *crème de la crème* of body-fat tests is dual photon x-ray absorptometry. A highly accurate, total-body scan, it calculates fat-to-muscle ratio as well as the mineral content of the entire body, a plus for women worried about osteoporosis.

Top-flight athletes use fitness testing to forecast how they'll perform in competition. At the U.S. Olympic Training Center in Colorado Springs, Colo., Carl Lewis wanna-be's can undergo the Wingate test of anaerobic capacity to assess their training program. (During activities like sprints, which require short, intense bursts of energy, the body fuels itself anaerobically—literally, without oxygen—using energy stored inside the muscles.) Sprinters pedal a stationary bike as hard as possible for 30 seconds, then get a reading of their power output. If necessary, training tactics will be altered to improve the numbers. A Wingate evaluation also makes sense for tennis players, cyclists and other athletes who rely on sudden bursts of speed.

For most people, however, the less medical— and less expensive— tests offered at health clubs work just fine. Be sure that whoever administers them is certified by an organization such as the American College of Sports Medicine. At Western Athletic Clubs in San Francisco, Sandy Minor, director of fitness operations, puts members through stretches to evaluate their range of motion, an abdominal crunch and pushup test to gauge muscular endurance, a body composition test with skin-fold calipers, and a bicycle or treadmill test of aerobic capacity.

The good news for the vast majority of Americans who aren't health club members is that many of these tests can be taken at home (see "Test Yourself," below). But since the average person lacks the knowledge of a trained exercise physiologist, self-tests are bound to be less accurate than those done at a fitness facility. And the standards against which your results are measured are estimates. But at-home tests are still useful, whether you're wondering if your regimen is actually improving your fitness or you're looking for an incentive to get active, perhaps for the first time in your life.

"Most people have some idea of their weaknesses—say, if they can't walk up a flight of stairs without gasping for breath," says Minor. "But having actual numbers gives you a starting point, so you can see your improvement in a tangible way."

Self-tests can also give you the information you need to tailor your regimen more specifically. If you discover that your cardiovascular endurance isn't up to par but your upper body strength is well above average, you obviously should do more aerobic activity. Don't become a slave to the numbers, however. "We have clients who get their body fat measured and then come back once a month for retesting," says James. "They expect immediate results, but significant changes take time."

In fact, some luxury clubs have shunned the numbers game altogether. Instead of taking the pulse of her clients, Laurie Cingle, director of health and fitness at the Houstonian Club in Houston. has them rate how hard they're working on a "perceived exertion scale" of zero to 10, based on how they're feeling. "If you're red in the face, nauseated and panting that's a 'nine,'" says Cingle, "a good sign you're working too hard!" For some of us, then, the only fitness test required may be tuning into our bodies. As Cingle puts it, "If people feel good and can get through the day without feeling sluggish, that's assessment enough."

Test Yourself

The following self-tests measure cardiovascular endurance, strength, flexibility and body composition, the primary components of fitness. To see whether you're improving, do the tests every three to six months; be sure to do them the same way every time, to reduce the possibility of error. If you've been sedentary or have a history of heart disease, diabetes or other health problems, see a doctor before self-testing or starting an exercise program.

Three-Minute Step Test

This measures your immediate postworkout heart rate, which is a rough estimate of your VO_2 *max*, or how much oxygen you consume during exercise. What you'll need: a 12-inch bench or stair, a metronome to set the pace, and a timer, a stopwatch or a watch with a second hand. What to do:

1. Set the metronome at 96 beats per minute and the timer for three minutes.

2. Start the metronome and the timer. Keeping pace with the metronome, step up on the bench with your left foot and right foot, respectively, then step down on the floor, left foot first, then the right one. Keep going until the time is up.

3. Sit down quickly and take your pulse for one minute.

4. Compare your heart rate with the YMCA standardized norms on p. 17 (numbers indicate beats per minute).

One-Minute Pushup Test

This measures your upper body endurance. What you'll need: a timer, a stopwatch or a watch with a second hand. What to do:

1. Warm up with the following stretches.

    Doorway stretch: Stand in a doorway and place your right forearm against the outside of the door-frame. Twist your body away from your forearm until you feel a stretch; hold for 30 seconds. Switch sides and repeat.

    Shoulder stretch: Standing erect, place your left hand on your right shoulder. Gently cup your left elbow with your right hand and bring it as far across your chest as possible, holding the stretch for 30 seconds. Switch sides and repeat.

Triceps stretch: Standing erect, place your right hand behind your head and point your elbow toward the ceiling. Cup your right elbow with your left hand and press down gently to extend the stretch. Hold for 30 seconds; switch sides and repeat.

2. Set the timer for one minute.

3. Get into the pushup position, resting your weight on your knees, of you're a beginner or your toes if you're more advanced. Keep your hands directly under your shoulders and your fingers facing forward.

4. Start the timer. Keeping your back straight, lower your chest almost to the floor, then push yourself up. continue lowering and pushing up, remembering to breathe and to count the number of repetitions, until one minute is up.

5. Compare the number of pushups you can do with the American College of Sports Medicine (ACSM) standardized norms on p. 18, reprinted from the *ACSM Fitness Book* (Leisure Press, 1992).

One-Minute Sit-Up Test

This test measures your abdominal and hip flexor muscular endurance, which correlates loosely with your total-body muscular endurance. What you'll need: an exercise mat and a timer, a stopwatch or a watch with a second hand. What to do:

1. Set the timer for one minute.

2. Lie on your back on the mat with your knees bent, your feet flat on the floor and your arms folded across your chest.

3. Start the timer. Do as many sit-ups as you can for one minute, alternately touching one elbow to the diagonally opposite knee for each repetition. Your shoulders should touch the mat each time you come down.

4. Compare the number of sit-ups you can do with the YMCA standardized norms on p. 19.

Sit-and-Reach Test

1. This test measures your lower back and hamstring flexibility, which loosely correlates with your total-body flexibility. What you'll need: a yardstick and masking tape. What to do:

2. Tape the yardstick to the ground with the zero mark closest to you. Tape the stick at the 15-inch mark; the tape should be perpendicular to the stick.

3. Sit with the yardstick between your legs and your heels even with the 15-inch mark. Your feet should be 10 to 12 inches apart.

4. Slowly reach forward and down with both hands, exhaling and dropping your head to extend the stretch as far as possible. Don't lead with one hand or bend your knees. Note the farthest point you can reach on the stick with your fingertips. Repeat two more times. 4. Compare your best score to the ACSM standardized norms on p. 20 (numbers given are in inches).

Body-Fat Risk Test

People who carry excess weight around their waist have a greater incidence of heart disease than those who accumulate flab on their hips and thighs. This test gauges your waist-to-hip ratio, one indication of whether your figure is putting you at risk. What you'll need: a tape measure and a calculator. What to do:

1. Measure your waist and your hips at their widest point.

2. Divide your waist measurement by your hip measurement.

For men, the result should be no greater than one; for women, it should be no greater than .8 or .85.

What your score means: If your waist-to-hip ratio is in the unhealthy range, lower your dietary fat intake and step up exercise. As a general rule, walking or running one mile burns 100 calories; strength training will help boost your metabolism so that you burn more calories throughout the day.

Sizing Up Your Numbers

Three-Minute Step Test

MEN

Ages	18-25	26-35	36-45	46-55	56-65	66+
Excellent	70-78	73-79	72-81	78-84	72-82	72-86
Good	82-88	83-88	86-94	89-96	89-97	89-95
Above average	91-97	91-97	98-102	99-103	98-101	97-102
Average	101-104	101-106	105-111	109-115	105-111	104-113
Below average	107-114	109-116	113-118	118-121	113-118	114-119
Poor	118-126	119-126	120-128	124-130	122-128	122-128
Very Poor	131-164	130-164	132-168	135-158	131-150	133-152

WOMEN

Ages	18-25	26-35	36-45	46-55	56-65	66+
Excellent	72-83	72-86	74-87	76-93	74-92	73-86
Good	88-97	94-97	93-101	96-102	97-103	93-100
Above average	100-106	103-110	104-109	106-113	106-111	104-114
Average	110-116	112-118	111-117	117-120	113-117	117-121
Below average	118-124	121-127	120-127	121-126	119-127	123-127
Poor	128-137	129-135	130-138	127-133	129-136	129-134
Very Poor	142-155	141-154	143-152	138-152	142-151	135-151

What your score means: If your cardiovascular fitness is no better than below average, do some type of aerobic exercise three to five times a week for 15 to 60 minutes at a time. Work at 55% to 90% of your maximum heart rate, which is roughly 220 minus your age multiplied by .55 and .9.

One-Minute Pushup Test

MEN

Ages	20-29	30-39	40-49	50-59	60+
High	45+	35+	30+	25+	20+
Average	35-44	25-34	20-29	15-24	10-19
Below Average	20-34	15-24	12-19	8-14	5-9
Low	<19	<14	<11	<7	<4

WOMEN

Ages	20-29-	30-39	40-49	50-59	60+
High	34+	25+	20+	15+	5+
Average	17-33	12-24	8-19	6-14	3-4
Below Average	6-16	4-11	3-7	1-5	1-2
Low	<5	<3	<2	0	0

What your score means: If your upper body muscular endurance is low or below average, do 10 to 15 repetitions each of exercises that target the chest and the triceps muscles, two to three times a week. Try pushups and triceps dips at home, or the chest press and the triceps extension machines at the gym.

One Minute Sit-Up Test

MEN

Ages	18-25	26-35	36-45	46-55	56-65	66+
Excellent	50-60	46-55	42-50	36-50	56-65	29-40
Good	45-48	41-45	36-40	29-33	26-29	22-26
Above average	40-42	36-38	30-34	25-28	21-24	20-21
Average	36-38	32-34	28-29	22-24	17-20	16-18
Below average	32-34	29-30	24-26	18-21	13-16	12-14
Poor	26-30	24-28	18-22	13-17	9-12	8-10
Very Poor	12-24	6-21	4-16	4-12	2-8	2-6

WOMEN

Ages	18-25	26-35	36-45	46-55	56-65	66+
Excellent	44-55	40-54	34-50	28-42	25-38	24-36
Good	37-41	33-37	27-30	22-25	18-21	18-22
Above average	33-36	29-32	24-26	18-21	13-17	14-16
Average	29-32	25-28	20-22	14-17	10-12	11-13
Below average	25-28	21-24	16-18	10-13	7-9	6-10
Poor	20-24	16-20	10-14	6-9	4-6	2-4
Very Poor	4-17	1-12	1-6	0-4	0-2	0-1

What your score means: If your muscular endurance is no better than below average, do 10 to 15 repetitions each of moves that work the abdominals—such as crunches—two to three times a week. Do lunges and squats for the lower body, or try the leg press and leg curl machines at the gym.

Sit-and-Reach Test

MEN

Ages	20-29	30-39	40-49	50-59	60+
High	19+	18+	17+	16+	15+
Average	13-18	12-17	11-16	10-15	9-14
Below Average	10-12	9-11	8-10	7-9	6-8
Low	9	8	7	6	5

WOMEN

Ages	20-29	30-39	40-49	50-59	60+
High	22+	21+	20+	19+	18+
Average	16-21	15-20	14-19	13-18	12-17
Below Average	13-15	12-14	11-13	10-12	9-11
Low	12	11	10	9	8

What your score means: If your flexibility is no better than below average, set aside 10 to 15 minutes at the end of your workout to stretch your major muscle groups. (It's best to stretch *after* you've exercised, when your muscles are already warm and pliable.) Shoulder rolls, hamstring stretches and lunges are good ones to try.

Chapter 3

Getting Fit Your Way: A Self-Paced Fitness Guide

Introduction

Exercise Has a Lot to Offer

Many individuals have set exercise goals, done what they intended, and have gotten results—results such. as having their bodies become firmer, having more energy to do the things they enjoy, and being more mentally alert. By being successful, they feel more in command of their lives. They have proven that they can set a goal and succeed.

You may be just starting regular exercise, or you may have been exercising, but need to do more. Perhaps you have tried exercising but have stopped. Exercising regularly is not easy.

This chapter will show you how to prepare for a strong start. It will help you to avoid the pitfalls along the way and keep your exercise program going strong. It will also show you how to make exercise a part of your daily routine that you can live with.

The only way to get the important benefits of exercise is to exercise at least three times a week. You may think that you are already in good shape because you played sports in school, or because you exercise on weekends, or because you are young and slim.

You may not be as fit as you think. Why not check it out. Turn to **Stage 1: Two Weeks for Making a Winning Game Plan** (see be-

---

Maryland Department of Health and Mental Hygiene. Used by permission.

low) to see how fit you really are. Maybe a few small changes in your current exercise will make a difference in how you feel.

You may want to excuse yourself from regular, vigorous exercise because you smoke cigarettes or you are overweight. While exercise may be a little harder if you smoke or are overweight, you can still exercise and receive the benefits. In fact, for many people, exercise has been a good first step to losing weight or kicking the smoking habit.

Whoever you are, this booklet can help you build an exercise routine that you can do to help you look and feel your best. It will show you how to be successful and make your efforts really count. But the booklet can not do it for you.

It Takes Effort on Your Part

This chapter is about exercising your heart and building stamina. Exercising your heart will give you benefits, such as having more energy and a feeling of being in charge of your life.

Exercise and a strong heart have a lot to offer you, but you will have to do some work to get the benefits. During the first few weeks of the program, you will have to do more exercise than probably you are used to. Then, once your program is started, you will need to keep it going by exercising every week. But you do not have to be superhuman to do regular, vigorous exercise. All you have to do is give it a good, solid try. *Getting Fit Your Way* will show you how to make that try go a long way towards success.

Quick Checklist

Exercise is a safe activity for most people. Some people, however, should see a doctor before starting an exercise program. To decide if you are one of those people, take a few minutes to check any of the following statements that are true for you. Do this even if you think you are healthy, and if you already exercise. It is very important.

❑   Your doctor said you have heart trouble or a heart murmur.

❑   You have had a heart attack.

❑   You often have pains or pressure in the left or mid-chest area, left neck, shoulder, or arm, during or right after you exercise.

❑   You frequently feel faint or have spells of severe dizziness.

❑   You experience extreme breathlessness after mild exertion.

❑   Your doctor has said your blood pressure was too high and is not under control.

❑   You do not know whether or not your blood pressure is normal.

❑   Your doctor has said that you have bone or joint problems, such as arthritis.

❑   You are over 50 and not used to vigorous exercise.

❑   You have a family history of premature coronary artery disease.

❑   You have a medical condition, not mentioned here, which might need special attention in an exercise program (for example, insulin-dependent diabetes).

If you did not check any of the above statements, go to Stage 1 and start planning your own successful exercise program.

If you checked one or more of the above statements, see your doctor before starting to exercise. The chances are good that you will be able to begin exercising, but your doctor can help you get started safely.

If you have not completed the above checklist. . . STOP. Take five minutes and do it now. It is important.

Stage 1: Two Weeks for Making a Winning Game Plan

After using the checklist to make sure that exercise is safe for you, begin the two weeks of Stage 1. *Stage 1 is your chance to organize and prepare your winning game plan for exercise.* After learning the three exercise guidelines, you will be making decisions about which exercises are right for you, when you want to do them, and how to fit them into your normal, daily routine. Then, after thinking it over, you will be asked to make a commitment to exercise for three weeks.

You may be tempted to skip Stage 1 and start exercising right away. This is not a good idea. To get the full benefit of exercise, you have to exercise regularly. Exercising regularly is easier when it becomes an accepted part of your regular schedule. That way, you do not have to make a decision each time. It becomes a habit, like brushing your teeth. So do not take a chance on wasting your valuable time and energy by starting off on the wrong foot. Just as a good carpenter measures before he cuts, be sure you plan before you start your exercise program.

Exercising Your Heart

Your heart is a muscle just like an arm or a leg muscle. And, just like arm and leg muscles, your heart needs to exercise to be strong and work at its best. When you exercise your arm and leg muscles, they get stronger and, perhaps, bigger. When you exercise your heart, its new strength pumps more blood through your body with less effort. A stronger heart can help you wake up rested, looking forward to your day. It can also give you more energy.

Exercising your heart is simple. All it takes is moving your body until your heart beats faster than it does normally. But there is a little more to helping your heart get stronger and do its best than just that. There are three guidelines that your exercise must meet to give your heart enough and the right kind of exercise:

---

3   You need to exercise (get your heart to beat faster) a minimum of three times a week with no more than two days of rest between exercise sessions.

ZONE   You need to have your heart rate in your ZONE.

20   You need to have your heart rate in your ZONE a minimum of twenty minutes straight.

Together, these three guidelines for exercising your heart are called 3 ZONE 20: exercising three times a week with your heart rate in your ZONE for at least twenty minutes. These guidelines represent the minimum. You have to do at least this much to exercise your heart and to look and feel your best.

You do not have to do any more than this. 3 ZONE 20 exercise will give you a good level of fitness. You do not have to swim across an ocean or run a marathon to get the full benefits from your exercise. Each of these guidelines will be explained more fully later.

In one minute a heart, strengthened by exercise, can pump the same amount of blood in 45 to 50 beats that it takes an average heart 70 to

75 beats to pump. That adds up to 36,000 more times per day, 13.1 million more times per year. Exercise your heart and save a heart beat.

What Happens to Your Body When You Exercise

- The lungs expand and can take in more oxygen.

- The number of tiny blood vessels or capillaries that deliver blood throughout the body increases.

- The total amount of blood increases.

- The ability of the blood to carry oxygen increases.

- As a result of the above, the heart has to work less, and the resting heart rate and recovery rate after exercise decrease.

How You Feel When You Exercise

- More alert

- More self-confident

- More relaxed

- More alive and energetic

How You Look When You Exercise

- Slimmer

- Stronger

- More attractive

Understanding 3 ZONE 20 Exercise

Scientific studies show that when more than two days go by without the heart getting exercise, it begins to become less conditioned. This means that if you exercise on Monday, you will need to exercise again by at least Thursday. By Friday you will have begun to lose the good effect of the work you have done. So, at least three exercise sessions a week are needed to get your heart fit and to keep it that way.

To get enough exercise, your heart has to beat somewhat faster than it usually beats during your normal day. But it should not beat too much faster because that can be unsafe. The area between "not fast enough" and "too fast" is called your heart rate zone or ZONE for short.

25

For example, a man 30 years old might have a resting heart rate of 70 beats a minute, and his ZONE would be from 115 beats to 160 beats a minute. To exercise his heart he would need to get his heart beating somewhere between 115 and 160 beats a minute, as shown below.

The most accurate way to tell if you are in your ZONE is to take your pulse. But, there are other ways to tell. When you are in your ZONE, you will breathe more quickly and more deeply. You will sweat. For the most part, you will feel comfortable and be able to keep going for twenty minutes without stopping.

If you are moving too slowly to have your heart rate in your ZONE, you will not breathe hard or sweat much. You will not feel as though you are putting out much effort. If your heart rate is higher than your ZONE, you will be so tired and winded that you will have to stop to

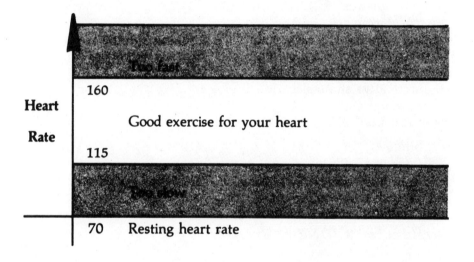

catch your breath. Think of a stroll, a brisk walk or jog, and a 40-yard wind sprint to catch the bus. Later in Stage 2, you will learn how to find your personal ZONE.

Many exercises will raise your heart rate. But some are better than others at keeping it high enough to be in your ZONE for twenty straight minutes. These exercises tend to call for constant, rhythmic movement.

Running is a good example of this. So is swimming. They both keep your body constantly moving and are such that you can get a good "rhythm," or pace, going. Although not as rhythmic as swimming, basketball does call for constant movement. It is a good exercise for keeping your heart rate in your ZONE for twenty minutes straight. The exercises that meet these guidelines are discussed below.

Meeting the Guidelines

You may have noticed that the "3" of 3 ZONE 20 deals with only how often you exercise a week. The ZONE 20 deals with the type of exercise that will make your heart stronger. So as you decide which exercises you want to do, ask yourself two questions:

- Will the exercise raise your heart rate high enough, but not too high?

- Will you be able to do the exercise for twenty minutes without stopping?

If you can answer "yes" to both of these questions, the exercises you are considering are probably good ones for your heart. Almost all activities that move your body exercise both your heart and your body's other muscles. But some exercises are better than others for making your heart strong.

Using ZONE 20, these are some examples to see if an activity is a good exercise for your heart:

Running Sprints

Heart rate high enough but not too high?

"*No*. My heart-rate will be too high. I will definitely have to stop and catch my breath."

Twenty minutes without stopping?

"*No*. I cannot run sprints for 20 straight minutes."

Probably not good exercise for your heart.

Bowling

Heart rate high enough, but not too high?

"*No*. My heart rate will not be high enough. I will not breathe that hard or sweat very much. I usually share a lane and spend time waiting anyway."

Twenty minutes without stopping?

"Yes. Given the chance, I can certainly bowl for 20 minutes without a rest."

Probably not a good exercise for your heart.

Walking

Heart rate high enough, but not too high?

"Maybe. Whether I breathe hard and break into a sweat depends on how hard I walk or if I am going up a hill. If I am taking a pleasant evening stroll, my heart rate does not get high enough to be in my ZONE. But if I am walking to work, I think it does get high enough."

Twenty minutes without stopping?

"Yes. I can certainly walk for 20 minutes without a rest."

May be good exercise for your heart.

Basketball

Heart rate high enough, but not too high?

"Maybe. If I play a lazy half-court game, I do not breathe that hard, so sometimes my heart rate might not get high enough. On the other hand, if we play a tough full-court game, I will have to stop to catch my breath. So sometimes my heart rate might be too high. But certainly sometimes I can play with my heart rate in my ZONE."

Twenty minutes without stopping?

"Maybe. Whether I can move constantly for 20 straight minutes depends on how hard I play. If I go all out, I have to stop ant rest. But if I take it a little easy, I can go the whole 20 minutes."

May be a good exercise for your heart.

An exercise can be too hard (sprints) or too easy (bowling) to give your heart the solid but safe exercise it needs to give you the full benefits of your efforts. The effects of other exercises, such as walking and jogging, depend on how you do them. In some cases, your level of fitness will also affect whether or not an activity is good exercise for your heart.

Meet ZONE 20 guidelines

Cross-country skiing
Hiking (uphill)
Ice hockey
Jogging
Jumping rope
Running in place

May meet ZONE 20 guidelines

Bicycling
Downhill skiing
Basketball
Calisthenics
Handball
Racquetball
Soccer
Swimming
Tennis (singles)
Walking
Stationary cycling

Do not meet ZONE 20 guidelines

Baseball
Bowling
Football
Golf (on foot or by cart)
Softball
Volleyball

For example, when you first start exercising, jogging two and a half miles in 20 minutes might be too hard. Your heart rate might go too high to remain in your ZONE. But after several months of 3 ZONE 20 exercise, your heart would be stronger, more fit, and you might well be able to jog the two and a half miles in 20 minutes with your heart rate comfortably within your ZONE.

Look at the chart above to see whether the exercises listed will help to condition your heart. The chart is based on the exercises being done by average individuals, not professional athletes. For example, a pickup football game is not going to be good exercise for your heart because there are too many breaks, time-outs, and not enough constant, vigorous movement. The professionals who play football, however, are certainly in good shape, and their playing football may be good exercise for their hearts.

As mentioned earlier, most activities exercise both your heart and your body's other muscles. If you swim to make your heart strong and to get the benefits that type of exercise can give, your arms, chest, back, and legs will also get stronger.

Choosing Your Exercises

Look at the list of exercises in the previous section. Think about the sports you play and the exercises you do now. Think about the exercises your friends do, that you have seen done, or that you always wanted to try. Then, choose at least three exercises that meet the 3 ZONE 20 guidelines so that you can have fallback exercises and some variety. As you choose, consider these two issues:

- **Is it fun?** Will you really enjoy doing this activity? If you like to exercise alone, do not pick a team sport. If you do like to exercise with other people, choose activities that people do in groups, or clubs, or exercises that friends or family will do with you.

- **Is it convenient?** Does the exercise require equipment? If it does, can you afford the equipment cost? Make sure there is a shower available. If traveling is involved, do not underestimate the extra time and effort involved. Make exercise as convenient and reasonable for yourself as possible.

If you have chosen three exercises that are fun, convenient, and meet the guidelines, great! These are your foundation. You are on your way to building a solid and successful exercise program. Go to the next section. If you have not picked out your three exercises. . . STOP. Do it now. It is important.

Fitting Exercise into Your Schedule

How you fit exercise into your normal daily schedule can make or break your program. It is that important. The goal is to find times in your daily life where exercise can fit easily and become an accepted part of your everyday routine. That way, you make the best possible use of the time, discipline, and work you are putting in. Exercise that does not fit your schedule is likely to take two or three times the amount of work.

You can find times in your life when exercise will take a reasonable effort, not a superhuman one. Just be honest with yourself and do not try to change your basic nature. Decide where exercise fits for you.

By using the **Activity Chart** in this section:

- Block out the time that is already taken by work, chores, favorite TV programs, etc.

- Plan for at least three exercise sessions a week with no more than two days between any of the sessions. Look also for backup times.

- A session, including time to change clothes and shower, will take about an hour.

Consider the following issues to be sure you chose the best times for you:

Does your exercise plan fit you?

Think about what kind of person you are, what you like and do not like, how you feel during different times of the day. If you are a night person, maybe exercising after work will help to relieve stress from your job. If you are an early riser, perhaps exercise will help you to get a good start on your day.

Does the plan fit your family and friends?

If you want to exercise with a friend, you will have to find a time that is good for both of you. The same goes for team sports. Your family may have feelings about when you exercise. Your spouse may not want the alarm clock going off an hour earlier in the morning. On the other hand, your spouse may like to exercise with you but can do that only in the evening.

How hungry are you?

Exercising right after eating can be uncomfortable. But, if you have not eaten for hours, you may not have much energy for your exercises. Wait at least one hour after a meal to exercise. Try eating a little fruit or a snack one to two hours before exercising.

31

Activity Chart

	Monday	Tuesday	Wednesday	Thursday	Friday	Saturday	Sunday
5-6							
6-7							
7-8							
8-9							
9-10							
10-11							
11-12							
12-1							
1-2							
2-3							
3-4							
4-5							
5-6							
6-7							
7-8							
8-9							
9-10							
10-11							
11-12							

What are you going to do when you miss a day?

You cannot always keep to a schedule. Most people cannot. There are always interruptions and unexpected happenings. A friend may drop in. It may rain or snow. To become a part of your routine, exercise needs to adapt to such changes.

One common way to make an exercise program adaptable is to schedule exercise for every other day. If you miss a day, just do the exercises the next day and there will still be no more than two days between sessions.

If, after completing the **Activity Chart,** you have decided where at least three exercise sessions will fit into your regular schedule, good! By deciding what is going to work for you, you have made great strides toward a successful exercise program. Go to the next section.

If you have not yet fit exercise into your life. . . STOP. Do not risk wasting your hard work. Go back and plan your exercise program.

Making a Commitment

Since you have read this far, you have probably thought about the pro's and con's of exercise. But before making a commitment, look closely at your reasons for exercising. Use the **Pro and Con Chart** below:

Pro and Con Chart

If I exercise to make my heart stronger and gain the benefits that exercise can give me, these are the things that will happen for me.

Good things for me   **Negative things for me**

_____   _____
_____   _____
_____   _____
_____   _____

**Good things for others
close to me**   **Negative things for others
close to me**

_____   _____
_____   _____
_____   _____
_____   _____

If there are more con's than pro's and you still want to exercise, try to change some of the negative things and to strengthen positive aspects. If your chart confirms your desire to exercise, make a commitment to "test drive" your exercise program for three weeks. Fill out the **Commitment Form** below. This three-week period will give you a chance to see how your scheduling works out.

Not all of you will want to fill out the Commitment Form. even if you are committed to giving exercise a try. However, experience has shown that the chance to succeed will be better if you fill out a commitment form.

Your chances are even better if you complete the form and post it on your refrigerator (or somewhere else where you can see it) to remind you of your firm decision to exercise. Go ahead. You can do it.

Take the first step toward a lifetime of feeling and looking your best. Give exercise a try for three weeks.

COMMITMENT FORM

I will exercise on

Monday

Tuesday

Wednesday

Thursday

Friday

Saturday

Sunday

for 3 weeks with my heart rate in my ZONE, which is between _____ and _____, for at least 20 minutes straight. My starting date is

_____ .

Remind yourself of your commitment to 3 ZONE 20 exercise; complete the pullout form in the center of the booklet and post it where you will see it every day.

Stage 2: Three Weeks for Getting a Good Start

The three weeks of Stage 2 will give you a chance to "test drive" exercise. Stage 2 will show you:

- How to get off to a gentle and reasonable start;
- How to warm up and cool down;
- How to avoid getting stiff, sore, and uncomfortable;
- How to tell if you are exercising hard enough, or too hard; and

- How to reward yourself for completing the three weeks of Stage 2.

Regular, vigorous exercises can help you to feel great, but usually you do not feel all that great right away. Stage 2 will help you make a strong and comfortable start that will launch you well into a lifetime of exercise.

Avoiding Injury and Soreness

Being injured or even stiff, sore, and uncomfortable is not a fun or helpful way to start your exercise program. Below are explained four ways you can make sure your first three weeks are as pleasant as they can be. These include starting slow and easy, warming up and cooling down, stretching, and gradually changing the speed at which you do your exercises.

Start Slow and Easy

The single most important thought for the short three weeks of Stage 2 is this, GO SLOWLY. This is not a crash program. There is no hurry. You are trying gradually to make exercise a part of your daily routine. In time you will get fit.

Going slow and easy may be difficult for some of you. You may have the mistaken idea that you have to always go harder and faster. You may remember those old sayings: "No pain, no gain," and "You have to work until it hurts." When it comes to 3 ZONE 20 exercise, these sayings are not only wrong they can be harmful. They are partly true for strength building exercises, such as pushups, sit-ups, and weight lifting but even here there are limits.

The three main reasons that the "No pain, no gain" approach is wrong are listed below:

- Your muscles get fit slowly. If you push too hard or try to go too fast, your muscles will let you know—you will be stiff and sore the next day.

- A painful program is usually a short program. Most people tend to give up exercise and the benefits it offers in order to avoid the pain.

- Exercise does not have to hurt to make your heart and body stronger. Pain is unnecessary. In fact, if you are in a lot of pain, your heart rate may be too high and you should slow down.

So, increase your activity levels slowly to give your muscles the time they need to get into shape. You want to get fit, not sore. Build your exercise program a little at a time so that it can help you feel and look your best for a lifetime. Do your 3 ZONE 20 exercise slow and easy.

To help you keep it slow and gentle during the three weeks of Stage 2, try the following:

Keep your heart rate in the lower half of your ZONE. That way, you will be working hard enough to make your heart stronger, but not pushing yourself.

Measure your exercise by time only. If you measure your exercise by both time and distance, it encourages hurrying. While you might start with something reasonable, each day you would be tempted to push to go further or faster. So try just going out to exercise for 20 minutes and do not worry about how far you go. Just watch your heart rate and put in your time.

Slow down or rest if you need to. Some of you will find that you cannot keep going the entire 20 minutes. That is fine. The idea is to get stronger, and you will get stronger if you simply keep your body moving the entire 20 minutes. For example, if you get tired after 10 minutes of bicycling, walk for a while. Build up to the 20 minutes. If you swim, float for a while to rest and then try swimming again.

Do not worry if you are not up to 20 minutes at the beginning. The important thing is to keep going. If you stick with it, your heart will soon get stronger and you will be able to go the whole 20 minutes.

Listen to your body. Occasional minor stiffness the morning after exercise is to be expected. It is a sign that you are getting into shape. Soreness, however, tells you that you overdid it. You need to cut back a little, to go slow and easy. Listen to your body and you will get into shape in time.

Warm-up and cool-down

Like an engine on a cold morning, your body needs a chance to warm up. A warm-up gradually prepares your muscles for exercise. Warming-up is especially important for exercise that requires quick bursts of effort, such as basketball or racquet sports. Rather than plunging into exercise, take five minutes to gradually get your heart and breathing going faster. Start your normal exercise slowly and pick up the pace gradually until you are in your ZONE.

Also, before exercising, some people like to stretch. Some think it is better to stretch at other times. Some do both. Do what feels best to you. Stretching exercises are provided below.

When you finish your 3 ZONE 20 workout, your body needs a chance to cool down slowly. This means you should slow your heart rate down gently. Do not stop abruptly by standing still, sitting, lying down, or bending over with your hands on your knees. Your heart needs to come gradually back to the resting rate. Keep moving but at a slower pace to cool down.

Stretch Your Muscles

You need to stretch your muscles at each major joint in your body at least three times per week. This will keep them flexible so you are likely to avoid strains.

The main reasons for stretching your muscles are to avoid "pulled muscles" and to increase your range of motion. Exercise makes you stretch your muscles beyond the usual length they are used to when not exercising. If the muscle cannot easily meet the demand for more length or for more force, there is a danger of strain. Routinely stretching your muscles and building your muscle fitness slowly decreases your chances of straining them.

Below are suggested stretches for each major muscle group. Feel free to add your own. Schedule time to do these stretches at least three times a week (before and/or after exercise, at another time, both). Do what feels best for you. All stretching should be done in the following manner:

- Stretch until you feel tension in your muscles, not pain or discomfort.

- Hold your stretch for 30 seconds or so.

- Do not bounce. Bouncing tends to overextend the muscles and increase the likelihood of strain.

- Go gently and slowly.

Gluteus Maximus (Buttocks) Stretch. Lie on your back. If you can, keep your head on the floor and pull your right leg toward your chest. Hold for 30 seconds and then switch legs. Stretch gently and steadily.

Thigh Stretch. Hold your right foot in your left hand. Slowly pull the heel of your left foot toward your buttocks. Use your right hand to keep your balance. Stretch gently, steadily and do not bounce. Hold for 30 seconds and then switch legs.

Hamstring Stretch. Stand with your feet at shoulders width apart and pointed straight ahead. Bend slowly forward. With your knees slightly bent, stretch gently, steadily and do not bounce. Relax your neck and arms. Hold for 30 seconds.

Calf Stretch. Face a wall. Rest your forearms on the wall with your forehead on the back of your hands. Bend one knee and move it toward the wall. The back leg should be straight with the foot flat and pointed straight ahead. Move your hips forward until you feel the stretch. Stretch gently and steadily. Do not bounce: Hold for 30 seconds and then switch legs.

Side and Arm Stretch. Stand with your knees slightly bent. Gently pull your elbow behind your head as you bend to the side. Hold for 10 seconds and then switch sides. Stretch gently.

Shoulder Stretch. Put your hands together behind your back. Lift your arms up. Hold for 30 seconds. Stretch gently.

Just as an added tip: try a few stretches on breaks if you work in an office. Especially try stretching your hamstrings, back, and shoulders (by bending). This feels good and gives you energy.

Make Any Changes in Your Exercise Speed Gradually

If you try doing some activity harder or faster than normal so that you increase the usual range of motion or force demanded of your muscles, your muscles will get sore. For example, if you run sprints or run a lot faster than your normal 3 ZONE 20 pace, your leg muscles will be sore in the morning.

Muscles are very specialized. If you train them to run in a certain range of motion and exert a certain level of force, when you go beyond that range, you are likely to get sore. How sore? It depends on how large an increase in the range of motion or force demanded and for how long.

To increase your speed or your ability for quick action, go slowly.

Stretching will not prevent soreness here. Muscles change condition slowly. Play your first game of basketball or racquet sports at less than full force. Volley for fun, not to win. Gradually change and you will avoid unnecessary pain.

Finding Your Heart Rate Zone

Use the ZONE chart to find your ZONE. The area between not fast enough and too fast is your heart rate ZONE for giving your heart the good exercise it needs. Your heart beats at a certain speed, or rate, during a normal day. To exercise your heart, you have to make it beat faster than its normal rate, but not so much faster that it is unsafe.

For example, for a thirty-year-old man the ZONE is 115 heart beats a minute to 160 heart beats a minute. In other words, for a thirty-year-old man to get the full benefit of his exercise, his heart needs to beat at least 115 times a minute, but no more than 160 times a minute. Find your own heart rate ZONE on the ZONE chart.

There are two ways to tell whether or not you are in your ZONE. You should learn to use both of them: The first way is to take your pulse. To take your pulse:

- Use a watch with a second hand.

- Stop exercising.

- Immediately after stopping your exercise, place one or more fingers just to either side of your Adam's apple or inside your wrist at the base of your thumb. Find your heart beat.

- Count your heart beats for six seconds. Add a zero to that number to get your heart rate. (Thirteen beats in six seconds would be 130 beats a minute.)

ZONE CHART

AGE	20	25	30	35	40	45	50	55	60	65
too fast										
	170	165	160	160	155	150	145	140	135	130
Your ZONE										
	120	120	115	110	110	105	100	100	100	95
too slow										

	70	resting heart rate

Complete the next sentence. My heart rate ZONE is between _____ beats a minute to _____ beats a minute. Find a way to help yourself remember your ZONE. Perhaps the numbers will remind you of something else. You could also write your ZONE on a piece of paper to take with you during your first few weeks of exercise.

Take your pulse often during the three weeks of Stage 2, perhaps once in the middle of your exercise session and again immediately afterwards.

As you exercise and take your pulse, you will gradually learn the second way to tell if your heart rate is in your ZONE—by experience. After a while, you will know if you are in your ZONE by how your body feels. When you are in your ZONE, you will be breathing hard, breaking into a sweat, but feeling good and be able to go for 20 minutes.

If your heart rate is too low to be in your ZONE, you will not feel as if you are working very hard. If it is too high to be in your ZONE, you will have to stop to catch your breath and rest your muscles. When you have a good sense of how it feels to be in your ZONE, you probably will not need to take your pulse more than once or twice a week.

If you follow the guidelines, exercise will help you to look and feel your best.

Keeping a Record

Keeping a record of when and how much you have actually exercised is important. You will feel good looking back and seeing all the exercise that you have done and how successfully you have followed through on your program.

If you should have any problems, the record will show you where they were and help you decide what you might do about them. Each time you return from an exercise session, fill out the record chart below (see page 42). Try not to wait. If you are like most people, it will be hard to remember what you did if you do not fill out the record right away.

You may wish to continue filling out your record for a long time, but try using it at least for the first three weeks of your program in Stage 2. It will help you to become a successful exerciser.

Rewarding Yourself

Exercise can make you feel great, but probably not in the first three weeks of the program. The rewards of exercise come a little later. So, for now, provide your own rewards.

You are giving the new program your best for three weeks. If you meet your commitment, you will deserve a reward. Think about what it could be. Make it immediate and real. "A vacation next year" is too far away. "Something nice" is too vague. How about new jogging shoes, a dinner out, a tune-up for your bicycle, or a weekend away. Give yourself the reward you deserve and be successful.

Dealing with Excuses

Now and then everybody uses excuses to miss a session. ("I'm too tired.", "I need the sleep.", "I have a tough day tomorrow.", "I do not have the time.")

What are your excuses likely to be? When will you want to use them? Think about these questions ahead of time and do not let excuses get the better of you. Be in charge of your program and yourself.

Stage 3: Nine Weeks for Building an Exercise Habit

You have finished three full weeks of exercise. Before going on to Stage 3, find out how you did starting your exercise program in Stage 2. Review your exercise record, and answer these questions:

- Did you exercise at least nine times in the three weeks?

Date	Warm-up	Time with heart rate in your ZONE	Type of exercise	Strength exercise	Cool-down	Com-ments
Monday						
Tuesday						
Wednesday						
Thursday						
Friday						
Saturday						
Sunday						

- For all nine times, did you keep your heart rate in your ZONE for at least 20 minutes?

- Did you start slowly by keeping your pulse in the lower part of your ZONE, measuring your exercise by time alone, and by avoiding pain?

- Did you warm up and cool down at each session?

- Did you stretch at least three times a week?

If you answered "yes" to all five questions above, you should feel good about yourself. You have started on the road to success. Stage 3 will show you how to stay on that road.

If you answered the first two questions "yes" but one or more of the last three questions "no," you were able to get a good start on your 3 ZONE 20 exercise program. But why make it harder than it needs to be?

Starting fast and pushing yourself further and faster may look good now, but in the long run it can hurt you. All that effort will not matter much if you burn yourself out. Start slowly and increase your activity gradually. Build an exercise program that can last a lifetime.

Neglecting your warm-up, cool-down, and stretching may not have caused problems yet, but exercise is a lifetime program. Warming up helps prepare the body for exercise. Cooling down lets your heart rate slow down gradually. And stretching keeps you flexible. So take care of your body and warm up before and cool down after each session. Stretch at least three times a week.

If you answered "no" to either of the first two questions, do not feel too bad about it. You probably gave it your best shot, but you had a few problems. Do not worry. It happens to everyone. If you keep trying, you will succeed.

The important thing now is to figure out your problems. Did you schedule exercise for inconvenient times? Was the place for exercise too far away? Turn to **Handling Some Common Exercise Problems** on page 50, for some suggestions to help you get started again.

When you think you have your problems worked out and are ready to go on, return to Stage 2 and make a new commitment to exercise for three weeks within the guidelines. Good luck. If you keep trying, you can do it.

Building an Exercise Habit

Now that you have made your start, in the nine weeks of Stage 3, you will learn how to keep your program going so that you can build it into a normal part of your everyday routine. Usually, it is during this stage that you will slowly begin to feel stronger and more eager to exercise. Your exercise will become easier to do. You will begin to feel a sense of pride in what you have done and are going to do.

You may also run into a few minor problems. Stage 3 is a time when excuses start to sound a little better. Small problems seem larger. A single missed session can mean the end of an entire program, the loss of weeks of effort and discipline.

Stage 3 will show you how to deal with your excuses and with missing a day. You will see how to use goals, reminders, a record of your exercise, and your friends and family to help you keep your program going strong for a commitment of nine more weeks.

The challenge of Stage 3 is to keep your exercise program going until it becomes a self-sustaining habit and an enjoyable part of your everyday routine.

Handling Problems Immediately

Most exercise problems are minor and easily fixed. But, sometimes people try to put up with them, or they think they can tough it out. Why not make it easy for yourself. See what the problem is and fix it.

Do not let yourself get stuck with something that does not feel right for you. You made the decisions about your program in the first place. You can change them until you find the exercises and the times to exercise that make exercising easy for you.

Setting Your Goals and Tracking Your Progress

Working toward a goal can help keep your motivation high. Make your goals specific and reasonable. ("I will be able to run for 25 minutes without stopping on an outdoor track by September 30.", "By June 15, I will be able to bicycle Cliff Street hill without stopping or walking.") When you do reach a goal, be sure to enjoy your success. Celebrate. Reward yourself.

Another way to feel successful is to watch your progress. As your heart becomes stronger, it will be able to push more blood through your body with fewer beats. So, as your heart works better, your heart rate will go down.

You will be able to see this change by keeping a record of your resting heart rate. Each week take your pulse in the morning when you wake up. You may not see a change from week to week, but your pulse will gradually get slower.

You can also watch how far you go in your 20 minutes. As you become stronger and more fit, you will need to swim or pedal faster, run or walk more quickly to reach your ZONE. It will not feel as if you are working harder. Being in your ZONE will usually feel about the same. But you will have to move more quickly to get your pulse up and into your ZONE.

As your pace goes up, so will your distance. If, when you started you could swim 15 laps in 20 minutes, after six weeks you may find yourself going 20 laps. You do not have to push yourself to go further. Just notice improvements that come naturally from your regular 3 ZONE 20 exercise.

Rewarding Yourself

Just as in Stage 2, rewards are important. Exercise itself is probably not a powerful enough reward yet. Until it becomes one, you need to reward yourself. Do not wait the entire nine weeks to do it. Do something special to celebrate six straight weeks of exercise, a goal reached, or progress made.

Having an Answer for Your Excuses

You are going to have excuses. Figure out what your excuses are likely to be or catch them as they happen. Then find an answer to them. For example:

Excuses	Answers
"It's too cold."	"I can run in place in the living room."
"I'm too tired."	"I really feel good after exercise."
"I can do it tomorrow."	"3 ZONE 20. . . If I don't exercise today I'll be wasting some of the work I did before."

Asking Your Friends to Help

Ask the people close to you (spouse, family, friends) to help you. Ask them to celebrate with you when you reach a goal, to exercise with you, or to help you realistically plan your schedule.

Tell them it is important to you and ask them to be interested and encouraging. Perhaps they would like to join you. It is easier to jump rope if other people are doing it too. It is easier to keep going when other people are rooting for you.

Keeping Up If You Miss a Day

Everyone misses a day once in a while. Do not waste time feeling that your program is over or that it will be too hard to exercise if a day has been missed. Just get restarted. A perfect record is not important. Just keep trying and you will do it.

Using Reminders

To remind yourself to exercise, put reminders out where you will see them in your home and at work. For example, put up a picture of a winning runner, breaking the tape and holding his hands high. Anything that reminds you of your commitment to being stronger and more fit will help to keep your motivation high until exercise becomes a habit.

Quitting Smoking and Losing Weight

Success breeds success. After three weeks of exercise, you have taken command. Now is a good time to think about taking charge of your smoking or excess weight.

Quitting smoking will help with your exercise routine, and your exercise routine will actually make it easier for you to quit smoking.

Losing weight and keeping it off is also aided by exercise. Combining exercise with changes in your eating routine will help you successfully lose your excess weight.

Making a Commitment

You have tried exercising for three weeks and made a good, solid start. You were a success. Now you are ready for the challenge of the nine weeks of Stage 3—keeping your exercise program going until it can build into a habit. Review your reasons for exercising and then take the next step. You can do it. Sign up below.

Commitment Form

I will exercise on	Type of Exercise	Time
Monday		
Tuesday		
Wednesday		
Thursday		
Friday		
Saturday		
Sunday		

for 9 weeks with my heart rate in my ZONE, which is between _____
and _____ for at least 20 minutes straight. My starting date is

_____ .

You are now on your way to a successful nine weeks of exercise. If during the nine weeks of Stage 3 you have any problems, return to this book and read **Handling Some Common Exercise Problems.** Good luck and enjoy yourself.

Stage 4: Lifetime of Exercise

How did you do in Stage 3? Review your exercise record and answer these questions:

- Did you exercise at least 27 times in the nine weeks (three times a week for nine weeks)?

- During each of the 27 sessions, did you keep your pulse in your ZONE for at least 20 minutes?

- Do you know what your ZONE is?

- Do you know the three guide lines for exercise?

If you answered "yes" to all of these questions, you now have 12 weeks of good, solid exercise behind you. You should be feeling good, confident. You are probably getting stronger, moving faster, and going longer.

Exercise is probably becoming more enjoyable. It is starting to become a habit. You are ready to go on to Stage 4 and have exercise as a normal part of your everyday life.

If you answered "no" to any of the questions, see what you can do to get back on the road to successful exercise. You had a few problems. That does not mean that you should give up.

Keeping exercise going can be difficult at first. Read the section on problem-solving on page 50. Work to make your exercise more reasonable and easier for you to do. Then go back to Stage 3 and make another nine week commitment. You can do it.

Enjoying a Lifetime of Exercise

Keeping your exercise going for a lifetime presents some new challenges. In Stage 4 you will learn how to handle missing a day, or even several. You will learn how to deal with "off days" when you go ahead and exercise, but just can't seem to do anything. You will discover ways of keeping the fun in your exercise.

Being Reasonable and Having Fun

Sometimes, as people begin to feel stronger and are able to go faster or longer, they go back to old exercise patterns. They start pushing too hard, instead of judging their exercise by the total time spent in their ZONE.

No matter what exercise you do, this exercise program is not a marathon. The goal is to feel good and be fit. If you always exercise in the lower part of your ZONE, you will still reach this goal. Do not push yourself. Be reasonable.

Try to vary your exercise, and let it be fun. Change your exercise patterns; swim at a different pool once in a while, run a new route. Try different exercises for variety. Exercise alone or with friends for a change of pace. Do not make exercise a job. Have fun.

Restarting Slowly After a Break

There will always be times when you cannot exercise (when you are ill, for example). Your body is used to exercise and will want to get back to it soon. Be sure to wait until you are really ready to start again. When you do restart, go slowly. Even though you will want to get back to running or swimming or bicycling as fast or as far as you were before, don't. Take your time. Let gentle 3 ZONE 20 exercise gradually get you back to your former pace.

Accepting Your Occasional Off Days

Every once in a while you will have a day when you just are not into it. Sometimes it will get better as you exercise, Sometimes it will not. When it does not, just relax and to what you can. Then call it a day. Accept your off days as a sign that your body is tired and needs rest more than exercise.

Making a Commitment

You have done 12 weeks of exercise. You should be entering Stage 4 where exercise becomes a normal, enjoyable part of your daily routine. Stage 4 lasts for the rest of your life—a long life of thinking and feeling better, of feeling strong and confident. But it is easier to make commitments for a shorter period of time than a lifetime. You decide. Do you want to sign up for six months of exercise? a year? Make your decision and complete the form below.

You are now on your way to a successful lifetime of exercise. Remember to continue to use this material when:

- You have a problem.
- You have missed exercising for a while and need to get restarted.
- You want to try another sport or exercise and you do not know whether or not it fits the guidelines.
- You cannot remember your ZONE.

Good luck!

Commitment Form

I will exercise on	Type of Exercise	Time
Monday		
Tuesday		
Wednesday		
Thursday		
Friday		
Saturday		
Sunday		

for _____ weeks with my heart rate in my ZONE, which is between _____ and _____, for at least 20 minutes straight. My starting date is _____.

Handling Some Common Exercise Problems

Problems are a normal part of life. You should expect to run into a few as you build your 3 ZONE 20 exercise habit. Most people do. But many of these common problems can be avoided. Those that cannot be avoided can often be minimized or overcome.

Do not let an occasional problem get you down or make you feel like a failure. You are in charge, and you can handle whatever comes up. Use your own common sense, your friends' ideas, and the suggestions below to successfully deal with any difficulties and keep your exercise program going strong.

Problem: "It takes too much time."

Suggestions:

A workout should take about an hour. This includes a five minute warm-up, at least 20 minutes with your heart rate in your ZONE, a five minute cool-down, and time to change and shower.

If your workouts are taking longer than an hour, then. . .

Make your workout shorter by figuring out which part of the workout is using extra time. If it takes 20 minutes just to get to your place of exercise, try to find something to do closer to home. If your warm-up takes 20 minutes, consider cutting back.

If your workouts are taking about an hour, but they seem to keep you from doing other things, then. . .

Consider making some changes in your exercise schedule. If you cannot get the shopping done or you are missing your favorite TV program because you are exercising, then exercise could easily seem to be taking up too much of your time. Do not stop your efforts. Try some different times until you find the time that fits you and your schedule.(See page 30 of Making a Winning Game Plan.)

Perhaps your enthusiasm is getting a little low and you need to raise it back up again. (See the suggestions below under, *"I do not have enough motivation or discipline."*)

Combine exercise with other activities. Spend time exercising with your friends and family. Walk to work. Bicycle to the store.

If your workouts are taking about an hour, but you are feeling that three hours a week is too much time to give to exercise now, then. . .

You may need to reexamine your commitment to exercise. Try re-doing the Pro and Con Chart on page 33 of Making a Winning Game Plan. If your chart comes out on the negative side, maybe this is a poor time for you to be starting an exercise program.

Perhaps you are changing jobs or moving. If so, wait and begin your program later. If your chart is on the positive side, review your reasons for exercising and make a new and firm commitment to 3 ZONE 20 exercise. (See the Introduction and page 34 of Making a Winning Game Plan.)

Problem: "Exercise is boring."

Suggestions:

If you are in Stages 2 or 3 (0-9 weeks of exercise) then. . .

Try giving exercise a little more time. As you become stronger, you may find that exercise in general and the specific exercise that you are doing will become more fun and less boring.

If you are in Stage 3 (10 weeks or more of exercise) then. . .

Add variety to your exercise schedule. Try different exercises that meet the 3 ZONE 20 guidelines. Try exercising with family or friends some of the time and alone some of the time. Exercise in new places or at a different time once a week.

Problem: "I do not seem to have enough motivation or discipline."

Suggestions:

If you are in either Stage 2 or early Stage 3 exercise, then. . .

You may wish to consider starting your program later. Perhaps there are other important things going on in your life now. If you are starting a new job, moving, or have some other change occurring in your life, you may not have enough energy left to start a 3 ZONE 20 program. Wait until the crisis is over and then start again when you can give exercise your full attention.

You may be pushing yourself harder than you need to. Always trying to go faster and further can make exercise painful and unpleasant. This can cause you to rapidly use up your motivation and discipline. Remember, you have to do only 3 ZONE 20 to get the full benefit of your exercise. (See page 35 in Getting a Good Start.)

Be sure to do your warm-up and cool-down. It is normal for your body to be a little uncomfortable and sore when you start a new exercise program. Warming up before and cooling down after exercise can help keep the discomfort down and your motivation up. (See page 37 in Getting a Good Start.)

If you are in Stage 4 or late Stage 3 exercise and you are not absolutely sure you have made exercise as easy as it can be, then. . .

Be sure that your choice of exercises, and of time to do those exercises, make your exercising easy. Nothing will sap your motivation like trying to do an exercise you do not like or exercising at the wrong time. (See Making a Winning Game Plan.)

Be careful not to push yourself too hard. As you get stronger, you may be tempted to push yourself to go further and faster than needed. This only saps your motivation and discipline. Your body will naturally get stronger, go further and faster just by doing your 3 ZONE 20 exercise. Progress is natural. Enjoy it. Do not force it. (See page 48 in A Lifetime of Exercise.)

If you are in Stage 4 or late Stage 3 exercise, and you are absolutely sure that you have made your exercise as easy as it can be, then give one or more of the following a try. . .

- Setting personal goals.

- Keeping a record of your exercise.

- Tracking your progress.

- Rewarding yourself for reaching goals or making progress.

- Reminding yourself of your commitment to exercise.

- Taking charge of your excuses.

- Seeking help from your friends.

(See page 41 in Getting a Good Start and pages 44-46 in Building an Exercise Habit.)

Problem: "I am uncomfortable when I exercise and sore afterwards."

Suggestions:

If you are in Stage 2, the first three weeks of exercise, then. . .

You may be pushing for too much, too soon. Relax and do 3 ZONE 20 exercise. Progress will come naturally.

You should expect some discomfort and soreness. Your body is adapting to a new level of activity. You are doing more than you usually do; Some discomfort and soreness is normal.

Sometimes feelings and sensations that now seem rather intense may later become an accepted part of exercising. For example, dur-

53

ing the first few days of exercising the feelings in your legs might seem to say "I'm hurt—maybe even crippled." Later, the same feelings in your legs will just mean that your legs are working hard and working well. (See page 35 in Getting a Good Start.)

If you are in Stages 3 or 4 and often feel this way, then. . .

Chances are good that you are either pushing yourself too hard or not doing the same exercise three times a week. If so, go easier and more routinely. If you are not pushing and are stretching regularly but continue to have pain and soreness, you may have strained a muscle and need to rest for a while until it feels better. If rest does not help, check with your doctor to see what is wrong. (See page 35 in Getting a Good Start.)

If you are in Stage 3 or 4 and you only occasionally feel sore days after exercising, then. . .

You may be trying to do an exercise that you are not used to. Muscles stay in condition only for what they routinely do. So do your 3 ZONE 20 exercise routinely. When you do plan to do something different, or your routine exercise faster, build up to it gradually. In special events or races, do not overexert yourself and do expect some soreness for the few days afterward. If you occasionally feel uncomfortable when exercising, then you may just be having an off day. It happens to all of us. Do what you can and then call it a day. (See page 48 in A Lifetime of Exercise.)

Problem: "I'm not making any progress."

Solution:

If you are in the early stages of your exercise program (Stages 2 and 3), then. . .

Relax. If you keep doing 3 ZONE 20 exercise, your heart will get stronger and progress will come. Concentrate on making exercise easy and on letting it become a habit. Do not get caught up in pushing for progress. Progress will come on its own.

If you are in Stage 4 exercise, then. . .

Many exercisers find that they have plateaus or periods during which they make little progress. You might, for example, be able to swim faster and faster for the first six months of your exercise program. Suddenly, however, you are not making any progress. Then, after a period of time, you begin to make progress again. This is normal. After your first improvements, progress often comes in fits and starts. The important thing is to do your 3 ZONE 20 exercise, strengthen your heart, and look and feel your best.

You cannot always make progress. Everyone has his limits. The point of 3 ZONE 20 exercise is not to become an Olympic medal winner or a professional athlete. The point is to be confident, alert, energetic. (See page 44 in Building an Exercise Habit.)

Problem: "I do not know what to do when the weather is bad or I am traveling."

Suggestions:

Try out several exercises that you can do indoors with a minimum of equipment. For example, try jumping rope, running in place, or moving athletically to music. Find an exercise that fits your needs and have it ready when the plane leaves or the snows come.

Additional Resources for Getting Fit Your Way.

1. Anderson, Robert A. *Stretching*. Bolinas, CA: Shelter Publications, 1980.

2. Maryland Commission on Physical Fitness. *Employee Office Exercise Program*. Baltimore, Maryland.

A poster describing and demonstrating exercise that can be done in the office. A free copy may be obtained from:

Maryland Commission on Physical Fitness
201 W. Preston Street
Baltimore, Maryland 21201
(301) 383-4040

3. Cooper, Kenneth H. *The Aerobics Way*. New York, NY: Bantam Books, 1977.

4. National Heart, Lung and Blood Institute. *Exercise and Your Heart.* Bethesda, Maryland: NIH, NHLBI, May 1981.

5. Maryland Department of Health and Mental Hygiene, Health Education Center, Healthy People Project. *Look Better, Feel Better, and Enjoy Life Longer: 9 Ways to Help You.* Baltimore, Maryland: MDHMH, September 1982.

Items (4) and (5) may be obtained free from:

Health Education Center
Maryland Department of Health and Mental Hygiene
300 W. Preston Street, Room 410
Baltimore, Maryland 21201

Chapter 4

Exercise and Weight Control

Just about everybody seems to be interested in weight control. Some of us weigh just the right amount, others need to gain a few pounds. Most of us "battle the bulge" at some time in our life. Whatever our goals, we should understand and take advantage of the important role of exercise in keeping our weight under control.

Carrying around too much body fat is a major nuisance. Yet excess body fat is common in modern-day living. Few of today's occupations require vigorous physical activity, and much of our leisure time is spent in sedentary pursuits.

Recent estimates indicate that 34 million adults are considered obese (20 percent above desirable weight). Also, there has been an increase in body fat levels in children and youth over the past 20 years. After infancy and early childhood, the earlier the onset of obesity, the greater the likelihood of remaining obese.

Excess body fat has been linked to such health problems as coronary heart disease, high blood pressure, osteoporosis, diabetes, arthritis and certain forms of cancer. Some evidence now exists showing that obesity has a negative effect on both health and longevity.

Exercise is associated with the loss of body fat in both obese and normal weight persons. A regular program of exercise is an important component of any plan to help individuals lose, gain or maintain their weight.

The President's Council on Physical Fitness and Sports

Overweight or Overfat?

Overweight and overfat do not always mean the same thing. Some people are quite muscular and weigh more than the average for their age and height. However, their body composition, the amount of fat versus lean body mass (muscle, bone, organs and tissue), is within a desirable range. This is true for many athletes. Others weigh an average amount yet carry around too much fat. In our society, however, overweight often implies overfat because excess weight is commonly distributed as excess fat. The addition of exercise to a weight control program helps control both body weight and body fat levels.

A certain amount of body fat is necessary for everyone. Experts say that percent body fat for women should be about 20 percent, 15 percent for men. Women with more than 30 percent fat and men with more than 25 percent fat are considered obese.

How much of your weight is fat can be assessed by a variety of methods including underwater (hydrostatic) weighing, skinfold thickness measurements and circumference measurements. Each requires a specially trained person to administer the test and perform the correct calculations. From the numbers obtained, a body fat percentage is determined. Assessing body composition has an advantage over the standard height-weight tables because it can help distinguish between "overweight" and "overfat."

An easy self-test you can do is to pinch the thickness of the fat folds at your waist and abdomen. If you can pinch an inch or more of fat (make sure no muscle is included) chances are you have too much body fat.

People who exercise appropriately increase lean body mass while decreasing their overall fat level. Depending on the amount of fat loss, this can result in a loss of inches without a loss of weight, since muscle weighs more than fat. However, with the proper combination of diet and exercise, both body fat and overall weight can be reduced.

Energy Balance: A Weighty Concept

Losing weight, gaining weight or maintaining your weight depends on the amount of calories you take in and use up during the day, otherwise referred to as energy balance. Learning how to balance energy intake (calories in food) with energy output (calories expended through physical activity) will help you achieve your desired weight.

Although the underlying causes and the treatments of obesity are complex, the concept of energy balance is relatively simple. If you eat more calories than your body needs to perform your day's activities, the extra calories are stored as fat. If you do not take in enough calories to meet your body's energy needs, your body will go to the stored fat to make up the difference. (Exercise helps ensure that stored fat, rather than muscle tissue, is used to meet your energy needs.) If you eat just about the same amount of calories to meet your body's energy needs, your weight will stay the same.

On the average, a person consumes between 800,000 and 900,000 calories each year! An active person needs more calories than a sedentary person, as physically active people require energy above and beyond the day's basic needs. All too often, people who want to lose weight concentrate on counting calorie intake while neglecting calorie output. The most powerful formula is the combination of dietary modification with exercise. By increasing your daily physical activity and decreasing your caloric input you can lose excess weight in the most efficient and healthful way.

Counting Calories

Each pound of fat your body stores represents 3,500 calories of unused energy. In order to lose one pound, you would have to create a calorie deficit of 3,500 calories by either taking in 3,500 less calories over a period of time than you need or doing 3,500 calories worth of exercise. It is recommended that no more than two pounds (7,000 calories) be lost per week for lasting weight loss.

Adding 15 minutes of moderate exercise, say walking one mile, to your daily schedule will use up 100 extra calories per day. (Your body uses approximately 100 calories of energy to walk one mile, depending on your body weight.) Maintaining this schedule would result in an extra 700 calories per week used up, or a loss of about 10 pounds in one year, assuming your food intake stays the same.

To look at energy balance another way, just one extra slice of bread or one extra soft drink a day—or any other food that contains approximately 100 calories—can add up to ten extra pounds in a year if the amount of physical activity you do does not increase.

If you already have a lean figure and want to keep it you should exercise regularly and eat a balanced diet that provides enough calories to make up for the energy you expend. If you wish to gain weight you should exercise regularly and increase the number of calories you consume until you reach your desired weight. Exercise will help ensure that the weight you gain will be lean muscle mass, not extra fat.

The Diet Connection

A balanced diet should be part of any weight control plan. A diet high in complex carbohydrates and moderate in protein and fat will complement an exercise program. It should include enough calories to satisfy your daily nutrient requirements and include the proper number of servings per day from the "basic four food groups": vegetables and fruits (4 servings), breads and cereals (4 servings), milk and milk products (2-4 depending on age) and meats and fish (2).

Experts recommend that your daily intake not fall below 1200 calories unless you are under a doctor's supervision. Also, weekly weight loss should not exceed two pounds.

Remarkable claims have been made for a variety of "crash" diets and diet pills. And some of these very restricted diets do result in noticeable weight loss in a short time. Much of this loss is water and such a loss is quickly regained when normal food and liquid intake is resumed. These diet plans are often expensive and may be dangerous. Moreover, they do not emphasize lifestyle changes that will help you maintain your desired weight. Dieting alone will result in a loss of valuable body tissue such as muscle mass in addition to a loss in fat.

How Many Calories?

The estimates for number of calories (energy) used during a physical activity are based on experiments that measure the amount of oxygen consumed during a specific bout of exercise for a certain body weight.

The energy costs of activities that require you to move your own body weight, such as walking or jogging, are greater for heavier people since they have more weight to move. For example, a person weighing 150 pounds would use more calories jogging one mile than a person jogging alongside who weighs 115 pounds. Always check to see what body weight is referred to in caloric expenditure charts you use.

Energy Expenditure Chart

	Energy Costs Cals/Hour*
A. Sedentary Activities	
Lying down or sleeping	90
Sitting quietly	84
Sitting and writing, card playing, etc.	114
B. Moderate Activities	**(150-350)**
Bicycling (5 mph)	174
Canoeing (2.5 mph)	174
Dancing (Ballroom)	210
Golf (2-some, carrying clubs)	324
Horseback riding (sitting to trot)	246
Light housework. cleaning, etc.	246
Swimming (crawl, 20 yards/min)	288
Tennis (recreational doubles)	312
Volleyball (recreational)	264
Walking (2 mph)	198
C. Vigorous Activities	**(More than 350)**
Aerobic Dancing	546
Basketball (recreational)	450
Bicycling (13 mph)	612
Circuit weight training	756
Football (touch, vigorous)	498
Ice Skating (9 mph)	384
Racquetball	588
Roller Skating (9 mph)	384
Jogging (10 minute mile, 6 mph)	654
Scrubbing Floors	440
Swimming (crawl, 45 yards/min)	522
Tennis (recreational singles)	450
X-country Skiing (5 mph)	690

*Hourly estimates based on values calculated for calories burned per minute for a 150 pound (68 kg) person.

(Sources: William D McArdle. Frank I. Katch. Victor L Katch. "Exercise Physiology: Energy, Nutrition and Human Performance" (2nd edition). Lea & Febiger, Philadelphia, 1986; Melvin H. Williams, *"Nutrition for Fitness and Sport,"* William C. Brown Company Publishers. Dubuque. 1983.)

Exercise and Modern Living

One thing is certain. Most people do not get enough exercise in their ordinary routines. All of the advances of modern technology—from electric can openers to power steering —have made life easier, more comfortable and much less physically demanding. Yet our bodies need activity, especially if they are carrying around too much fat. Satisfying this need requires a definite plan, and a commitment. There are two main ways to increase the number of calories you expend:

1. Start a regular exercise program if you do not have one already.

2. Increase the amount of physical activity in your daily routine.

The best way to control your weight is a combination of the above. The sum total of calories used over time will help regulate your weight as well as keep you physically fit.

Active Lifestyles

Before looking at what kind of regular exercise program is best, let's look at how you can increase the amount of physical activity in your daily routine to supplement your exercise program.

- Recreational pursuits such as gardening on weekends, bowling in the office league, family outings, an evening of social dancing, and many other activities provide added exercise. They are fun and can be considered an extra bonus in your weight control campaign.

- Add more "action" to your day. Walk to the neighborhood grocery store instead of using the car. Park several blocks from the office and walk the rest of the way. Walk up the stairs instead of using the elevator; start with one flight of steps and gradually increase.

- Change your attitude toward movement. Instead of considering an extra little walk or trip to the files an annoyance, look upon it as an added fitness boost. Look for opportunities to use your body. Bend, stretch, reach, move, lift and carry. Time-saving devices and gadgets eliminate drudgery and are a bonus to mankind, but when they substitute too often for physical activity they can demand a high cost in health, vigor and fitness.

These little bits of action are cumulative in their effects. Alone, each does not burn a huge amount of calories. But when added together they can result in a sizable amount of energy used over the course of the day. And they will help improve your muscle tone and flexibility at the same time.

What Kind Of Exercise?

Although any kind of physical movement requires energy (calories), the type of exercise that uses the most energy is "aerobic" exercise. The term "aerobic" is derived from the Greek word meaning "with oxygen." Jogging, brisk walking, swimming. biking, cross-country skiing and aerobic dancing are some popular forms of aerobic exercise.

Aerobic exercises use the body's large muscle groups in continuous, rhythmic, sustained movement and require oxygen for the production of energy. When oxygen is combined with food (which can come from stored fat) energy is produced to power the body's musculature. The longer you move aerobically, the more energy needed and the more calories used. Regular aerobic exercise will improve your cardiorespiratory endurance, the ability of your heart, lungs, blood vessels and associated tissues to use oxygen to produce energy needed for activity. You'll build a healthier body while getting rid of excess body fat.

In addition to the aerobic exercise. supplement your program with muscle strengthening and stretching exercises. The stronger your muscles. the longer you will be able to keep going during aerobic activity, and the less chance of injury.

How Much? How Often?

Experts recommend that you do some form of aerobic exercise at least three times a week for a minimum of 20 continuous minutes. Of course, if that is too much, start with a shorter time span and gradually build up to the minimum. Then gradually progress until you are able to work aerobically for 20-40 minutes. If you need to lose a large amount of weight, you may want to do your aerobic workout five times a week.

It is important to exercise at an intensity vigorous enough to cause your heart rate and breathing to increase. How hard you should exercise depends to a certain degree on your age, and is determined by measuring your heart rate in beats per minute.

The heart rate you should maintain is called your target heart rate, and there are several ways you can arrive at this figure. The simplest is to subtract your age from 220 and then calculate 60 to 80 percent of that figure. Beginners should maintain the 60 percent level, more advanced can work up to the 80 percent level. This is just a guide however, and people with any medical limitations should discuss this formula with their physician.

You can do different types of aerobic activities, say walking one day, riding a bike the next. Make sure you choose an activity that can be done regularly, and is enjoyable for you. The important thing to remember is not to skip too many days between workouts or fitness benefits will be lost. If you must lose a few days, gradually work back into your routine.

The Benefits of Exercise in a Weight Control Program

The benefits of exercise are many, from producing physically fit bodies to providing an outlet for fun and socialization. When added to a weight control program these benefits take on increased significance.

We already have noted that proper exercise can help control weight by burning excess body fat. It also has two other body-trimming advantages: 1) exercise builds muscle tissue and muscle uses calories up at a faster rate than body fat; and 2) exercise helps reduce inches and a firm, lean body looks slimmer even if your weight remains the same.

Remember, fat does not "turn into" muscle, as is often believed. Fat and muscle are two entirely different substances and one cannot become the other. However, muscle does use calories at a faster rate than fat which directly affects your body's metabolic rate or energy requirement. Your basal metabolic rate (BMR) is the amount of energy required to sustain the body's functions at rest and it depends on your age, sex, body size, genes and body composition. People with high levels of muscle tend to have higher BMRs and use more calories in the resting stage.

Some studies have even shown that your metabolic rate stays elevated for some time after vigorous exercise, causing you to use even more calories throughout your day.

Additional benefits may be seen in how exercise affects appetite. A lean person in good shape may eat more following increased activity, but the regular exercise will burn up the extra calories consumed. On the other hand, vigorous exercise has been reported to suppress appetite. And, physical activity can be used as a positive substitute for between meal snacking.

Better Mental Health

The psychological benefits of exercise are equally important to the weight conscious person. Exercise decreases stress and relieves tensions that might otherwise lead to overeating. Exercise builds physical fitness which in turn builds self-confidence, enhanced self-image, and a positive outlook. When you start to feel good about yourself, you are more likely to want to make other positive changes in your lifestyle that will help keep your weight under control.

In addition, exercise can be fun, provide recreation and offer opportunities for companionship. The exhilaration and emotional release of participating in sports or other activities are a boost to mental and physical health. Pent-up anxieties and frustrations seem to disappear when you're concentrating on returning a serve, sinking a putt or going that extra mile.

Tips to Get You Started

Hopefully, you are now convinced that in order to successfully manage your weight you must include exercise in your daily routine. Here are some tips to get you started:

1. Check with your doctor first. Since you are carrying around some extra "baggage," it is wise to get your doctor's "OK" before embarking on an exercise program.

2. Choose activities that you think you'll enjoy. Most people will stick to their exercise program if they are having fun, even though they are working hard.

3. Set aside a regular exercise time. Whether this means joining an exercise class or getting up a little earlier every day, make time for this addition to your routine and don't let anything get in your way. Planning ahead will help you

get around interruptions in your workout schedule, such as bad weather and vacations.

4. Set short term goals. Don't expect to lose 20 pounds in two weeks. It's taken awhile for you to gain the weight, it will take time to lose it. Keep a record of your progress and tell your friends and family about your achievements.

5. Vary your exercise program. Change exercises or invite friends to join you to make your workout more enjoyable. There is no "best" exercise—just the one that works best for you.

It won't be easy, especially at the start. But as you begin to feel better, look better and enjoy a new zest for life, you will be rewarded many times over for your efforts.

Tips to Keep You Going

1. Adopt a specific plan and write it down.

2. Keep setting realistic goals as you go along, and remind yourself of them often.

3. Keep a log to record your progress and make sure to keep it up-to-date.

4. Include weight and/or percent body fat measures in your log. Extra pounds can easily creep back.

5. Upgrade your fitness program as you progress.

6. Enlist the support and company of your family and friends.

7. Update others on your successes.

8. Avoid injuries by pacing yourself and including a warmup and cooldown period as part of every workout.

9. Reward yourself periodically for a job well done!

Part Two

Fitness for Specific Age Groups

Chapter 5

Kids in Action: Fitness for Children 2-17

The challenge for parents is to find ways to encourage their children to be physically active. This chapter contains some ideas for activities that you and your child can do together.

There are two sections in this chapter. The first section contains activities for children ages 2—6 years. The second section describes the President's Council on Physical Fitness and Sports' tests for measuring the physical fitness of children 6 to 17 years.

Initially some activities may be more difficult than others. With practice most activities will become easier. Activity variations are suggested to accommodate children's different abilities.

Children 2-6

1. Over-Under-Around

Adult sits on floor, legs apart. Child moves around parent going over legs. Parent forms a bridge. Child goes under and around.

Variations: Lower or raise height of body. Have child roll ball over-under-around. Have child form bridge.

President's Council on Physical Fitness and Sports.

2. Twister

Child takes a pole and holding it with both hands, steps through the triangle formed by the arms and pole. The child then should be able to step foot by foot forward and backward without letting go of the stick.

3. Jump the Stick

Parent holds a pole just above the floor and child jumps over.

Variations: Change the height of the pole. Move the pole back and forth. Vary the speed of pole.

4. Jump the Brook

Use a towel or mark the sidewalk with the "banks of the brook." Child stands on one of the brook and attempts to jump the brook without "falling in."

Variations: Increase the width of the brook.

5. Simon Says

Simon says: "Can you touch your toe to your chin?" Select body parts that encourage stretching.

Variations:

Touch your ear to your shoulder
Touch your toe to your elbow
Touch your knee to your ankle
Touch your knee to your elbow
Touch your nose to your knee

6. Wall Push-ups

Stand about arms distance away from a wall with your legs together. Place your hands on the wall just a little wider than your shoulders. Lean forward and touch your nose to the wall and push back to your starting position. Be sure to keep your body in a straight line and your heels on the floor. How many can you do?

7. *Jumping Beans*

Hold the child's hands in yours. Child starts bouncing, then jumping up and down. Stop, rest and start again.

Variations: Hop on one foot then the other. Vary the speed (fast, slow).

8. *Beanbag Balance*

Place a beanbag (or soft toy) on the child's head. Ask the child to walk from one place to another without dropping the beanbag. To make it easier, have the child hold the beanbag in place.

Variations: Place the beanbag on other body parts (e.g., back of hand, shoulder, elbow). Use a different toy or more than one toy. Walk around or under things.

9. *Row, Row, Row Your Boat*

Parent sits with legs apart, child sits opposite with legs in the middle. Grasp the child's hands. Child leans back as if "rowing a boat", then pulls to upright sit. Repeat. Sing "Row, row, row your boat."

10. *Wheelbarrow*

Child lays face down on the floor. Parent grasps child's ankles and lifts upward. Ask the child to push up with arms until arms are straight. With head up, walk the hands forward. Child's body should not sag.

11. *Toe-Walking*

Walk around on your toes.

Variations: Carry an object. Swing your arms.

12. *Statues*

Can you balance on one foot for the count of "4 alligators"? (One alligator, two alligators...)

Variations: Count more alligators Balance in different postures (i.e., statues).

13. One-Foot Balance Game

Place 5 small objects on an unbreakable dish near another container. Child stands on one foot in front of the dish and container. Ask the child to move the objects one at a time from the dish to the container without losing balance.

Variations: Vary the distance between the dish and container. Time the game.

14. Inch Worm

Child bends over, placing both hands on the floor. The feet are kept stationary while the hands walk forward as far as possible. Then the hands remain stationary while the feet walk forward as close to the hands as possible. Repeat the cycle.

15. Egg Roll

Sit on the floor with the legs drawn up to the body and the knees spread outward. Holding the feet with the hands, roll over to the right, across the back to left, and return to the sitting position. Keep the hands around the feet throughout.

16. Somersault

Teach your child to roll backwards and forwards. Make sure the child's chin is close to the chest and that weight rests on shoulders and not on head. Be sure to practice on a sofa or cushions.

17. Up-Up-Down-Down

Repeat the cadence, "up-up-down-down" as parent and child step up (right), step up (left), step down (right), step down (left) on the first step of the stairs.

18. Clutch ball

Child sits on floor and holds a ball tightly between legs with hands above head. Parent lifts child in the air by the arms and child tries to keep ball from dropping.

19. Around the World

Child sits on the floor with legs crossed. Lift ball high over head. Reach forward to place ball as far in front as possible. Reach as far to the right and to the left without lifting body from the floor.

20. Catch

Parent and child stand 2-3 yards apart. Bounce ball so that each can catch without leaving their place. If child has difficulty with catching a ball, use a balloon (mylar)—it travels much slower.

Variations: Clap your hands before catching (or spin around). Throw and catch without a bounce. Two bounces rather than one.

21. Throw

Can you fly a paper airplane? Child practices throwing paper airplane.

Variations: Throw ball made of newspaper or old pantyhose. Throw objects upstairs (How for up the stairs can you throw ball?)

Young People 6-17

Being physically fit is important for everyone. When you are physically fit, your muscles, heart and lungs are strong and your body is firm and flexible. To help you measure your physical fitness, the President's Council on Physical Fitness and Sports has developed fitness tests for youngsters ages 6 to 17 years. The five test items included in the President's Challenge Test battery are:

Challenge Item	Primary Fitness Component Measured
One-mile run/walk	heart/lung endurance
Curl-ups	abdominal strength/endurance
V-Sit Reach (or sit and reach)	lower back/hamstring flexibility
Shuttle Run	leg strength/endurance/power/agility
Pull-ups	upper body strength/endurance

Each test and the score for the 50th and 85th percentiles for boys and girls are described in this chapter.

Instructions for the President's Challenge Test items.

Before performing these test items, read the directions carefully so that they are performed correctly. The medical status of a child should be reviewed to identify medical, orthopedic or other health problems that should be considered prior to participation in physical activities, including testing. For information on adapting the test items to youths with special needs, call the President's Council on Physical Fitness and Sports toll free number, 1 -800-258-8146.

What Does Percentile Mean?

The standards for the President's Challenge test are based on the fitness scores of thousands of students in the United States. If you score at the 85th percentile or above, you have scores in the top 15 percent of your age group. If you score at the 50th percentile or above, it means that you have scored in the top half among the youngsters in your age group who have taken this test.

1. Curl Ups

Objective: To measure abdominal strength/endurance by maximum number of curl-ups performed in one minute

Rules: "Bouncing" off the floor is not permitted. The curl-up should be counted only if performed correctly.

Testing: Have student lie on cushioned, clean surface with knees flexed and feet about 12 inches from buttocks. Partner holds feet.

Arms are crossed with hands placed on opposite shoulders and elbows held close to chest. Keeping this arm position, student raises the trunk curling up to touch elbows to thighs and then lowers the back to the floor so that the scapulas (shoulder blades) touch the floor, for one curl-up. To start, a timer calls out the signal "Ready? Go!" and begins timing student for one minute. The student stops on the word "stop."

Curl Ups (Timed one minute)

			Percentile			
	Boys				**Girls**	
Age	**50th**	**85th**		**Age**	**50th**	**85th**
6	22	33		6	23	32
7	28	36		7	25	34
8	31	40		8	29	38
9	32	41		9	30	39
10	35	45		10	30	40
11	37	47		11	32	42
12	40	50		12	35	45
13	42	53		13	37	46
14	45	56		14	37	47
15	45	57		15	36	48
16	45	56		16	35	45
17	44	55		17	34	44

2. Shuttle Run

Objective: To perform shuttle run as fast as possible.

Testing: Mark two parallel lines 30 feet apart and place two blocks of wood or similar object (approximate size of 2"x2"x4") behind one of the lines. Students start behind opposite line. On the signal "Ready? Go!" the student runs to the blocks, picks one up, runs back to the starting line, places block behind the line, runs back and picks up the second block and runs back across starting line.

Rules: Blocks should not be thrown across the lines. Scores are recorded to the nearest tenth of a second.

Shuttle Run (seconds)

Percentile

| | Boys | | | Girls | |
Age	50th	85th	Age	50th	85th
6	13.3	12.1	6	13.8	12.4
7	12.8	11.5	7	13.2	12.1
8	12.2	11.1	8	12.9	11.8
9	11.9	10.9	9	12.5	11.1
10	11.5	10.3	10	12.1	10.8
11	11.1	10.0	11	11.5	10.5
12	10.6	9.8	12	11.3	10.4
13	10.2	9.5	13	11.1	10.2
14	9.9	9.1	14	11.2	10.1
15	9.7	9.0	15	11.0	10.0
16	9.4	8.7	16	10.9	10.1
17	9.4	8.7	17	11.0	10.0

3. One Mile Run/Walk

Objective: To measure heart/lung endurance by fastest time to cover a one-mile distance.

Testing: On a safe, one-mile distance, students begin running on the count "Ready? Go!" Walking may be interspersed with running. However, the students should be encouraged to cover the distance in as short a time as possible.

Rules: Before administering this test, students' health status should be reviewed. Also, students should be given ample instruction on how to pace themselves and should be allowed to practice running this distance against time. Sufficient time should be allowed for warming up and cooling down before and after the test. Times are recorded in minutes and seconds.

One-Mile Run (minutes/seconds)

	Boys			Girls	
Age	50th	85th	Age	50th	85th
6	12:36	10:15	6	13:12	11:20
7	11:40	9:22	7	12:56	10:36
8	11:05	8:48	8	12:30	10:02
9	10:30	8:31	9	11:52	9:30
10	9:48	7:57	10	11:22	9:19
11	9:20	7:32	11	11:17	9:02
12	8:40	7:11	12	11:05	8:23
13	8:06	6:50	13	10:23	8:13
14	7:44	6:26	14	10:06	7:59
15	7:30	6:20	15	9:58	8:08
16	7:10	6:08	16	10:31	8:23
17	7:04	6:06	17	10:22	8:15

4. Pull-Ups

Objective: To measure upper body strength/endurance by maximum number of pull-ups completed.

Testing: Student hangs from a horizontal bar at a height the student can hang from with arms fully extended and feet free from floor, using an overhand grasp (palms facing away from body). Small students may be lifted to starting position. Student raises body until chin clears the bar and then lowers body to full hang starting position. Student performs as many correct pull-ups as possible.

Rules: Pull-ups should be done in a smooth rather than jerky motion. Kicking or bending the legs is not permitted and the body must not swing during the movement.

Flexed-Arm Hang: Alternative to pull-ups for National Physical Fitness Awards.
Students who cannot do one pull-up may do the flexed-arm hang in order to qualify for the National Physical Fitness Awards. To qualify for the Presidential Award, students are required to do pull-ups.

Objective: To maintain flexed-arm hang position as long as possible.

Testing: Using same hand position as in pull-ups, student assumes flexed-arm hang position with chin clearing the bar. Students may be lifted to this position. Student holds this position as long as possible.

Rules: Chest should be held close to bar with legs hanging straight during hang. Timing is stopped when student's chin touches or falls below the bar.

Pull-Ups

				Percentile			
	Boys				**Girls**		
Age	**50th**	**85th**			**Age**	**50th**	**85th**
6	1	2			6	1	2
7	1	4			7	1	2
8	1	5			8	1	2
9	2	5			9	1	2
10	2	6			10	1	3
11	2	6			11	1	3
12	2	7			12	1	2
13	3	7			13	1	2
14	5	10			14	1	2
15	6	11			15	1	2
16	7	11			16	1	1
17	8	13			17	1	1

Flexed-Arm Hang (seconds)

	Percentile		
Boys		**Girls**	
Age	**50th**	**Age**	**50th**
6	6	6	5
7	8	7	6
8	10	8	8
9	10	9	8
10	12	10	8
11	11	11	7
12	12	12	7
13	14	13	8
14	20	14	9
15	30	15	7
16	28	16	7
17	30	17	7

5. V-Sit Reach

Objective: To measure flexibility of lower back and hamstrings by reaching forward in the V position.

Testing: A straight line two feet long is marked on the floor as the baseline. A measuring line is drawn perpendicular to the midpoint of the baseline extending two feet on each side and marked off in half-inches. The point where the baseline and measuring line intersect is the "0" point. Student removes shoes and sits on floor with measuring line between legs and soles of feet placed immediately behind baseline, heels 8-12 inches apart. Student clasps thumbs so that hands are together, palms down and places them on measuring line. With the legs held flat by a partner, student slowly reaches forward as far as possible, keeping fingers on baseline and feet flexed. After three practice tries, the student holds the fourth reach for three seconds while that distance is recorded.

Rules: Legs must remain straight with soles of feet held perpendicular to the floor (feet flexed). Students should be encouraged to reach slowly rather than "bounce" while stretching. Scores, recorded to the nearest half-inch are read as plus scores for reaches beyond baseline, minus scores for reaches behind baseline.

V-Sit Reach (inches)

		Percentile				
	Boys				**Girls**	
Age	**50th**	**85th**		**Age**	**50th**	**85th**
6	+ l.0	+ 3.5		6	+ 2.5	+ 5.5
7	+ 1.0	+ 3.5		7	+ 2.0	+ 5.0
8	+ 0.5	+ 3.0		8	+ 2.0	+ 4.5
9	+ 1.0	+ 3.0		9	+ 2.0	+ 5.5
10	+ 1.0	+ 4.0		10	+ 3.0	+ 6.0
11	+ 1.0	+ 4.0		11	+ 3.0	+ 6.5
12	+ 1.0	+ 4.0		12	+ 3.5	+ 7.0
13	+ 0.5	+ 3.5		13	+ 3.5	+ 7.0
14	+ l.0	+ 4.5		14	+ 4.5	+ 8.0
15	+ 2.0	+ 5.0		15	+ 5.0	+ 8.0
16	+ 3.0	+ 6.0		16	+ 5.5	+ 9.0
17	+ 3.0	+ 7.0		17	+ 4.5	+ 8.0

Awards

If you were able to reach the 85th percentile on all 5 items for your age group, you may qualify for the President's Physical Fitness Award. Or, if you achieved the 50th percentile on all 5 items, the National Physical Fitness Award. For more information on the Presidential Physical Fitness Awards program write:

President's Council on Physical Fitness and Sports
Kids in Action
701 Pennsylvania Ave., NW, Suite 250
Washington, D.C. 20004

Chapter 6

Get Fit!

How to get in shape to meet the President's Challenge

Introduction

American youth have participated in the Presidential Physical Fitness Award Program or the "President's Challenge" since 1966. The program includes all young people from the ages six through 17, including those student with special needs.

In addition, two awards have been added to go with the prestigious Presidential Physical Fitness Award for outstanding achievement. The National Physical Fitness Award was introduced in 1987 and is for those who reach a basic yet challenging level of fitness. A new award called the Participant Physical Fitness Award, introduced in the Fall of 1991, is for those who attempt the President's Challenge but don't qualify for a Presidential or National Award.

You should strive for either the Presidential or National Physical Fitness Awards, and to become as physically fit as you can be. This booklet will help you. On the following pages you will learn how to get in shape, how to practice for each of the events in the "President's Challenge" and how to improve on those events which are giving you trouble so that you can increase your chances of earning either of the President's Challenge awards.

Everyone can become physically fit. All it takes is some determination, some time and a serious commitment. Don't be discouraged if you can't do EVERY exercise immediately. Do what you can and go on to the next exercise. By following the directions in this booklet, you'll soon be on the way to improvement.

It's important to remember, however, that you shouldn't try to do too much too soon, because you could injure yourself. Getting in shape requires time. If you feel pain or exhaustion, ease off and tell your parent or instructor. A workout should be challenging, but not painful. As you get in better shape you'll also find it fun and exhilarating.

Motivational tips from the PCPFS

Don't make the mistake of thinking that just because you are active, you are physically fit already. It takes specific exercises to build fitness—exercises for flexibility, strength and endurance. That's where this chapter will help. It's also fun to learn how your muscles work. You may want to read a book on fitness or on the human body to increase your knowledge.

It's also important and fun to set goals. Record your weekly progress in a personal log or notebook. Keep track of the number of pull-ups and curl-ups you do and how far you can stretch. Keep track of the number of miles jogged. You may want to chart them on a map and plot a cross-country, imaginary trip. It's also fun to make exercise a part of your daily life and to try to include friends and family members in your physical activities—walking, bicycling, swimming, skating, skiing, just to mention a few.

Even with a busy schedule, you can find time to exercise. Try to set aside a specific time each day. Maybe you can cut down on the amount of time you spend watching TV. Or you can find exercises you can do while watching your favorite programs. The important thing is to make the commitment to get fit. Even if you don't earn an award this year, you'll know that you've tried and that you are heading in the right direction. No one can expect more of you than that.

What is Physical Fitness?

Being physically fit means having the energy and strength to perform daily activities vigorously and alertly without getting "run down," and to have energy left over to enjoy leisure time activities or meet emergency demands. When you are physically fit, your heart, lungs and muscles are strong and your body is firm and flexible. Your weight and percent body fat are within a desirable range.

Physical fitness will help you control your weight and cope with stress. You'll feel and look better, and that often means success in anything you want to do, such as work, sports, dance, and other recreational activities. You may even do better in school.

Getting in shape is important for your future. You'll be healthier both now and as an adult, and that means a more enjoyable and active life.

How do you Measure Physical Fitness?

Physical fitness can be broken down into three main parts: endurance, strength and flexibility. Each one can be measured and there are specific exercises to improve each area.

Endurance is the ability to keep moving for long periods of time. There are two types of endurance:

- *Cardiorespiratory endurance* means that your heart and lungs are in good shape and are able to supply your muscles with lots of oxygen and nutrients. "Aerobic" exercises like running, walking, jumping rope and cycling build endurance in your heart and lungs. How fast you can run or walk a mile is one test of heart/lung endurance.

- *Muscular endurance* means that your muscles are strong enough to move for long periods of time. Exercises such as push-ups, leg raises, and curl-ups build muscular endurance and strength. How many curl-ups you can do is a test of abdominal muscle strength and endurance.

Why Build Endurance? With high levels of endurance you have more energy and are able to last longer when you play sports or games. You don't get out of breath easily and your muscles are firm and trim. When your heart and lungs are in good shape you're healthier and less likely to develop some forms of disease. Also, doing "aerobic" exercises burns extra calories and helps keep your weight under control.

Strength is how much force you can exert with your muscles. You can measure this by seeing how much weight you can hold in place (static strength), how much weight you can move (dynamic strength), or how fast you can move a weight (power). This weight can refer to your own body weight or special equipment such as a barbell or strength training machine. Always make sure you talk to someone who knows a lot about strength training before you use special equipment.

Why Build Strength? When you are strong you don't need to rely on others to do the "heavy" work and you are less likely to injure your muscles. You can do things like lift your body weight and move heavy objects. Hard jobs become easier and you'll also do better in sports, games and other activities

Flexibility means that you can move your muscles and joints through their "full range of motion." Stretching exercises increase flexibility. Seeing how close you can come to touching or reaching beyond your toes is one measure of flexibility.

Why Build Flexibility? When your muscles are flexible you can reach, bend and stretch more easily. You are less likely to injure your muscles and joints. Stretching helps decrease tension and stress, and makes your body feel good.

Other factors that will affect how well you do in the "President's Challenge" are Speed, Agility, and Coordination. These factors also will help improve your performance in your daily activities.

Body Composition

People who are physically fit have a well-balanced body shape and good body composition. Body composition means how much of your body is fat compared to lean body mass, which includes muscles, bones, tissues and organs.

Exercise gives muscles their shape, and muscles give shape to your body. People who exercise are more likely to have less body fat than those who are not in shape. Boys tend to have less body fat than girls.

You are healthier when your weight and body fat are in the right range.

The scale is not always a good indicator of fitness particularly for athletes. Since muscle weighs more than fat, you could have good body composition yet appear to weigh too much on the scale or, you could weigh the right amount but have too much fat on your body. If you want to know whether your body composition is good ask your physical education or health teacher, or a fitness instructor, to measure your percent body fat.

How to Improve

To improve your fitness level, you must follow the P.R.O.S.—the principles of exercise. They are PROGRESSION, REGULARITY, OVERLOAD, SPECIFICITY, and here's what they mean:

Progression—Gradually increase how hard, how long and how many times you do an exercise over a period of time. It takes six to eight weeks for physical improvements to be seen, but you'll feel better right away. For example, don't try to go from 5 curl-ups to 50 curl-ups overnight, but add a few more every week until you've reached your goals.

Regularity—Set up a regular schedule and work out every day, or at least 3-4 times each week. It's not good to take too much time off between workouts—what you don't use, you lose.

Overload—For a muscle to get stronger it must work harder than it does at rest. This means making your heart beat faster and your breathing increase during aerobics, doing more repetitions of an exercise or lifting more weight. If an exercise feels too easy it probably is, and chances are you won't improve. But remember, don't overdo it. "No pain, no gain" is a myth!

Specificity—Exercise is specific. For example, aerobic exercises won't build flexibility. And, stretching exercises won't make your muscles stronger. To be flexible you have to stretch, and to be strong you have to make your muscles work hard. And, to be good at a certain sport you have to practice that sport.

How to Meet the "President's Challenge"

Since 1966, American youngsters have taken part in the Presidential Physical Fitness Award program or the President's Challenge. Those youngsters reaching the 85th percentile or above on all five items of the test became eligible to receive the Presidential Physical Fitness Award for outstanding achievement.

To help motivate many more young people to exercise regularly and improve their fitness, two awards were added to complement the long-standing Presidential Physical Fitness Award. The National Physical Fitness Award was added in 1987 and recognizes those youngsters who score at or above the 50th percentile on the same five test items. The Participant award, introduced in the Fall of 1991, recognizes boys and girls who attempt all five test items but whose scores fall below the 50th percentile on one or more of them. (Note: Students who cannot do one pull-up may substitute the flexed arm hang and its standards in order to qualify for the National or Participant Physical Fitness Award.) All three awards are now available to boys and girls with special needs based on the criteria outlined on page 97 of this chapter.

Challenge Item	Primary Fitness Component Measured
One-mile run/walk	heart/lung endurance
Curl-ups	abdominal strength/endurance
V-Sit Reach (or sit and reach)	lower back/hamstring flexibility
Shuttle Run	leg strength/endurance/power/agility
Pull-ups	upper body strength/endurance

What Does Percentile Mean? The standards for the President's Challenge test are based on the fitness scores of thousands of students like yourself in the United States. If you score at the 85th percentile or above, you have scored in the top 15 percent of your age group. If you score at the 50th percentile or above, it means that you have scored in the top half among the youngsters in your age group who have taken this test.

When you qualify for the Presidential Physical Fitness Award you are eligible to receive a Presidential certificate of achievement and a **blue** emblem. The emblem may be purchased with or without the number of years the award has been won.

When you qualify for the National Physical Fitness Award you are eligible to receive either a National certificate of achievement, a **red** emblem or both.

When you qualify for the Participant Physical Fitness Award (**new**) you are eligible to receive either a Participant certificate of achievement, a **white** emblem or both.

The program is conducted in schools, park and recreation departments, YMCA's, Jewish Community Centers and other youth organizations. Ask your teacher for more information on the program.

Winning an award is something of which to be proud. We encourage you to strive to do better and if you qualify for the white emblem this year, go for the red next year; if you win the red, go for the blue. But remember, you're all winners in fitness!

These are the exercises you will be asked to do to qualify for the Presidential, National or Participant Awards. Check your scores against the chart on pages 89–90.

Curl-ups

Sit on the floor with your knees flexed feet about 12 inches from your buttocks. Place hands on opposite shoulders, arms close to chest. A partner will hold your feet and count each curl-up. Raise your trunk up to touch elbows to thighs. A complete curl-up is counted each time you lie back and touch your shoulders to the floor. The goal is to do as many curl-ups as you can in one minute.

Pull-ups

Grasp a bar with an overhand grip. Small children can be lifted to this position. Feet should not touch the floor and legs should hang straight.

Begin by hanging with your arms straight. Pull your body up with a steady movement until your chin is over the bar and extend back down. Do as many pull-ups as you can. There is no time limit and the pull-ups must be done with straight legs.

Shuttle Run

Two blocks of wood or similar objects are placed behind a line drawn 30 feet from where you start. On the signal "Ready, Go!" you run to the blocks, pick one up, bring it back and place it behind the starting line. You then run and pick up the second block and bring it back across the starting line. Your fastest time is recorded.

One Mile Walk\Run

At the signal "Ready, Go" you begin running one mile on a track or safe area marked off to the correct distance. Walking is permitted. However, the goal is to complete the mile as fast as possible.

V-sit Reach

Take off your shoes and place your feet directly behind a line marked on the floor. Your feet should be 8-12 inches apart. This is the baseline. A measuring line is placed between your legs. Clasp your thumbs so that your hands are together with palms down and place them on the measuring line. A partner will hold your legs straight. Keeping your toes pointing upward (feet flexed) reach forward as far as possible along the measuring line. Exhale as you reach forward. Reaches beyond baseline are "plus" scores, behind baseline are "minus." Baseline equals "0." You'll have three practice tries and the fourth reach will be recorded.

Option: Sit and Reach

A specially designed box is used for this flexibility test. You sit on floor with legs straight and feet held flat against end of box. A measuring line is on top of the box with 23 centimeters marked at the level of the feet. You place your hands evenly along measuring line, one hand on top of the other, and reach as far as you can. Three practice tries are allowed and the fourth reach is recorded. Scores are recorded in centimeters.

Can You Meet the President's Challenge?

On the following pages are some exercises you can do to get in shape for the "President's Challenge". How you do these exercises is very important so be sure to follow the directions carefully. If you are unsure about what to do or would like some different exercises, ask your physical education teacher or someone knowledgeable about physical fitness. Remember, exercising comes easier to some kids than others. Work hard but don't make getting in shape a contest. Progress at your own pace and you will soon see and feel the benefits.

If you score at or above these scores for your age and sex on **all five** events you qualify for the **Presidential Physical Fitness Award.**

The Presidential Physical Fitness Award

Qualifying Standards

Boys

Age	Curl-Ups (Timed one minute)	Shuttle Run (seconds)	V-Sit Reach or Sit And Reach (inches)	(centimeters)	One-Mile Run (minutes/seconds)	Pull-Ups
6	33	12.1	+3.5	31	10:15	2
7	36	11.5	+3.5	30	9:22	4
8	40	11.1	+3.0	31	8:48	5
9	41	10.9	+3.0	31	8:31	5
10	45	10.3	+4.0	30	7:57	6
11	47	10.0	+4.0	31	7:32	6
12	50	9.8	+4.0	31	7:11	7
13	53	9.5	+3.5	33	6:50	7
14	56	9.1	+4.5	36	6:26	10
15	57	9.0	+5.0	37	6:20	11
16	56	8.7	+6.0	38	6:08	11
17	55	8.7	+7.0	41	6:06	13

Girls

Age	Curl-Ups (Timed one minute)	Shuttle Run (seconds)	V-Sit Reach or Sit And Reach (inches)	(centimeters)	One-Mile Run (minutes/seconds)	Pull-Ups
6	32	12.4	+5.5	32	11:20	2
7	34	12.1	+5.0	32	10:36	2
8	38	11.8	+4.5	33	10:02	2
9	39	11.1	+5.5	33	9:30	2
10	40	10.8	+6.0	33	9:19	3
11	42	10.5	+6.5	34	9:02	3
12	45	10.4	+7 0	36	8:23	2
13	46	10.2	+7.0	38	8:13	2
14	47	10.1	+8.0	40	7:59	2
15	48	10.0	+8.0	43	8:08	2
16	45	10.1	+9.0	42	8:23	1
17	44	10.0	+8.0	42	8:15	1

The National Physical Fitness Award

Qualifying Standards

Boys

Age	Curl-Ups (Timed one minute)	Shuttle Run (seconds)	V-Sit Reach or Sit And Reach		One-Mile Run (minutes/seconds)	Pull-Ups or Flexed-Arm Hang	
			(inches)	(centimeters)			(seconds)
6	22	13.3	+1.0	26	12:36	1	6
7	28	12.8	+1.0	25	11:40	1	8
8	31	12.2	+0.5	25	11:05	1	10
9	32	11.9	+1.0	25	10:30	2	10
10	35	11.5	+1.0	25	9:48	2	12
11	37	11.1	+1.0	25	9:20	2	11
12	40	10.6	+1.0	26	8:40	2	12
13	42	10.2	+0.5	26	8:06	3	14
14	45	9.9	+1.0	28	7:44	5	20
15	45	9.7	+2.0	30	7:30	6	30
16	45	9.4	+3.0	30	7:10	7	28
17	44	9.4	+3.0	34	7:04	8	30

Girls

Age	Curl-Ups (Timed one minute)	Shuttle Run (seconds)	V-Sit Reach or Sit And Reach		One-Mile Run (minutes/seconds)	Pull-Ups or Flexed-Arm Hang	
			(inches)	(centimeters)			(seconds)
6	23	13.8	+2.5	27	13:12	1	5
7	25	13.2	+2.0	27	12:56	1	6
8	29	12.9	+2.0	28	12:30	1	8
9	30	12.5	+2.0	28	11:52	1	8
10	30	12.1	+3.0	28	11:22	1	8
11	32	11.5	+3.0	29	11:17	1	7
12	35	11.3	+3.5	30	11:05	1	7
13	37	11.1	+3.5	31	10:23	1	8
14	37	11.2	+4.5	33	10:06	1	9
15	36	11.0	+5.0	36	9:58	1	7
16	35	10.9	+5.5	34	10:31	1	7
17	34	11.0	+4.5	35	10:22	1	7

The Participant Physical Fitness Award

Boys and girls who attempt all five test items but whose scores fall below the 50th percentile on one or more of them are eligible to receive the new Participant Award.

Getting in Shape to Meet the President's Challenge

Always warm up your body first for about five minutes to get your muscles and joints ready for action. You'll know you are warmed up when you start to sweat and breathe heavier. Warm-up exercises actually raise your body's temperature and make your muscles more limber. After you've warmed up your body and mind are ready for more vigorous activity. The four exercises that follow are warm-up exercises.

Deep Breather

Stand tall with knees slightly bent. Rise on your toes and slowly circle your arms inward and upward, until arms are straight overhead. Inhale deeply. Continue circling your arms backward and downward while lowering your heels and exhaling. This exercise should be done slowly and smoothly. Repeat 5 times.

Swinging March

Stand up straight with feet shoulder-width apart, hands at your sides. Alternate right and left arms in forward circle motions as if you were doing the forward "crawl" swimming stroke. At the same time, lift your opposite knee so that when your right arm is circling forward your left knee is raised; right knee is raised while left arm is moving forward. Do 10 complete circles with each arm and then switch arms to do the "backstroke." repeat 10 full circles with each arm.

The Pendulum Push

Stand straight with arms at your side. Step to right, bending your right knee. Raise arms overhead and push towards the ceiling. At the same time, rise on your right toes and lift your left leg off the ground, keeping all your weight on the right foot. Put your left leg back on the ground, bending both knees and placing hands on shoulders. Repeat to the left side by pushing off on your left foot, pushing palms towards the ceiling and lifting your right foot off the ground. Repeat 10 times on each side.

Jumping Jacks

Stand straight with feet together. Jump up and land with your feet shoulder-width apart as you swing: arms to shoulder height. Jump back to starting position while clapping your hands over your head. Jump up and land with feet apart while bringing; your arms back to shoulder height. Jump back to starting position while lowering arms to your sides. Repeat this 4-part jumping jack 10-20 times at a slow, controlled pace.

Stretching

Stretching helps prevent your muscles and joints from getting injured. Stretching makes your body more flexible so you are able to move easily and do your best in your activities.

When you stretch, relax and breathe comfortably. Don't bounce or jerk. Hold each position for about 10 seconds. If it hurts ease up a little. As you improve, hold each stretch for 30 seconds. Stretching also helps you relax when you're feeling tense. Always remember to stretch muscles after they've been warmed up.

The following are just a few of the stretches you can do every day to improve your flexibility.

Back Scratch Stretch

You can do this stretch standing or sitting. Raise your right hand in the air with your palm facing to the back. Bend your elbow and place the palm of your hand on your back between your shoulders. Bring your left hand behind your back and try to touch your right hand. Hold 10-30 seconds. Repeat two times on each side. Don't force this stretch; you may find one side easier than the other!

Knee-Hi Stretch

While standing, lift left knee toward your chest. Place left hand under your knee and pull leg up to stretch the back of your leg and your lower back. Keep standing leg slightly bent. Hold for 10-30 seconds. Repeat twice on each side.

Thigh Stretch

Keeping body upright, grasp left foot behind you with left hand. Slowly pull leg back so that your knee moves away from your body until you feel a stretch in front of your leg. Hold 10-30 seconds. Repeat twice with each leg.

Calf Stretch

Lean against a wall and put right leg behind you. Keep right heel on the floor and very slightly bend the right knee. Lean forward until you feel a pull in your calf and behind your ankle. Hold 10-30 seconds. Repeat twice with each leg.

Cardio-Respiratory Exercises

Every exercise program should include aerobic activities to strengthen your heart and lungs. Aerobic exercises require lots of oxygen and make your heart beat faster. Walking, swimming, running and aerobic dancing are examples of this type of exercise. Since the President's Challenge includes a one-mile run/walk, it's a good idea to practice running as your aerobic activity.

After you've warmed up and stretched you're ready to run. And, don't forget the P-R-O-S (page xx).

First, find an area where a one-mile distance can be marked off. Four times around a school track is usually one mile. If you've never run a mile before, follow the Beginner program. If you're a pretty good runner, but haven't been following a regular running routine, follow the Intermediate program. If you've done a lot of running and are ready to time yourself for the one-mile, follow the Advanced program.

Beginner:—Jog 2 minutes/walk 1 minute for a total of 15 minutes. Repeat. Do this at least three times a week for 2 weeks. Don't worry about the distance yet.

Intermediate:—Jog 4 minutes/walk 1 minute. Do this for about 15-20 minutes at least three times a week. After about two weeks, reduce the amount of walking time to 30 seconds. Gradually build up to about 30 minutes using this pattern.

Advanced:—Continuously jog for 20 minutes. Of course, there is no limit here. If you find jogging is for you, you can run longer distances. Once a week, time a one-mile run for speed and work up to the score you need to meet the "President's Challenge."

Training Tips for a Jogging Program

- Wear good running shoes with plenty of cushion and support.

- Land on your heel, roll through your feet and push off from the ball of your foot. Running on your toes can make your calves feel very tight.

- Keep your shoulders relaxed and your elbows slightly bent. Look straight ahead, not at your feet.

- Breathe steadily and deeply, with mouth open. If you have trouble catching your breath, slow down a little.

- Run with good form. Let your arms swing naturally, and alternate arms and legs. Your right arm and left leg should be moving forward at the same time and your left arm and right leg at the same time.

- Always warm up (start gradually) and cool down (stop gradually). Stretch your muscles before and after you jog.

- *Never* stop abruptly or lie down after your jog. When you're ready to stop, gradually slow down and walk for about 3 minutes before coming to a complete stop.

Muscular Strength and Endurance Exercises

These exercises will help you get in shape to do Curl-Ups, Pull-Ups, and Shuttle Run for the "President's Challenge." They will help develop your muscle strength and endurance. Do these exercises and practice the specific "Challenge" items as well.

Curl-Ups:

Lie on your back with knees bent at 90 degrees, feet flat on the floor. Place your arms across your chest, hands on opposite shoulders. Slowly curl your head, shoulders and upper back off the floor bringing elbows to thighs. Breathe out as you curl up and then return to starting position while breathing in. Start with 10 repetitions.

Gradually add 2 curl-ups each week until you've reached the 85th percentile score needed for your age and sex. Practice these curl-ups at least 3 times each week. In addition, have someone time you once a week to see how many curl-ups you can do in one minute. Eventually, you'll reach your goal! You can do it with enough practice.

Modified pull-ups

Place a strong pole or pipe on the seats of two chairs placed about four feet apart. Make sure the ends of the bar are secure. Lie on your back, slide under the bar and grasp it with two hands, palms facing away from your body and hands about shoulder width apart. Pull your chest up to the bar keeping your body straight from head to feet. Do this 10 times. If it is easy, find a higher bar. Eventually, work up to a horizontal bar where your body can hang completely off the ground. Practice holding your chin above the bar or doing pull-ups at least three times each week. Work up to the number you need to do to meet the "President's Challenge."

Push-ups

Get down on your hands and knees and position yourself so that your back is straight, head in line with your spine. Hands should be placed slightly outside your shoulders, fingers pointed forward, feet on the ground. Slowly lower your body until your chest touches the floor. Return to starting position. Once you can do 20-25 with your knees bent, advance to the straight-leg position on your hands and toes. Try to do 10 repetitions again to start!

Coffee Grinder

Support your body (turned sideways) on your right hand and arm and both feet. Keep your right arm and both legs fully extended, with feet slightly apart. Now "walk" your body in a circle using your right arm as a pivot. Repeat using your left arm. Repeat 10 times on each side.

Crab Walk

Sit on the floor with knees bent, feet flat on the ground and hands placed behind you on the floor. Raise your body up so that it is supported by your hands and feet. Walk forward on hands and feet for 5 steps, then backward for 5 steps. Add one step each way every week. Build up to 20 steps in each direction.

The Hoop Hopper

Cut out circles of paper or mold circles out of wire about 12-15 inches in diameter. Stagger 12 hoops in two rows of six with 12 inches separating the hoops from one another. Run through hoops, alternating right and left, with right foot going through hoops on right side, and left foot going through left hoops. Lift your knees high. Once you get good at this, time yourself and try to get faster.

The Wall Jump

Stand sideways next to a wall and extend your arm up. Mark, mentally or with a piece of tape, the spot one yard away from your fingers. Drop your arm, bend your knees and leap up and try to touch that mark. Repeat 10 times on each side.

Cooling Down

After you have done your "aerobic" or "muscular conditioning" work, you're ready to " cool down". Just as you had to "warm up" your body before exercising vigorously, you should "cool it down" to get your breathing back to normal. Cooling down helps keep your muscles from becoming sore and stiff.

Before you do your cool-down stretches, walk around for a few minutes to make sure your breathing is back to normal and your heart is not beating fast. You should be feeling slightly relaxed by the time you're ready to do stretches.

You can choose stretching exercises you've done in your warm-up or add others. The important thing to remember is to stretch all major joints and muscle groups, especially those you have used during your workout. This is the time when you really can work on your flexibility, since it's easier to stretch warm muscles.

When you're done, see how many questions you can answer correctly in the fitness quiz that follows . . . you're on the road to physical fitness!

PRESIDENT'S COUNCIL ON PHYSICAL FITNESS AND SPORTS
New Statement of Policy
and
Criteria for Qualifying Students with Special Needs for the Presidential, National and Participant Physical Fitness Awards

Students with special needs have the right to an individualized physical fitness program and the President's Council on Physical Fitness and Sports (PCPFS) includes this important element in guidelines for quality physical education. The Council also believes these students can be motivated to develop lifetime habits of appropriate exercise through recognition of achievement in physical fitness. The modified award criteria listed below have been prepared to permit boys and girls ages 6-17 with special needs to qualify for the Presidential, National or the Participant Awards in the President's Challenge Awards Program.

Qualified instructors who verify they have followed the criteria presented may qualify students with special needs who do not reach PCPFS printed standards on one or more of the five test items in the awards program.

These Modifications Apply To All Awards.

Criteria for qualifying students with special needs for the Presidential, National or Participant Awards:

1. The instructor has reviewed the individual's records to identify medical, orthopedic or other health problems which should be considered prior to participation in physical activities including physical fitness testing.

2. The individual has been participating in an appropriate physical fitness program that develops and maintains cardiorespiratory endurance; muscle strength, endurance and power; and flexibility.

3. The individual has one or more disabilities which directly affects performance in physical fitness activities.

4. The individual has on file an Individual Education Program (IEP) as defined under The Education of all Handicapped Children Act (Public Law 94142) and The Rehabilitation Act of 1973, Section 504 (Public Law 93-112) or is certified by a qualified instructor as possessing a physical disability which affects performance in physical fitness activities.

5. The instructor has administered the following five test items according to the provided program instructions allowing for modifications of or substitutions for those items necessary to accommodate the individual's condition: (1) one mile walk/run, (2) abdominal-curl, (3) pull-ups or flexed-arm hang, (4) shuttle run, and (5) V-sit reach or sit and reach.

6. The instructor judges that the individual has performed each of the five test items and/or necessary modifications or substitutions at his/her Fitness Award age group qualifying standards or at a level equivalent to a Presidential, National, or Participant level of performance for a boy or girl this age with this condition.

Fitness Quiz

1. Stretching exercises will help:
   A. Build strength
   B. Avoid injuries
   C. Burn calories
   D. None of these

2. Joints and muscles are prepared for vigorous exercise by:
   A. Jogging and weight training
   B. Warm-ups and stretching
   C. Rope climbing and sit-ups
   D. Pushups and jumping rope

3. Muscle endurance is:
   A. The ability to move a heavy weight once
   B. The ability to stretch
   C. The ability to move something many times
   D. The ability to jump high

4. Jogging for 20 minutes will improve:
   A. Flexibility
   B. Muscle strength
   C. Heart/lung endurance
   D. None of these

5. The best heart/lung (aerobic) endurance exercise is:
   A. Short, fast runs
   B. Long, slow runs
   C. Tumbling
   D. Basketball

6. Muscle strength is the ability to:
   A. Move a heavy weight once
   B. Play sports
   C. Move something many times
   D. Run fast

7. Which athlete will probably require the most heart/lung (aerobic) endurance during a game:
   A. Soccer goalie
   B. Softball fielder
   C. Basketball guard
   D. Football quarterback

Fitness Quiz (continued)

8. Cooling down after a workout is important because:
   A. It gives your body time to return to its normal level
   B. It helps reduce your chance of injury
   C. It lowers your pulse and breathing rate slowly
   D. All of the above

9. The ratio of lean body mass to fat is:
   A. Body size
   B. Body type
   C. Body fitness
   D. Body composition

10. Physical fitness is important for:
    A. Health
    B. Physical performance
    C. Mental well-being
    D. All of the above

(Adapted from "Fitness for Living," Walt Disney Educational Media Company in cooperation with the PCPFS)

Answers to Fitness Quiz

1. B	6. A
2. B	7. C
3. C	8. D
4. C	9. D
5. B	10. D

Chapter 7

Physical Education: A Performance Checklist

How good is the physical education program in your child's school? It's possible—even likely—that you've never asked yourself that question before. Some parents tend to take physical education for granted, and others simply don't consider it important enough to merit concern. They are vitally concerned about the three R's—Reading, 'Riting and 'Rithmatic—but they don't realize that the fourth R, Regular Physical Activity, is just as important.

That attitude is reflected in the poor physical condition of much of today's youth. Recent reports indicate that American children and adolescents aren't getting enough vigorous activity to develop a healthy heart and lungs, and fewer young people are able to achieve minimum standards of fitness than in past surveys.

The problem is twofold:

- Only one child in three participates in a daily program of physical education (at least one school period of vigorous physical activity) as recommended by the President's Council on Physical Fitness and Sports and leading medical authorities, and some have no programs at all.

- Some schools place little emphasis on activities I that develop physical fitness and useful skills.

President's Council on Physical Fitness and Sports, OM 85-0053.

What about your children? Are they getting the kind of physical education that they need? The answer is important to their future— physically fit young people are likely to grow up to be physically fit adults.

Regular, vigorous exercise is essential to physical and emotional development, and studies show that children's self-confidence and self-mastery grow as their fitness level rises. Childhood experiences also help shape adult behavior. The boy or girl who develops skills and learns to enjoy physical activity has a headstart on good health and happiness throughout life.

This chapter is intended to help you assess the quality of the physical education program in your schools. You owe it to yourself and your child to know the answer.

The Other Half Of Education

Physical education has been called "the other half of education."

Most school subjects are designed to train the mind, but physical education helps students develop and learn to use their bodies. Since physical education is the only subject that concerns itself with the complex organism that houses and supports the mind, its importance should be evident.

Basically, physical education in the school has three objectives:

- To produce physically fit youth;

- To educate young people concerning the essential nature of physical activity and its relationship to health, physical fitness and a more dynamic, productive life;

- To give students the skills, knowledge and motivation to remain fit.

How does your child's program measure up?

The checklist below has been prepared to help you find out. If you can answer "yes" to each of the questions asked, the program probably is a good one. If not, you will want to see what can be done to strengthen the program.

Remember: Your child has a right to good health and fitness. Exercise it!

A Performance Checklist For Your Schools

Not all good physical education programs are exactly alike, but experience has shown that those which fulfill the three objectives described in the previous section tend to have certain features in common. These are reflected in the checklist that follows.

We urge you to check the program in your school against this yardstick. Your interest could make the difference between a program that meets your child's needs and one that falls short.

A Performance Checklist

YES   NO

☐ ☐ Physical fitness is not a part-time thing. Does your school provide at least one period per day of instruction in vigorous physical activity?

☐ ☐ Play alone won't develop physical fitness. Is a part of each physical education period devoted to activities like running calisthenics, agility drills and weight training?

☐ ☐ Skill in sport is a valuable social and health asset. Does your school program offer instruction in lifetime sports like tennis, swimming, golf, skiing and jogging?

☐ ☐ Most physical problems can be alleviated if discovered early enough. Does the school give a screening test to identify those students who are weak, inflexible, overweight, or lacking in coordination?

☐ ☐ All children can improve with help. Are there special physical education programs for students with special problems such as the retarded/ the handicapped, and the underdeveloped?

☐ ☐ Testing is important to measure achievement. Are all students tested in physical fitness at least twice a year?

What to do to change the "No" answers to "Yes"—

First: Make sure you know what your local school code says about physical education, and what is specified in state laws or regulations.

Then:

1. Speak to the physical education instructor in your child's school. You will find him or her very cooperative and willing to answer your questions.

2. If the physical education instructor can't help, speak to the school principal.

3. If significant changes are needed in the school's priorities or scheduling try to encourage your parent/teacher organization to support a regular physical education program with an adequate emphasis on physical fitness.

4. It the problem is one of policy in the entire school district take up the issue with your local Board of Education.

5. If your school is doing all it can at this time make certain your child gets at least one-half hour of vigorous physical activity every day before or after school.

For additional information or help in setting up a program of vigorous physical activity for your child write:

The President's Council on Physical Fitness And Sports
Washington, D.C. 20001

Chapter 8

Fit Kids, Smart Kids

New research confirms that exercise boosts brainpower.

By Eric Olsen

At a time when school systems all over the United States are reducing "frills" in order to concentrate on "basics," one of the classic candidates for cutting back has been recreation—specifically, physical-education classes and after-school athletics. According to a recent national study, only 36.3 percent of schoolchildren in the United States even have daily phys-ed classes on their schedule.

Related to this surprising statistic is another finding, made by the American Academy of Pediatrics, that fewer than half of all schoolchildren get enough exercise to develop healthy hearts and lungs. Moreover, 40 percent of all children in the United States between ages 5 and 8 have at least one risk factor for heart disease.

It is sad enough that the decreasing role of recreation in our schools is taking its toll on our children's bodies. What makes it doubly unfortunate is the toll it is taking on their minds. New data from a variety of studies have provided a solid foundation for what had been a largely unproven notion: that kids spending time in phys-ed classes or after-school recreation programs—or simply playing, running, jumping, swinging, hopping, and generally giving themselves a good aerobic workout—reap the results both physically and academically.

In fact, that is precisely what Roy J. Shepard, M.D., Ph.D.—professor of applied physiology, and a child-fitness expert, at the Univer-

---

Parents Magazine,

sity of Toronto—found out back in the 1970s while studying more than 500 Canadian children. The students who spent an extra hour each day in gym class—an hour that reduced the amount of time for academics—performed notably better on exams than less active children.

In a confirmation of Shepard's findings, recent studies are uncovering a direct physical link between fitness and intelligence. One such study was conducted by Robert Dustman, Ph.D., director of neuropsychology research at the Veterans Affairs Medical Center, in Salt lake City. Dustman recently gave a series of mental and physical tests to a group of relatively inactive men and women in their 50s and 60s, then put the subjects on a four-month aerobic-training program of regular brisk walking. Following the training course, their performance on a series of mental tests jumped by 10 percent.

In a similar study, Brad Hatfield, Ph.D., a professor of kinesiology at the University of Maryland at College Park, and several colleagues compared the beta-wave activity—which researchers have associated with mental stamina and clarity of mind—of two groups of men similar in age, education, income, and socioeconomic status. One of Hatfield's groups regularly ran as much as six miles per day; the other group did no cardiovascular conditioning or training. Hatfield, like Dustman, found that the men who participated in aerobic activities did significantly better on tests of mental performance, including concentration, arithmetic and spatial problems, and reaction times.

Of course, both of these studies look at adults, not children. Researchers maintain, however, that if these findings demonstrate the importance of aerobic exercise to a well-functioning adult mind, then they are probably even more significant for children, whose brains are still developing. Dan Landers, Ph.D., a professor of exercise science and physical education at Arizona State University, has looked Closely at 13 different studies on the exercise-brainpower link, and he says that in every one of those studies, "we found that the biggest effects were in the young—under 16—and in the elderly. Exercise stimulates the growth of developing brains and prevents the deterioration of older brains."

What is the connection between aerobic exercise and intelligence? The answer, according to Dustman, can be summed up in one word: "oxygen." "The brain depends on oxygen to function properly," he says, "and a healthy cardiovascular system gets more oxygen to the brain. Improve the function of the heart and lungs, and you get smarter."

That claim is certainly supported by the laboratory work of William Greenough, Ph.D., professor of neuroscience at the University of

Illinois, and James Black, M.D., Ph.D., professor-in-training at the University of Utah Medical Center. They found that rats put on an aerobic training program had 20 percent more blood vessels in their brains than sedentary rats had. Moreover, they found that rats trained in "acrobatic" activities—ones that require learning complex physical tasks—showed an increase in the number and complexity of connections between neurons. This is an indicator of improved brain efficiency.

According to Black, "I think that these findings apply to human beings as well, and they are particularly relevant to young children. The strongest effects we found were in young rats that were just weaned—about the equivalent of human toddlers."

But what is the best way to make sure that your child is getting her aerobic exercise? In the opinion of the experts, fitness begins at home. Says Roy Shepard. "When fitness is practiced by the whole family, children are more likely to take their fitness habits into adult life." (To find out what children's physical needs are at different ages, see below.)

Here are some simple things you can do to make physical activity a lifelong pursuit for your child:

- **Make it fun.** Whatever you do, avoid the boot-camp approach to fitness. A pushy parent can turn a child off to physical activity for life. Charles Kuntzleman, Ed.D., director of the Fitness for Youth program, in Jackson County Michigan, advises "Be a guest in your child's play, no matter what sport or activity is involved. Where there is interest, jump in. Where there is resistance, hold back. You want your child to be healthy *and* happy, and that happens when fitness is fun."

- **Set a good example.** Don't lecture your child on the importance of physical activity while sitting in a reclining chair. make sure that *you* are involved in a regular exercise program. Children of active parents are more likely to be more active themselves.

- **Emphasize aerobics.** Aerobic exercise includes brisk walking, jogging, cycling—anything that uses the larger muscles of the body, particularly the legs, gets the heart rate up, and keeps it up. Most fitness experts agree that for parents and school-age children, 30 minutes of aerobic exercise three or four times a week is the *minimum* amount necessary to foster physical (and intellectual) health. As for children, the

President's Council on Physical Fitness and Sports recommends a minimum of half an hour per day.

- **Include more challenging activities.** James Black suggests that aerobic conditioning is more effective when combined with activities that require learning and mental effort, such as gymnastics, tennis, and dance.

- **Emphasize activities that will last a lifetime.** Team sports can be great fun, but individual activities such as cycling, swimming, running, and cross-country skiing also develop fitness while at the same time providing the foundation for a lifetime of active living. Furthermore, they can be successfully pursued even by those who are not athletically talented; team sports, on the other hand, frequently offer chances to warm the bench for all but the most gifted.

What are Your Child's Exercise Needs?

Although it is tricky to generalize about children's physical requirements—each child develops at an individual pace, after all—there are some broadly defined stages of growth. Knowing what they are can help you and your child make the most of her playtime.

Birth to 2 Years.

It is too early to be thinking about structured physical activity. Plenty of physical contact between you and your child, however, can be the first step in fostering her love of exercise. Let your child be the guide as to how much she needs.

Two to 7 Years.

This is a time when children are intent on learning the basic vocabulary of sports skills—running, jumping, catching, skipping, and so on. Now is the perfect time for games in the backyard or mother-daughter "jogs." (Your child should set the pace.) In your games, stress effort and skill building over achievement and winning. And now, more than any other time in your child's life, is when you should emphasize the place of fun in physical activity.

Eight Years and Older.

Children are now generally entering the world of team sports. While these sports do foster virtues such as teamwork, you should also be encouraging your child's involvement in the "lifetime" sports, such as cycling, swimming, and running. Children are likely to get more out of these sports in terms of actual fitness.

Eric Olsen, a writer in northern California, specializing in health, is the author of the book, Lifefit *(Human Kinetics).*

Chapter 9

Nutrition and Sports Performance

A Guide for Physically-Active Young People

Eating well helps people of all ages to have better health, stamina and energy. Good nutrition is particularly important for young people who want to achieve and maintain top-notch athletic performance. Successful athletes are blessed with the right combination of heredity, training and coaching. But even the most talented athletes are unlikely to achieve their potential with poor nutrition. Physically-active people should eat a carbohydrate-based, moderate protein diet, similar to that recommended for average, healthy people. However, athletes generally require far more calories. How many calories they need will vary according to their height, growth rate, sex, age, type of sport and level of training.

Activity	Calories Burned Per Hour	
	Male	Female
Aerobics, moderate intensity	330	270
Basketball	720	600
Football, touch	490	410
Ice skating	380	320
Jogging (9-10 minute mile)	720	540
Running (7 minute mile)	890	730
Skiing, cross-country	660	540
Swimming, competitive	990	820
Swimming, fast	620	510
Weightlifting (heavy for males, light for females)	590	220

American College of Sports Medicine. Used by permission.

111

Active people may have varied calorie needs, depending upon their activity. But sprinting events, swimming, high jumps, weight lifting or other short duration events requiring power and strength require a carbohydrate-based diet, just as do all-day events or endurance sports, such as swim meets, cross-country skiing, soccer and long-distance running. For both power and endurance athletes, a daily carbohydrate-rich training diet is just as important as pre-event meals. A high-protein and high-fat diet during training can result in fatigue and may hurt performance. After all, how can athletes compete at their best if they can't train at their best?

A wholesome diet based upon carbohydrates (between 55 and 65 percent of daily caloric intake) including meat or protein-rich food as the "accompaniment" (10-15 percent of caloric intake) and fat for the remaining calories (about 25-30 percent of caloric intake) is appropriate for all young people to eat. This diet should include foods from the main food groups (at least 6-11 servings of breads, cereals, rices and pastas; 3-5 servings of vegetables; 2-4 servings of fruit; 2-3 servings from the meat, poultry, fish, dry beans, eggs and nuts group and 2-3 servings from the milk, yogurt and cheese group) that not only taste good, but are high in nutrients and are easy to digest. Young athletes and all young people need energy for growth as well as for extended activity and training. Concentrating on eating carbohydrate-rich foods is one way to meet that challenge.

Protein is necessary to build and repair muscle and other tissues; only a very small amount is used for energy needs. A small serving of protein-rich food (lean meat, poultry, seafood, dairy products and beans) at each meal 4 will support athletic performance and fulfill the body's basic requirements.

Carbohydrates come in two forms: simple and complex. Simple carbohydrates are found in fruits, juices, milk, frozen yogurt and candy, while complex carbohydrates are found in whole grains, vegetables, pasta, rice and breads. The body breaks down both forms of carbohydrates into glucose for immediate energy needs. Excess glucose is stored mainly in the muscles and, to a lesser degree, in the liver, as glycogen to fuel exercise. You need to eat wisely every day because you can deplete your glycogen stores in as little as 2-3 hours of moderate exercise. Depleted glycogen stores can cause fatigue and poor performance.

Fats carry vitamins through your system, are good for sustained energy, and add flavor to foods. Despite increased awareness of the health risks associated with a high-fat diet, consuming too little fat creates other problems, such as inadequate calorie intake. Some fat at each meal is appropriate, but avoid excessive amounts of fried, greasy, oily and buttery foods, which will fill the stomach but leave the muscles unfueled.

Fluids should be emphasized as a part of the diet, especially among athletes. You need fluids to regulate your body temperature and prevent over-heating. For example, if you lose 3-4 pounds during practice or training, you'll be less able to reduce body heat. This failure to regulate temperature will drastically hurt performance and can lead to medical problems. Fluids also transport energy, vitamins and minerals throughout the circulatory system and are necessary for all bodily functions. Everyone should drink at least six to eight glasses of fluids daily or until the urine is a clear color. Athletes should also drink liberal amounts of fluids before, during and after exercise. Frequent urination is a sign that you've had enough to drink. A simple way to determine how much fluid to drink is to weigh yourself before and after a workout or competition. The weight loss will be almost entirely fluids that should be replaced accordingly (1 lb. lost sweat = 2 cups fluid). Drinking more fluids rather than fewer can help prevent dehydration and over-heating. Fluids can include water, juices or sports drinks.

Young people who want to lose weight often resort to trendy or fad diets. These diets hurt not only their health but also their performance, due to inadequate calories and nutrients. Athletes who skip meals, eliminate food such as meat or milk, or lose excessive weight too quickly will find it difficult to sustain peak performance in their sport.

In spite of all the information that's generally available, sports nutrition myths prevail. The following questions and answers dispel some common misconceptions about nutrition and sports performance.

Q: Some of my son's teammates on the football team say it's important to eat lots of steak and take protein supplements to build muscle. Is their information correct?

A: No. If your son eats too much protein and too little carbohydrate (i.e., a big steak with a small potato or extra chicken with only a little rice), he'll deny his muscles the energy they need to perform well.

Try to develop a wide assortment of carbohydrate-rich food choices for your family at home—cereals, casseroles, pastas, breads. Spending some extra time in the weight room rather than eating excessive protein also will help your son to better achieve his goals because exercise, not eating extra protein, builds muscle. Although some protein is necessary to build all body cells, including muscles, excess protein is broken down and stored as body fat. There is no valid scientific evidence that protein supplements are necessary if your son eats a balanced, varied diet. Vitamin and mineral supplements do not provide the body with any additional energy. Do note that athletes should be sure to monitor their calorie and iron intakes. Teens who do not eat red meat should pay careful attention to other dietary iron sources and make the effort to combine iron-rich vegetable sources, such as beans, with the intake of vitamin C to ensure maximum absorption. Calcium-rich foods...milk, yogurt and cheese (preferably low fat) should be consumed 2-3 times a day.

Q: My daughter's lunch period is at 11 a.m. and basketball practice starts at 4 p.m. She claims that she's not supposed to eat before practice, but I worry that going too long without food is unwise. Would a snack hurt her performance?

A: No. Your daughter's performance could benefit from eating a snack sometime before practice. A banana, for example, is a carbohydrate-rich snack that would supply her with a number of key vitamins and minerals. Other popular snacks include fruit, juice or confectionery (containing simple carbohydrates), and bagels, crackers, or half a sandwich (containing complex carbohydrates).

Q: I'm on the high school swim team and want to lose about five pounds. My friend lost weight fast by eating nothing but fruit one day and high-protein foods like chicken the next day. Is this a good idea?

A: Definitely not. First, discuss with a registered dietitian or your family doctor how much—weight if any—you should try to lose. If losing five pounds is a reasonable expectation, eat smaller portions of a well-balanced diet that emphasizes a variety of foods. By cutting back on fat (butter, mayonnaise, salad dressing), you will reduce calories safely, without reducing energy needs for your sport. Nutrition experts recommend you lose no more than 1-2 pounds per week. If you lose weight faster, you'll lack energy to exercise, lose some muscle, and probably regain the weight very quickly. Rather than go on a restrictive crash diet, simply consume smaller portions at meals and snack times.

Q: My son wants to fast to make weight on his wrestling team. He also believes that carbohydrates are fattening and would prevent him from making the wrestling team. What can I tell him?

A: Fasting or restricting carbohydrates will hurt your son's performance, not enhance it. Carbohydrates are essential for fueling the muscles. Although an athlete may think carbohydrates are fattening, they are not. Excess fats are fattening —i.e., butter, mayonnaise, fried foods, etc. Encourage your son to enjoy high-carbohydrate foods like potatoes, rice and pasta, which will also provide the energy to sustain his performance. To cut back on calories, he can simply go easy on the added fats, like butter and cheese. He should enjoy an adequate breakfast (cereal/fruit/ juice) and lunch (sandwich, soup, milk, fruit), then eat smaller-than-usual portions at dinner so that he'll have energy during the day to study and train.

Menu Plan For Active People

	Male (2,800 kcal)	**Female (12,200 kcal)**
Breakfast	¾ cup bran cereal ½ banana 1 cup 1% milk 6 oz. orange juice 1 slice toast 1 tsp. margarine* 1 tsp. jam	½ cup bran cereal ½ banana 1 cup 1% milk 6 oz. orange juice
Lunch	1 cup minestrone soup roast beef sandwich: large roll, 3 oz. lean roast beef 2 tsp. mayonnaise* lettuce, tomato raw vegetables 1 apple 2 small oatmeal- raisin cookies 1 cup 1% milk 1 oz. pretzels	1 cup minestrone soup roast beef sandwich: large roll, 2 oz. lean roast beef 1 tsp. mayonnaise* lettuce, tomato raw vegetables 1 apple 1 small oatmeal- raisin cookie 1 cup 1% milk

Menu Plan for Active People (cont.)

	Male (2,800 kcal)	Female (12,200 kcal)
Afternoon Snack	6 oz. juice, 1 candy bar** or 1 slice of devil's food cake with frosting** (average slice 2.5 oz.)	6 oz. juice, 1 candy bar** or 1 slice of devil's food cake with frosting** (average slice 2.5 oz.)
Dinner	green salad with 1 tbs. low-cal dressing 1 whole grain roll 1 tsp. margarine* 1 chicken leg, no skin 1 ½ cup rice 1 cup broccoli sautéed in 1 tsp. olive oil* 1 orange 1 cup 1% milk	green salad with 1 tbs. low-cal dressing 1 whole grain roll 1 tsp. margarine* 1 chicken leg, no skin ¾ cup rice 1 cup broccoli sautéed in 1 tsp. olive oil* 1 orange 1 cup 1% milk
Evening Snack	1 cup vanilla low-fat yogurt	1 cup vanilla low-fat yogurt

* Small amounts of fat are a necessary pan of an overall low-fat diet.

** An overall wholesome diet can include some sweet snacks, such as cake and candy.

For more information, write to:

American College of Sports Medicine
P.O. Box 1440
Indianapolis, IN 46206-1440
Tel: 317-637-9200
Fax: 317-634-7817

Chapter 10

Play It Safe!

A Guide to Preventing Sports-related Injuries in Young Athletes.

We all want kids and teens to grow up healthy and happy. That's why we put together these materials—we're going to show you the best ways to keep kids active and in the game.

Safety First

Healthy kids are active kids. Traditional sports like baseball, football and basketball have never been more popular. And, new ones are popping up every day—in-line skating, snowboarding, rollerhockey. Encouraging kids to participate in sports will help them become fit, coordinated, and confident, *and* teach them the spirit of teamwork.

With all that activity, injuries *can* happen. And, sports injuries are no fun. You can play an important role today to help prevent injuries from happening tomorrow. Experts estimate that 50% of all sports injuries are preventable. Here are five simple steps to help young athletes play it safe. By the way, these steps will help keep you safe, too, so don't forget to follow them yourself!

Step 1: Get Involved

Whether you're a parent, coach, athletic trainer, or medical professional, *you* are responsible for the safety of the kids and teens under your care. Let's take a look at each role:

American College of Sports Medicine. Used by permission.

Parents: Here are three easy ways to help keep kids on the road to safety and good health. Parents should:

- Check the qualifications of prospective coaches, athletic trainers and doctors *before* letting a young athlete participate.

- Pay close attention to their child's medical needs. This includes watching for signs of over-exertion. (Your health care provider can give you more details on these signs.)

- Keep a positive, upbeat attitude...especially when the competition is fierce and the emotions are running high. Never pressure kids to play a sport they don't want to play. Reinforce the ones they do like to play.

Coaches: Coaches need to know the basics of skills development, rules, equipment maintenance, first aid, training methods, and appropriate coaching behaviors, no matter what level. Check out helpful information through programs such as the National Federation of Interscholastic Coaches Association (NFICA) 816-464-5400 or National High School Athletic Coaches Association (NHSACA) 800-COACH-95.

Athletic Trainers: Trainers can help an athlete stay in the game, or get back into the game (both physically and mentally), by working closely with the athlete, parents, coaches and doctors. By working as a team, you'll not only fix injuries that have already occurred, but you'll also help to prevent future injuries.

Medical Personnel: It's critical that health care providers stay involved with the athlete's life. Start with the pre-season check-up. Then, keep medical supplies and equipment on site at sporting events and be there for assistance should an injury occur.

Step 2: Get a Pre-Season Check-Up

A comprehensive check-up will help the doctor spot medical problems early and help prevent new ones from happening.

Here's what to expect from a comprehensive check-up:

A complete physical exam. The doctor will get vital information from the athlete's physical examination and use it to help keep him or her safe and healthy. For example, the doctor may prescribe special treatment or specific training programs to best help the young athlete with a pre-existing condition participate in sports activities. Or, the doctor may suggest alternative activities if a condition stops the athlete from participating.

A strength and flexibility exam. From this exam, the doctor can identify the strength and flexibility of the athlete's muscles and the alignment and range of motion in the major joints. A doctor can also spot weaknesses and prescribe special training to strengthen them or correct abnormalities. All of this information can be used to bolster a young athlete's confidence and self-esteem.

A discussion on nutrition, drug use, and mental attitude. This part of the exam gives the doctor a chance to reinforce that playing sports is supposed to be a fun and healthy experience. A doctor should ask questions to find out how the athlete feels about playing sports, explain the dangers of drug use, encourage a well-balanced diet, and stress the importance of drinking plenty of fluids.

Step 3: Train the Right Way

It's vital that young athletes follow the rules and keep safety first.

Proper training methods can be fun *and* help prevent injuries at the same time. But first, let's talk about what we mean by training.

A proper training program results in a progressive improvement in performance capacity. The coach or athletic trainer should work closely with athletes to monitor progress of the training program, and keep them on a schedule to help them achieve peak performance.

If an athlete doesn't use proper training methods, he or she may run the risk of getting two types of injuries: acute and overuse. An acute injury comes from a sudden, single trauma, like pulling a muscle or breaking a bone.

As the name implies, overuse injuries may result from the cumulative effects of heavy workouts.

It's important to remember that both overuse and acute injuries are preventable. That in mind, here are a few simple guidelines to help avoid both types of injuries. *Remember, these are only guidelines.* A doctor, coach, or athletic trainer can provide specific methods to suit an athlete's personal needs.

Always have warm-up and cool-down sessions. Allow plenty of time for stretching tight muscles. Warm up before playing any sport or doing any exercise. Also, spend plenty of time cooling down when practice or games end. A coach or athletic trainer should be able to provide proper guidelines.

Progress gradually. As time is needed to allow for adaptation to the demands of training, a young athlete's training program should not progress rapidly. It's back to the idea that building muscle and endurance should be a gradual process. Again an athletic trainer can provide more specific information based on an athlete's personal needs.

Employ proper weight training techniques. For many sports, weight training with professional instruction and proper supervision is a great way to build strength safely. Especially with young athletes, the concentration should be on lifting light weights for a high number of repetitions to build strength. The stronger the athlete, the less likely injuries will occur.

Modify training for different climates. For example, it takes an athlete's body time to adjust to training in the eat. Take frequent breaks on hot, humid days. Ideally, training sessions should be scheduled to avoid times of peak heat stress.

Drink plenty of fluids. Adequate fluid intake is necessary for an athlete's peak performance and avoidance of heat injuries. So it's crucial to drink fluids before, during and after physical activity. Don't let young athletes get dehydrated. For example, athletes involved in continuous activity should drink approximately 1½ cups of water or sports drinks every 15 minutes to help prevent dehydration. Having athletes drink on a schedule, not just when they're thirsty, will help prevent problems. Be sure to have lots of water or sports drinks available at sporting events and training sessions.

Step 4: Use the Right Equipment and Proper Facilities

Being safe and using the right equipment go hand in hand. If you're a parent, coach, or athletic trainer, it's your responsibility to provide safe equipment and proper facilities. Here's a checklist you can use to ensure safe sports:

- Be sure to have *all* of the proper equipment. You don't want an in-line skater skating with knee pads but not wrist guards, or a football player with a helmet and no mouth guard. For safety's sake, have a complete set of equipment.

- Be sure the equipment fits correctly. For example, a helmet that is too big may not protect the head to the level it's supposed to. Equipment manufacturers usually specify the correct fittings.

- Inspect playing surfaces and facilities before an activity gets underway. For example, gymnastic equipment should be secure. For playing softball after dark, make sure the field is well lit. You get the idea...safety first.

- Maintain athletic equipment. Keeping equipment in top-notch condition helps to prevent injuries. Look for products with set rules for maintenance, servicing and safety, and follow the instructions.

- Wear appropriate clothing. What an athlete wears can help or hinder their performance. For example, a tennis player wearing a fleece sweat suit to a tennis match may not perform as well as an opponent in shorts and a t-shirt. Wear loose, lightweight and lightly colored clothing in hot weather. And wear warmer, yet breathable, clothes in layers in cold weather.

Step 5: Play By the Rules

Sporting events have rules to help keep players and their teammates safe. Here are some tips to keep in mind:

- To be safe, familiarize athletes with the rules for their sports. And if you see ways to make activities even safer, talk with other parents, coaches and athletic trainers about them.

- Encourage teamwork and good sportsmanship. One way to help prevent injuries is to encourage players to have fun and be a good sport while they compete.

More Ways to Play it Safe

Sports and games are supposed to be fun, teach teamwork, increase confidence, and build strength. All participants from young players to parents can enjoy safety in sports by taking a few simple steps today.

As we've shown you here, injuries don't have to be a part of sports when you play it safe.

If you're looking for more information on how you can play it safe, send a self-addressed, stamped envelope (first-class postage) to:

Play it Safe
American College of Sports Medicine
P.O. Box 1440
Indianapolis, IN 46206-1440

ACSM will send you information about joining ACSM's Fit Society$_{SM}$

Chapter 11

Better Health and Fitness Through Physical Activity: Guidelines for Teens

What exactly is physical fitness? Being fit means you have more energy to do daily tasks, can be more active, and do not tire as easily during the day. Being ht also helps you build a positive self-image and feel better about yourself.

You do not have to spend hours in a gym to be physically active. Every time you throw a softball, swim a lap, or climb up a flight of stairs you are improving your health and fitness level.

The American Academy of Pediatrics has developed the following material to help you understand what physical fitness is and to give you ideas on how you can become more physically active.

Benefits of Physical Activity

Physical activity has many proven benefits. When you are physically fit, you feel and look better, and you stay healthier. Physical activity can help you to:

- Prevent high blood pressure
- Strengthen your bones
- Ward off heart disease and other medical problems
- Relieve stress

American Academy of Pediatrics: HE0090, 1996.

123

- Stay active as an adult

- Maintain or achieve an appropriate weight for your height and body build

A major benefit of physical activity is that it helps reduce stress. Learning to cope with stress is an important part of healthy living. Family problems, conflicts with friends, and school pressures can cause stress. Major changes in your life, such as moving to a new home or breaking up with someone, are also sources of stress. Exercise helps you relax by causing physical changes inside your body that help it react to and handle stress.

Physical activity also has many other health benefits, such as helping to ward off heart disease. Coronary heart disease is the leading cause of death in the United States. Research has shown that your risk factors as an adult for developing heart disease start during your childhood. A lack of physical activity is one of the major risk factors influencing heart disease, such as high blood pressure, and other medical illnesses.

Physical Fitness is a Balance of Many Areas

To be physically fit, you must work on all aspects of fitness, including the following:

Cardiorespiratory endurance (aerobic fitness) — This is the ability of the heart, lungs, and circulatory system to deliver oxygen and nutrients to all areas of your body. When you are active, you breathe harder and your heart beats faster so that your body is able to get the oxygen it needs. If you are not fit, your heart and lungs have to work extra hard during physical activity.

Body composition (body fat) — This is the percentage of body weight that is fat. Overweight people have more body fat in relation to the amount of bone and muscle in their bodies than do people who are physically fit Overeating, not exercising enough, or both often lead to more body fat. Being overweight increases your risk of diabetes, high blood pressure, and heart attacks.

Muscle strength and endurance — This is the amount of work and the amount of time that your muscles are able to do a certain activity before they get tired, such as lifting heavy objects or in-line skating.

Flexibility — Flexibility is the ability to move joints and stretch muscles through a full range of motion. For example, people who are very flexible can bend over and touch the floor easily. A person with poor flexibility is more likely to get hurt during physical activity.

What Can I Do to Become More Fit?

First, you have to make the commitment to become more physically active. Try to do some physical activity every day, whether it is through physical education classes in school or an activity on your own. Exercise should be a routine part of your day, just like brushing your teeth, eating, and sleeping. It may help to plan a physical activity with a friend or family member. Most people find that it is more fun to exercise with someone else. More importantly, though, is that you like the exercise or activity. You are more apt to stay in the habit of doing whatever activity you choose if it is one that you enjoy.

Now is a good time to pick a "life sport" that you enjoy. Unlike a competitive team sport like football or baseball, a life sport is any kind of physical exercise or activity that you can do throughout your life. Examples of life sports are:

- swimming
- tennis
- golf
- walking
- bicycling
- skating
- jogging

Regular exercise should include aerobic activity. Aerobic activity is continuous. It makes you breathe harder and increases your heart rate. This type of exercise increases your fitness level and makes your heart and lungs work more efficiently. It also helps you maintain a normal weight by burning off excess fat. Examples of aerobic activities are brisk walking, basketball, bicycling, swimming, in-line or ice skating, soccer, jogging, and taking an aerobics or step class. Baseball and football do not involve as much continuous exercise because you are not active the whole time.

In general, the more aerobic an activity, the more calories—and eventually fat—you will burn. The chart at the end of this chapter gives you an estimate of the aerobic level of many different activities. You will notice that all physical activities burn more calories than sitting does.

Choose any activity you enjoy. If you like the exercise, you will want to keep doing it. Anything that involves movement qualifies as exercise. You do not have to be on a sports team, have expensive athletic clothes or shoes, or be good at sports to become more fit. Any type of regular, physical activity is good for your body. Household chores, such as mowing the lawn, vacuuming, or scrubbing, involve exercise and may have fitness benefits depending on how vigorously you do the chores. The most important thing is that you keep moving.

Be sure to include stretching exercises in your daily routine. Before you do any physical activity, you should stretch out your muscles. This warms them up and helps protect against injury. Stretching makes your muscles and joints more flexible, too. It is also important to stretch out after you exercise to cool down your muscles. Exercise videotapes, programs on television, and magazines can show you examples of how to stretch out different muscle groups, as well as different exercises you can do.

Just about any physical activity will improve fitness. For example, walking is better than riding in a car, and using the stairs is better than taking an elevator. Making small changes like these in your everyday life can make you more physically fit.

Is it Safe to Train with Weights?

You may want to include strength training as part of your regimen of physical activity, along with some form of aerobic exercise. Strength training, also called "weight training" and "resistance training," is where you use free weights and/or weight machines to increase muscle strength and muscle endurance.

When you strength train, it is more important to focus on proper technique and number of repetitions than on the amount of weight you are lifting. If you decide to strength train or weight train, make sure you use the proper safety measures. You should always have a trained adult supervise you.

You should avoid weight lifting, power lifting, and body building until your body has reached full adult development (usually between the ages of 15 and 18) because these sports can result in serious injury. Your pediatrician can help determine your stage of development.

How Often Should I Exercise?

Make exercise a part of your lifestyle. Your goal should be to do some type of exercise every day, or at the very least, three to four times a week. Try to do some kind of aerobic activity that requires continuous physical activity without stopping for at least 20 to 30 minutes each time. Do the activity as often as possible, but do not exercise to the point of pain because that can lead to injury.

Like all things, exercise can be overdone. You may be exercising too much if:

- Your weight falls below what is normal for your age, height, and build

- It starts to interfere with your normal school and other activities

- Your muscles become so sore that you risk injuring yourself

If you notice any of these signs, talk with your parents or pediatrician before health problems occur.

Exercise is Only One Part of Living Healthy

Besides the physical and mental health benefits, regular physical activity can also help you become more self-confident, organize your time better, learn new skills, and meet people with similar interests. To make more time for exercise, limit the amount of time you watch television or play computer or video games. Whenever possible, eat three healthy meals a day, including at least two to four servings of fruit and three to five servings of vegetables each day. Limit your intake of fat, cholesterol, salt, and sugar. Also, get enough sleep and take time to do things you enjoy. For even better health, don't smoke, drink alcohol, or do other drugs.

Physical activity is just one important part of preventive health care, which should be a part of your daily lifestyle. The activities you decide to do should be enjoyable, use a variety of muscle groups, and include some weight-bearing exercises. If you are not exercising much now, increase your level of activity gradually and have fun! Exercise for a better today and a healthier tomorrow!

Fitness Activity Chart

Activity	Calories Burned During 10 Minutes of Continuous Activity	
	77-lb. Person (35 kg}	132-lb. Person (60 kg)
Basketball (game)	60	102
Cross country skiing	23	72
Bicycling (9.3 mph or 15 km/h)	36	60
Judo	69	118
Running (5 mph or 8 km/h)	60	90
Sitting (complete rest)	9	12
Soccer (game)	63	108
Swimming (30 m/min. or 33 yd)		
Breaststroke	34	58
Freestyle	43	74
Tennis	39	66
Volleyball (game)	35	60
Walking		
2.5 mph or 4 km/h	23	34
3.7 mph or 6 km/h	30	43

kg = kilogram; mph = miles per hour;
km = kilometer; m = meter.

Modified from Bar-Or O. *Pediatric Sports Medicine for the Practitioner*. New York, NY: Springer-Verlag; 1983: 349-350.

Ferguson J.M. *Habits, Not Diets*. Palo Alto. CA Bull Publishing Co.; 1988.

Chapter 12

Staying Fit Over Forty

Keeping Healthy with Exercise

"Physical Fitness"—If that term brings to mind the image of a toned and muscle-bound young Olympic athlete, think again. Becoming physically fit is attainable no matter what your age or previous level of activity. And even more important, the health benefits derived from getting fit are achievable for people of any age, including those over 40.

Mounting evidence has shown that by implementing a fitness program—even after age 40—you can lead a healthier and more energetic life in your older years.

Why begin now? With increasing age, our body undergoes many changes that unfortunately can increase the risk of chronic diseases, including heart disease, arthritis, and diabetes. By starting a regular exercise routine, you may help reduce your risk from these diseases, improve your health, and perhaps increase your life span.

Fitness has other benefits as well. Exercise helps maintain sturdier bones, and thereby helps reduce risk for osteoporosis, a debilitating chronic disease that occurs commonly in postmenopausal women. Fit individuals also tend to feel more self-confident. They report feeling more relaxed and less depressed than their sedentary counterparts.

American College of Sports Medicine. Used by permission.

The hardest part of exercise is getting started, but once you begin to feel the positive effects of exercise—feeling and looking good—you will want to stay with it. It's important to deep in mind that obtaining the health benefits of exercise doesn't require tremendous effort. Neither does it require that you join a health club or buy expensive equipment.

Even a daily activity such as walking up and down the stairs in your home can be transformed into an exercise program. With all the benefits of keeping fit, you can't afford not to begin an exercise program. And no time is better than now.

What Does it Mean to be Physically Fit?

To the doctors who study exercise and its effects on the body, achieving "physical fitness" means being able to do medium-to-difficult daily activities, such as raking leaves, shoveling snow, and cleaning windows, without becoming fatigued, and being able to maintain that ability throughout life. Becoming physically fit requires improving the function of your heart and lungs; keeping your muscles strong and your joints flexible; and maintaining an appropriate body weight.

Age-Related Changes

Aging can affect the body in many ways. For example, muscle strength normally declines gradually after the age of 40. The same is true for endurance. The heart may not pump blood as well as it used to, and blood pressure may rise. Weight may increase with age as a result of reduced physical activity. Bones can weaken and lose mass and structure.

Improving With Age

Many studies have shown that even moderate exercise can help prevent diseases associated with aging and prevent premature death. The following are some encouraging facts:

Fact: Exercise helps reduce risk for osteoporosis and bone fractures.

Regular, moderate weight bearing exercise is a vital ingredient in helping maintain good bone health and prevent osteoporosis, a loss of bone mass. Inactivity can hasten the process of bone loss.

Fact: Exercise may help reduce the risk for diabetes.

By prompting the body to use glucose (sugar) efficiently, exercise may help control diabetes associated with aging.

Fact: Exercise may help add extra years.

Active and fit middle-aged men and women have a lower risk of premature death than their sedentary and unfit counterparts.

Fact: Combined with a low-fat, low-calorie diet, exercise is effective in preventing obesity.

Obesity is associated with increased risk for such diseases as coronary heart disease, diabetes, and cancer.

Fact: Heart and lung function improve with exercise.

Aerobic exercise, which raises the heart rate through such activities as brisk walking, swimming, and bicycling, helps the heart deliver more oxygen-rich blood throughout the body.

Fact: Keeping fit strengthens the muscles that stabilize joints.

Strong muscles help support the joints, allowing you to bend and move freely. Walking, bicycling, swimming and other aerobic exercises help strengthen those muscles and thus improves the ability to carry out routine activities.

Fact: Regular exercise frequently helps reduce risk factors for heart attack.

Regular physical activity helps lower blood pressure, reduces the risk for diabetes, and decreases the likelihood of obesity. It also helps elevate the amount of HDL, the "good" cholesterol—important for warding off the nation's number one killer, heart disease.

How Much is Enough?

Consistency and moderation are the keys to achieving physical fitness. The rule of thumb is to build up slowly to exercising a total of 30 to 60 minutes for a minimum of three days per week. This amount of exercise may be taken in one exercise session or accumulated in multiple sessions during the day.

To help keep yourself exercising, choose an activity that you enjoy. Walking, hiking, swimming, bicycling, and stationary cycling are examples of popular moderate-intensity activities. When you begin an exercise program, you might want to avoid high-impact activities, such as jogging, aerobic dancing, and rope skipping, because they are more likely to cause injury.

And remember, it is far better to do a little exercise regularly than a lot of exercise once in a while. "Weekend athletes"—who exercise sporadically—are more susceptible to injury than people who exercise with regularity.

If you should become injured, however, you can take important steps to minimize the damage and promote healing by initiating R.I.C.E. (Rest, Ice, Compression, Elevation): Rest the injured area, apply ice immediately, wrap the area firmly with an elastic bandage or cloth, and elevate it above the level of the heart. Consult your physician if redness and/or swelling persists. You may want to consider taking an over-the-counter pain reliever such as an ibuprofen product, like Advil®. However, if you are taking any prescription medication or have any significant health problems, check with your physician before taking any pain reliever.

Although you need to exercise regularly to achieve and maintain physical fitness, don't worry if you miss a session now and then. An occasional lapse should not affect your total fitness. If you stop exercising altogether, however, you may begin to see a decline in fitness after just two weeks. To achieve the full benefits of exercise, it is best to commit yourself to a regular workout. Keep in mind that even a little exercise can go a long way. for instance, occasional low-intensity exercise such as a brisk walk is effective in helping to improve health and function.

Most sedentary, healthy individuals can safely begin a low-level exercise program such as walking or increasing daily activities. However, it is important to check with your physician before embarking on a more vigorous exercise program if you have any questions about increasing your activity level. This is especially true if you have any risks for cardiovascular disease, including: High blood pressure, high cholesterol, are overweight, smoke, have diabetes, or a family member with heart disease.

Get Up & Go

The time to start exercising is now. No matter your age or your previous activity level, you can become physically fit. Remember, whatever activity you choose, start slowly, progress gradual, and do it regularly. Gaining the health benefits of exercise does not require enormous effort, but it does require persistence. Walking instead of driving the car or riding the bus can be transformed into an exercise routine. With a little effort, you can get on the road to achieving physical fitness.

Checklist for Fitness

If you've decided to commit yourself to exercising regularly, congratulations! You're on your way to better health. Physical activity, done consistency, is an important component of a healthy lifestyle, particularly for people over age 40.

By reducing blood pressure, improving the function of the heart and lungs, and strengthening bones, exercise can help prevent or reduce the risk of many of the health problems associated with aging, including high blood pressure, coronary heart disease, and osteoporosis. And that's not all: moderate levels of physical fitness can be developed with as little as 30 to 40 minutes of brisk walking each day. Moderate physical fitness is associated with a reduced risk of death from all causes, particularly cardiovascular disease.

Although the benefits of exercise can be attained regardless of one's age, the guidelines for beginning an exercise program differ slightly for those over age 40. The following steps are designed to help people over age 40 start—and maintain—*a regular exercise program.*

Step 1: Most sedentary healthy individuals can safely begin a low level exercise program such as walking or increasing daily activities. However, it is important to check with your physician before embarking on a more vigorous exercise program if you have any questions about increasing your activity level. This is especially true if you have any risks for cardiovascular disease including: high blood pressure, high cholesterol, are overweight, smoke, have diabetes or a family member with heart disease.

Step 2: Pick an activity that you enjoy. That way, you'll be more likely to stick with it. It's far better to do a little exercise regularly than a lot of exercise once in a while.

Step 3: Try to make exercise part of your daily routine, and you'll be more likely to do it consistently.

Step 4: Find a place to exercise—and a partner if you can. Companionship can make exercise more enjoyable and help you stick to your program. Whether you select a gym, outdoor track, or health club, be sure that the spot you choose allows you to exercise year-round.

Step 5: Set realistic goals and approach them according to your skill and fitness level. Because growing older can be accompanied by a decrease in flexibility and aerobic capacity, it's important to start slowly and increase gradually so that the musculoskeletal system, heart, and lungs can adapt to new demands. Don't plunge into an intense training program too soon, or exercise too hard, too long, or too often. You'll obtain the most benefit if you build up slowly to exercising at least 30 minutes for a minimum of three days per week.

Step 6: Get the proper equipment. For example, without suitable shoes for walking or running you may be placing yourself at risk for injury.

Step 7: Walk slowly and then stretch for 5 to 10 minutes before exercising.

Step 8: Check the intensity of your workout. Being able to talk to your exercise partner while exercising, known as the "talk test," indicates that the intensity of exercise is probably appropriate. Another method of estimating exercise intensity is calculating your target heart rate. By first calculating your target heart rate and then comparing it with your actual exercising heart rate, you can determine if you need to pick up the pace or slow down.

To calculate your target heart rate:

- Subtract your age from 220

- Multiply that figure by 0.6 and by 0.9. Your target heart rate falls between the two figures.

If your exercising heart rate is below your target heart rate, you need to work harder. Try switching from a less strenuous activity to one that is more intense, or increase the intensity of your exercise activity.

Step 9: If it takes longer than five minutes for your pulse to slow down after exercise, reduce your exercise pace. Stop exercising immediately and seek medical advice if you develop any of the following: difficulty breathing, feeling faint, dizziness, nausea, confusion, chest pain, extreme fatigue, or leg pain.

Step 10: Complete your workout by cooling down for 5 to 10 minutes with stretching exercises.

Step 11: Follow the R.I.C.E. regimen—Rest, Ice, Compression, Elevation—if you injure a muscle or joint. Check with your physician if pain and/or swelling persists.

You may want to consider taking an over-the-counter pain reliever such as an ibuprofen product, like Advil®. However, if you are taking any prescription medication or have any significant health problems, check with your physician before taking any pain reliever.

Step 12: Enjoy the health benefits of being fit. These include increased stamina and energy, toned muscles, improved sleep, better mood, decreased body weight, a conditioned heart and lungs, and stronger muscles and bones.

Simple Steps for Injury Prevention

Never before has there been so much evidence that regular, moderate exercise can keep you fit and healthy. Exercise is beneficial for your heart, lungs, bones, and mental attitude no matter how old you are.

For people over age 40, regular moderate exercise is particularly beneficial, helping to prevent coronary heart disease, osteoporosis, and other diseases associated with growing older. If done improperly, though, exercise can result in injury. This is a particular concern for older individuals, who generally are not as flexible or as resilient to injury as younger people.

Injury is not limited to mature people beginning a regular exercise program. Even the most physically fit athletes are vulnerable to injury. You too can learn to reduce the likelihood of injury, and how to treat an injury if it occurs.

The guidelines outlined below will help you minimize your risk for injury and gain the most benefit from regular physical activity.

- Choose low- to moderate-impact activities such as walking, bicycling, or swimming instead of jogging, running, or aerobic dancing. Low-impact activities can provide you with cardiovascular benefits similar to those obtained through high-impact workouts but with less risk of muscle and joint injury. Postmenopausal women, in particular, who are at increased risk for bone fractures from osteoporosis, should select low-impact, weight-bearing activities, such as walking, that don't jar the body.

- Always warm up for 5 to 10 minutes before exercising to improve flexibility and prevent injury.

- Avoid exercising in extreme heat or humidity. This is particularly important for people over age 65, who can have a more difficult time ridding excess heat from their body.

- Never exercise to the point of pain. If pain persists, stop exercising immediately and see your doctor.

- Complete your exercise regimen by cooling down for 5 to 10 minutes with stretching exercises.

- If an injury to a muscle or joint should occur, you can take important steps to minimize the damage and promote healing by initiating R.l.C.E.* (See below)

You may want to consider taking an over-the-counter pain reliever such as an ibuprofen product, like Advil®. However, if you are taking any prescription medication or have any significant health problems, check with your physician before taking any pain reliever.

If an injury occurs, remember R.I.C.E.

Rest: Rest the injured part to promote healing

Ice: Apply ice (wrapped in plastic or cloth to prevent freezing of the skin) immediately to the injured area to help reduce swelling and pain

Compression: Wrap the injured area firmly, but not too tightly, with an elastic bandage or cloth to help reduce swelling

Elevation: Elevate the injured part above the level of the heart to reduce swelling and pain

If redness, swelling, or pain persists, or if you have any questions regarding these instructions, consult your doctor.

Walking Your Way to Fitness

Did you know that exercise doesn't have to be particularly strenuous or of high intensity to be beneficial? Even moderate low-impact activity is effective in providing health benefits. An added bonus is that moderate low-impact exercise is less likely than high-impact exercise to cause musculoskeletal injury—an important concern for those over age 40, who may be less flexible or resilient to injury.

Walking is an ideal activity for adults undertaking a regular exercise routine and can impart substantial health benefits. One study found that middle-aged men and women who engaged in moderate exercise tended to be less overweight and incurred benefits in cardiovascular risk factors. A routine walking program also helps to reduce the risk of osteoporosis and may help improve self-esteem and mood. Like walking, stair-climbing also is an excellent means of keeping fit.

Follow these steps to make walking a part of your healthy lifestyle.

Step 1: Be sure you are familiar with the recommendations in "Checklist for Fitness"(see above).

Step 2: Get proper, well-fitting walking shoes. Choose footwear made of durable material. Your shoes should have thick, flexible, shock-absorbing soles—essential for preventing injury. Because your feet swell during the day, it's best to purchase shoes in the afternoon.

Step 3: Find a place to walk. For outdoor walking select a park or other grassy area with a level, smooth soft surface. An indoor track at a school or health club, or a shopping mall are good choices for walking indoors.

Step 4: You may want to contact your local branch of the American Heart Association or the local YMCA to see if they offer community walking programs that you can join.

Step 5: If walking outdoors, dress appropriately. In winter, dress in layers that you can take off as you warm up. Wear warm socks, a hat, and gloves to keep out the cold and wind, and choose garments made from breathable fabrics, such as cotton, fleece-lined cotton, wool, or nylon. These materials allow sweat to evaporate and help keep you warm and dry. In summer, wear loose-fitting comfortable clothes made of cotton or other porous materials. Don't forget to add sunscreen to exposed areas.

Step 6: To obtain optimal health benefits from your exercise routine, you must walk at a brisk pace. This ensures that you are working hard enough to get fit but not so hard that you will become tired and have to stop after only a few minutes. Most likely, if you're walking at a brisk pace, you will meet the "talk test" and be within your "target heart rate." See "Checklist for Fitness" for more information about the "talk test" and how to calculate your "target heart rate."

In addition to preventing risk for many diseases, walking briskly also is an excellent way to burn calories. The faster you walk, the more calories you'll burn per minute. If you walk at a speed of two miles per hour, you'll burn between 150 and 250 calories per hour. By walking at a speed of three miles per hour, you'll burn between 200 and 300 calories per hour.

Step 7: As is true for any type of physical activity, it's important to warm up before your walk. Warm up by walking slowly for five minutes to get blood flowing to your muscles and prepare your body for vigorous exercise. Stretch for 5 to 10 minutes to limber up your muscles and joints.

Step 8: Don't forget to cool down. After 20 to 60 minutes of brisk walking, cool down by walking slowly for five minutes. Then stretch for 5 to 10 minutes to help keep your joints and muscles flexible.

Step 9: Congratulate yourself for making an effort to improve your health with walking.

Achieving a Healthy Lifestyle: Exercise and Proper Nutrition

Eating properly is just as important as exercising regularly. For people over age 40, exercise in combination with a change in eating habits is an excellent way to maintain good health and reduce some health risks like obesity and coronary heart disease.

To help reduce your risk for health problems associated with poor diet, and to keep yourself in the best nutritional condition for exercising, follow the steps outlined below.

- Maintain a healthy weight. Keep in mind that as you grow older, your body requires fewer calories per day. To avoid gaining excess pounds, you'll need to eat less than you did when you were younger. Ask your doctor to help you determine the desirable weight for your height and age.

- Eat a variety of foods, including those from the following food groups: vegetables and fruits; grains including breads, cereals, rice, and pasta; low-fat or non-fat milk and other dairy products; protein rich foods including lean meats, poultry without skin, and eggs in moderation.

- Limit fats in your diet and cut down on foods high in cholesterol. To accomplish this, limit your intake of butter, lard, shortening, egg yolks, salad dressings, mayonnaise, fatty cheeses, whole milk, fatty meats, poultry skin, olives, avocados, coconut, and processed foods made with coconut, palm kernel, or palm oils.

- Increase intake of carbohydrates in your diet. That means increasing your intake of vegetables, fruits, and grain products (e.g., breads, cereals, pasta, and rice). But don't douse your vegetables with butter or creamy sauces or you will lose some of the benefits.

- Keep your intake of protein foods (e.g., meat, dairy products, beans and peas) moderate. Most people eat sufficient protein to cover their needs. Protein supplements are not necessary for exercise.

- Increase your intake of foods rich in calcium to help protect your bones, which tend to lose calcium with age. Good sources of calcium that do not add excessive fat to your diet are skim milk, low-fat or non-fat yogurt, lowfat cottage cheese, and hard cheeses such as parmesan. Evaluate your diet to see if you can substitute some high-calcium foods. If such changes cannot be accomplished without compromising fat or total calorie intake, a calcium supplement may be required. Before taking any calcium supplement, check with your doctor.

- Use sugar in moderation. Limit table sugar, brown sugar, honey, molasses, and syrup. Rather than eating cakes, pies, puddings, and cookies for dessert, choose fruit and non-fat yogurt.

- If you drink alcoholic beverages, do so in moderation.

- To keep your body well-hydrated during vigorous exercise and to prevent heat injury, drink 20 oz. (2 ½ cups) of fluids (preferably cool) two hours before exercising, and another 12 oz. (1 ½ cups) 20 minutes before an exercise session. During exercise, drink 4 oz. (1/2 cup) of fluids every 15 minutes. Immediately following exercise, drink fruit juices or other beverages containing carbohydrate and salt to replenish some of the nutrients lost during exercise.

- Don't wait until you're thirsty to have a drink. Because the thirst mechanism decreases with age, dehydration can occur without warning. Avoid drinking soft drinks and other liquids containing large amounts of sugar immediately before or during exercise if you find they cause you distress.

If you're exercising for both fitness and weight loss, you'll need to exercise more often than if you are exercising for health benefit alone. You'll also need to decrease your intake of calories and fat, as exercise alone may have only a modest effect on body weight and weight loss.

Keep in mind that high-intensity activities, such as jogging, burn more calories than lower-intensity activities. If you jog for an hour at a speed of seven miles per hour, you'll expend between 600 and 900 calories per hour. If you walk at a speed of three miles per hour, you'll burn between 200 and 300 calories per hour.

Strength-training for Fitness

Muscular fitness is an important piece of the overall physical fitness picture. You may think that only athletes need to have muscle strength. But in fact, such daily activities as climbing stairs, lifting a child—even carrying groceries—require muscular fitness.

As you get older, keeping your muscles fit is particularly important. Muscle strength usually decreases 20 percent between the ages of 22 and 65; bone mass and flexibility also decrease with age. But regular strength-training—even at an older age—can increase muscle strength, bone mass, and flexibility. When your muscles are very fit, you can be more active.

To maintain muscular fitness, healthy adults should exercise at least three to five days each week, doing a minimum of the following:

- eight to ten exercises that condition the major muscle groups
- eight to twelve repetitions of each exercise

Once you've mastered 12 repetitions, slowly increase the number. And if you're using weights while you exercise, slowly increase the weight.

Some tips to remember with any strength-training exercise:

- Exercise slowly and bring each muscle group through a complete range of motion.
- Exhale on exertion and inhale when returning to the starting position.
- Stretch each muscle group before and after your workout.
- Stop any exercise that causes pain.

A few strength-training exercises you may want to try are described below. Remember, there are a variety of exercises that condition your muscles—ask your doctor or a certified health fitness instructor about the best program for you!

While holding small weights (these can be purchased in most sporting goods stores), extend your forearms in front of you. Bring the weights toward your body until they touch your shoulders, then return to original position. Repeat.

While lying on your back and holding weights out to your sides, bring both weights high over your chest, keeping your elbows slightly bent. Repeat.

While lying on the floor with your hands on your stomach and your chin on your chest, slowly curl up until the middle of your back no longer touches the floor. (Sitting up the whole way may strain your back.) Repeat.

While lying on your side with your arm extended underneath your head, slowly lift and raise the upper lea. Repeat with other side.

You may prefer to try strength-conditioning machines—another option in strength training. These machines use weights to automatically provide resistance that can be increased as your level of fitness improves. If you have never used strength-conditioning machines, ask a qualified instructor for assistance.

If you should injure a muscle or joint while exercising, you can take important steps to minimize the damage and promote healing by remembering R.I.C.E. (see above).

Exercising with Arthritis

Did you know that exercising on a daily basis is an important part of managing arthritis? With arthritis, joints can become stiff and muscles can get weak. But regular exercise can decrease pain and stiffness, build stronger muscles and bones, and promote flexibility.

Listed below are some helpful exercises for fun, flexibility, and fitness. You can work with your doctor to develop an exercise program that's best for you.

For flexibility, do strength and mobility exercise daily.

These exercises will help maintain joint movement, increase range of motion, and relieve stiffness. Remember to begin slowly—do one or two repetitions of each exercise twice daily, then gradually increase repetitions to 10 or 20, twice daily.

Touch your index finger to your thumb to form the letter "O", then straighten fingers. Repeat with each finger.

Lie on your stomach. Bend your knee, moving your ankle toward your back as far as possible, then straighten. Repeat with other leg.

Raise your arm so that it extends fully away from your body. Bend your elbow, bringing your hand to the top of your shoulder. Extend your arm outward again, then move it down to your side. Repeat.

To stretch the hips, lower back, and knees, lie on your back and bend each knee to your chest one at a time. Use your hands to help you if necessary. Next, pull both knees to your chest and hold for six seconds while gently rocking side to side. Repeat.

For fun and fitness, try aerobic exercise

Aerobic exercises—exercises that use the large muscles of your body in a continuous activity—are great for fitness and weight control. And if you have arthritis, it's important to help control your body weight to avoid excess stress on your joints.

- Before aerobic exercise, do about 10 to 15 minutes of strength and mobility exercises to loosen up.

- Exercise aerobically for at least 20 minutes.

- Gradually decrease your activity to cool down, and then stretch for five to ten minutes.

- Aerobic exercise should be done at least three days a week, taking every other day off if necessary.

Walking, swimming, and bicycling are the best aerobic exercises for individuals with arthritis. Avoid such activities as jogging and tennis, which can strain the joints.

With arthritis, some days are good and others are not so good. But even on days when you're not feeling your best, it's still important to exercise. On some days you may need to adjust your exercise program—cutting down on the number of repetitions or duration of exercise can help. Also, move joints more gently through their range of motion.

To relieve the minor aches and pains of arthritis, you may want to consider taking an over-the-counter ibuprofen-containing medication such as Advil®. Of course, if you are taking a prescription medication, check with your physician before taking any pain reliever.

Chapter 13

Pep Up Your Life

Fitness for Mid-Life and Older Persons

Exercise: The Key To The Good Life

The exciting news from recent scientific studies is that exercise benefits everyone—regardless of age. Exercise can help you take charge of your health and maintain the level of fitness necessary for an active, independent lifestyle. This booklet is designed to help you start a fitness program of exercise so you can maintain or improve your physical health.

Many people think that as we age, we tend to slow down and do less; that physical decline is an inevitable consequence of aging. For the most part, this is not true. According to The President's Council on Physical Fitness and Sports, much of the physical frailty attributed to aging is actually the result of inactivity, disease, or poor nutrition. But the good news is—many problems can be helped or even reversed by improving lifestyle behaviors. One of the major benefits of regular physical activity is protection against coronary heart disease. Physical activity also provides some protection against other chronic diseases such as adult-onset diabetes, arthritis, hypertension, certain cancers, osteoporosis and depression. In addition, research has proven that exercise can ease tension and reduce the amount of stress you feel.

American Association of Retired Persons, PF 3246(1193) D543. Used by permission.

To put it simply—exercise is one of the best things you can do for your health.

The exercise program described and illustrated on the following pages has been prepared specifically for you! It is a daily routine that takes 20 to 30 minutes. Take a minute to read the instructions carefully. Performing each exercise properly is as important as spending enough time on them.

You Are What You Eat

No matter what your age, a balanced, nutritious diet is essential to good health. Older adults need to eat a balanced diet with foods from all the food groups. Eating a variety of foods helps ensure adequate levels of vitamins and minerals in the body. The U.S. Dietary Guidelines also recommend that adults reduce the fat, saturated fat, cholesterol, sodium, and sugar in the foods they eat.

Some adults find they have problems being overweight as they age. This is generally due to overeating and inactivity. If you are overweight, the best way to lose body fat is to eat fewer calories, especially from saturated fats, and to participate in aerobic exercises.

Did you know that an excess of only 100 calories a day can cause a 10-pound gain in a year, and those extra calories can be burned up by a 20 to 30 minute brisk daily walk?

Sleep and Rest

Sleep and rest are great rejuvenators. As you grow older, your sleep patterns and need for sleep may change. Be sure to include rest periods in your daily exercise program, especially if you sleep fewer than eight hours each night. Exercise can help relieve problems with insomnia too. Mild exercise a few hours before bed, or during the day, helps many people get a restful night's sleep.

Balance and Agility

Balance and agility are important capabilities often taken for granted. Regular exercise can help to maintain or restore them. Older adults can sometimes lose their sense of balance, particularly if they wear bi-focal or tri-focal glasses. A well-maintained sense of balance can help make up for the dizziness sometimes caused by vision

146

changes. In addition, when muscles are not toned, the resulting weakness and unsteadiness can contribute to falls. Thus, it is important to maintain or restore physical agility through exercise which can help avoid the risk of injury from falls and accidents.

Preparing to Exercise

No matter at what age you begin to exercise, or how long you may have been inactive, proper exercise will always improve your physical condition. The exercises in this chapter can be done by people who have been inactive for some time.

Programs to improve flexibility, strength, and endurance are arranged in three levels of difficulty. It is important to begin any exercise program slowly and build up gradually. Remember, it may take several months to attain the minimal levels of physical fitness identified in Level I activities. Some people will take less time, others more.

Keep in mind your level of ability and endurance so that you don't risk discomfort or injury. In addition, before beginning an exercise program, have a physical examination and discuss the program with your doctor.

Stick with it, and you will see results!

Warming Up

Preparing the body for exercise is important for people at any age and all fitness levels. A warm-up period should begin with slow, rhythmic activities such as walking or jogging in place. Gradually increase the intensity until your pulse rate, respiration rate and body temperature are elevated, which is usually about the time that you break a light sweat. It also is advisable to do some easy stretching exercises (such as the ones on pages 149–150) before moving on to the strength and endurance activities.

Effective Exercising

Once you begin your daily exercise routine, keep these points in mind to get the best results:

- Always drink water before, during and after your exercise session.

- Make exercising a part of your daily routine. You may want to set a regular time to exercise each day and invite a friend to join you.

- Start gradually, about 5 to 10 minutes at first.

- Increase the amount of exercise each day, up to about 30 minutes.

- Breathe deeply and evenly during and between exercises. Don't hold your breath.

- Rest whenever it is necessary.

- Keep a daily written record of your progress.

- Exercise to lively music, TV or with friends for added enjoyment.

Cool Down

If you have been participating in vigorous physical activity, it is extremely important not to stop suddenly. Abrupt stopping interferes with the return of the blood to the heart and may result in dizziness or fainting. Simply reduce the intensity of the exercise gradually and end with a few slow stretches from the section on stretching.

Exercising from a Wheelchair

A number of the exercises in this booklet can be performed from a chair or a wheelchair. They are identified with the symbol: Ø.

Flexibility

Exercises in this category will help you maintain your range of motion. Through the normal aging process, muscles tend to lose elasticity and tissues around the joints thicken. Exercise can delay this process by stretching muscles to prevent them from becoming short and tight. It also helps slow down the development of arthritis, one of the most common and painful diseases associated with advancing age.

In addition to performing flexibility exercises, you should try to bend, move, and stretch every day to keep joints flexible and muscles elastic. Avoid reliance on push buttons and conveniences that take away the need for personal motion. And, compliment this program with such recreational activities as dancing, yoga, swimming, golfing, gardening, and housework.

Be sure to begin each workout with deep breathing and continue deep breathing at intervals throughout the session. You should work up to a total of 50 deep breaths per workout.

Flexibility Level I

- **Finger Stretching:** *to maintain finger dexterity.* With the palm of the right hand facing down, gently force fingers back toward forearm, using left hand for leverage; then place left hand on top and force fingers down. Suggested repetitions: 5 each hand. Ø

- **Hand Rotation:** *to maintain wrist flexibility and range of motion.* Grasp right wrist with left hand. Keep right palm facing down. Slowly rotate hand 5 times each clockwise and counter clockwise. Suggested repetitions: 5 each hand. Ø

- **Ankle and Foot Circling:** *to improve flexibility and range of motion of ankles.* Cross right leg over opposite knee, rotate foot slowly, making large complete circles. 10 rotations to the right, 10 to the left, each leg. Ø

- **Neck Extension:** *to improve flexibility and range motion of neck.* Sit up comfortably. Bend head forward until chin touches chest. You may want to stretch forward by simply jutting your chin out. Return to starting position and slowly rotate head to left. Return to starting position and slowly rotate head to right. Return to starting position. Suggested repetitions: 5.

- **Single Knee Pull:** *to stretch lower back and back of leg.* Lie on back, hands at sides. Pull one leg to chest, grasp with both arms and hold for five counts. Repeat with opposite leg. Suggested repetitions: 3-5.

- **Flexed leg Back Stretch:** *to maintain flexibility in torso, lower back and legs.* Sitting in a chair, allow your upper body to rest on your thighs, drape your arms at the side of the chair, and reach towards the floor. Hold for 10 to 15 counts. Suggested repetitions: 4-6.

149

- **Simulated Crawl Stroke/Back Stroke/ Breast Stroke:** *to stretch shoulder girdle.* Stand with feet shoulder-width apart, arms at sides, relaxed. Bend knees and alternately swing right and left arms backwards ...upward...and forward as if swimming. Suggested repetitions: 6-8 movements on each stroke.

- **Reach:** *to stretch shoulder girdle and rib cage.* Take deep breath, extend arms overhead. If standing, rise on toes while reaching. Exhale slowly, dropping arms. Can be done in a seated position. Suggested repetitions: 6-8.

- **Baskstretch:** *to improve the flexibility of the lower back.* Sit up straight. Bend far forward and straighten up. Repeat, clasping hands on left knee. Repeat clasping hands on right knee. Exhale while bending) 8 forward. Suggested repetitions: 4-6 over each knee. Ø

- **Chain Breaker:** *to stretch chest muscles.* Stand erect, feet about six inches apart. Tighten leg muscles, tighten stomach by drawing it in, shove hips forward, extend chest, bring arms up with clenched fists chest high, take deep breath, let it out slowly. Slowly pull arms back as far as possible keeping elbows chest high. Suggested repetitions: 8-10. Ø

Flexibility: Level II

- **Double Knee Pull:** *to stretch lower back and buttocks.* Lie on back, hands at sides. Pull legs to chest, lock arms around legs, pull buttocks slightly off ground. Hold for 10 to 15 counts. Suggested repetitions: 3-5.

- **Seated Pike Stretch:** *to stretch lower hack and hamstrings.* Sit on floor, legs extended forward, knees together. Exhale and stretch forward, slowly sliding hands down to ankles Stretch only as far as is comfortable and use your hands for support. Hold for 5 to 8 counts. Don't bounce. Return to starting position inhaling deeply. Suggested repetitions: 3-4.

- **Sitting Stretch:** *to increase flexibility of lower back and hamstrings.* Sit on floor with legs extended as far apart as is comfortable. Exhale and stretch forward slowly, sliding your hands down your legs. Reach as far as is comfortable and hold for 5-8 counts. Suggested repetitions: 3-4.

- **Chest Stretch:** *to stretch muscles in chest and shoulders.* Stand arm-length distant from a doorway opening. Raise one arm shoulder height with slight bend in elbow. Place hand against door jamb and turn upper body away so that the muscles in chest and shoulders are stretched. Suggested repetitions: 3-4 each arm.

Flexibility: Level III

- **Sitting Stretch:** *to increase flexibility of lower back and hamstrings.* Sit on floor with legs extended as far apart as is comfortable. Exhale and stretch forward slowly, sliding your hands down your legs. Reach as far as is comfortable and hold for 5-8 counts. Suggested repetitions: 3-4.

- **Seated Hamstring Stretch:** *to extend full spine and hamstrings.* Sit up straight on floor with Legs together extended in front of you. Tilting pelvis forward, lean gently forward until you feel a comfortable stretch in the back and legs. Relax back into the seated position. Suggested repetitions: 5-10.

- **Seated Stretch:** *to stretch lower back and hamstrings.* Sit on floor, one leg extended to your side and one leg bent comfortably in front of your body. Supporting your body weight with your hands and keeping your back straight, lean forward until you feel a comfortable stretch on the inside of your extended leg and hamstring. Hold the stretch for a few seconds, exhaling. Switch sides. Suggested repetitions: 3-5 each side.

- **Achilles Stretch:** *to stretch heel cord on back leg (Achilles tendon).* Stand facing wall 2 to 3 feet away. Extend arms, lean into wall. Move left leg forward ½ step, right leg backward ½ step or more. Lower right heel to floor. Lower body toward wall, stretching the heel tendon in the right leg. Hold 5 to 10 counts. Breathe normally. Reverse leg position and repeat. Suggested repetitions: 3-6 each leg.

- **Modified Seal:** *to stretch abdominal wall, chest, and front of neck.* Lie on the floor with arms extended, stomach down, feet extended, with toes pointed. While exhaling, slowly lift head and push up until arms are bent at right angles, with back arching gently. Keeping arms bent, hold for 5-10 counts. Return to starting position, inhaling deeply. Suggested repetitions: 4-6.

- **Half Bow:** *to stretch the top of the thigh and groin area.* Lie on left side. Grab ankle of right foot with right hand just above toes. Slightly arch back. Hold 5 to 10 counts. Suggested repetitions: 3-5.

Strength

Exercises designed to build strength can help prevent premature loss of muscle tissue and can improve muscle strength, size, and endurance at any age. The benefits of strength exercises also include improving reaction time, reducing the rate of muscle atrophy, increasing work capacity, and helping prevent back problems and injury.

The following program of muscle conditioning exercises for the whole body has been designed specifically for older adults. Calisthenics work muscles against resistance, enabling them to grow and maintain muscle tone. In addition to the strength exercises suggested in the next section, other physical activities that are essentially recreational can provide benefits to help maintain muscle integrity. Such activities include: bicycling, swimming, hiking, golfing, tennis, shuffleboard, and bowling.

Strength: Level I

- **Finger Squeeze:** *to strengthen the hands.* Extend arms in front at shoulder height, palms down. Squeeze fingers slowly, then release. Suggested repetitions: 5. Turn palms up, squeeze fingers, release. Suggested repetitions: 5. Extend arms in front, shake fingers. Suggested repetitions: 5. Ø

- **Shoulder Shrug:** *for the upper back, to tone shoulders and relax the muscles at the base of the neck.* Lift shoulders way up, then relax them. Suggested repetitions: 8-10. Ø

- **Touch Shoulders:** *to increase flexibility of the shoulders and elbows and tone the upper arm; can 6e done in a seated position.* Touch shoulders with hands, extend arms out straight. Bring arms back to starting position. Suggested repetitions: 10-15.

- **Leg Extensions:** *to tone the upper leg muscles.* Sit upright. Lift left leg off the floor and extend it fully. Lower it very slowly. Suggested repetitions: 10-15 each leg. Ø

- **Back leg Swing:** *to firm the buttocks and strengthen the lower back.* Stand up, holding on to the back of a chair. Keep your back parallel to the chair as you do the exercise. Extend one leg back, foot pointed towards the floor. Keeping the knee straight, lift the leg backwards approximately four inches and concentrate on squeezing the muscles in the buttocks with each lift. Be careful not to overextend your back as you raise your legs. Return to starting position. Suggested repetitions: 10 each leg.

- **Quarter Squat:** *to tone and strengthen lower leg muscles.* Stand erect behind a chair, hands on chair back for balance. Bend knees, then rise to an upright position. Suggested repetitions: 8-12.

- **Heel Raises:** *to strengthen the calf muscles and ankles.* Stand erect, holding a chair for balance if needed, hands on hips, feet together. Raise body on toes. Return to starting position. Suggested repetitions: 10.

- **Knee lift:** *to strengthen hip flexors and lower abdomen.* Stand erect. Raise left knee to chest or as far upward as possible. Return to starting position. Repeat with right leg. Suggested repetitions: 5 each leg.

- **Head and Shoulder Curl:** *to firm a stomach muscles and front of neck.* Lie on the floor, knees bent, arms at sides, head bent slightly forward. Reach forward with arms extended, until finger tips touch your knees. Hold for 5 counts. Return to starting position. Suggested repetitions: 10.

Strength: Level II

- **Arm Circles:** *to strengthen shoulders and upper back.* Sit or stand erect with arms at sides, elbows straight, head high. Rotate arms from shoulders in small circles, with palms of hands turned upward. Suggested repetitions: 10 forward, 10 backward.

- **Arm Curl:** *to strengthen arm muscles.* Use a weighted object such as a book or a can of vegetables (not more than 5 pounds). Stand or sit erect with arms at side, holding weighted object. Bend your arm, raising the weight. Lower it. Can be done seated. Suggested repetitions: 10-15 each arm. Ø

- **Arm Extension:** *to tone muscles in the back of the arm.* Sit or stand erect with arms at sides. Holding a weighted object of less than 5 pounds, extend your arm overhead. Slowly bend arm until weight is behind head. Slowly extend arm to original position. The arm curl and arm extension can be done separately or together, alternating arms. Can be done seated. Suggested repetitions: 10-15.

- **Modified Knee Push up:** *to strengthen upper back, chest, and back of arms.* Start on bent knees, hands on floor and slightly forward of shoulders. Lower body until chin touches floor. Return to start. Suggested repetitions: 5-10.

- **Calf Raise:** *to strengthen lower leg and ankle.* Stand erect, hands on hip or on back of chair for balance. Spread fee 6" to 12". Slowly raise body up to toes, lifting heels. Return to starting position. Breathe normally. Suggested repetitions: 10-15.

- **Alternate Leg Lunges:** *to strengthen upper thighs and inside legs.* Also stretches back of leg. Take a comfortable stance with hands on hip Step forward 18" to 24" with right leg while extending arms straight ahead. Keep left heel on floor. Shove off right leg and resume standing position. Suggested repetitions: 5-10 each leg.

- **Modified Sit up:** *to improve abdominal strength.* Lie on back, feet on the floor, with finger tips behind your ears. Look straight at the ceiling and lift head and shoulders off floor. Suggested repetitions: 10-15. Curl up to sitting position. Curl down to starting position. For best effect, secure feet under something stationary, such as a chair, to prevent them from lifting during exercise.

- **Side Lying Leg Lift:** *to strengthen and tone outside of thigh and hip muscles.* Lie on right side, legs extended. Raise leg four to five inches. Lower to starting position. Suggested repetitions: 10 each side.

Strength: Level III

Note: In Level III strength exercise, lightweight resistance equipment, such as the dumbbell, is introduced to overload the muscles. While equipment of this kind is low in cost and desirable, a number of substitutes can be used. These include a bucket of soil, a heavy household item such as an iron, a can of food. a stone, or a brick.

- **Alternate Dumbbell Press:** *to strengthen shoulders and upper back.* Sit comfortably on flat bench or chair. Hold dumbbells or weighted objects at shoulder height, using overhand grip. Extend right arm over right shoulder. Lower right arm while extending left arm over left shoulder. Suggested repetitions: 1 to 2 sets of 6-10 repetitions each arm.

- **Seated Alternate Dumbbell Curls:** *to strengthen biceps of upper arms.* Sit comfortably on a flat bench with arms at side. Hold a pair of dumbbells with an underhand grip, so that palms face up. Bending left elbow, raise dumbbell until left arm is fully flexed. Lower left dumbbell while raising right dumbbell from the elbow until right arm is fully flexed. Breathe normally. Suggested repetitions: 2 sets of 8-10 each arm. Ø

- **Dumbbell Fly:** *to strengthen chest muscles and improve lateral range of motion in shoulder girdle.* Lie on your back on a flat bench or floor if bench is not available. Grasp dumbbells in each hand over chest. Inhale and lower dumbbell to side with elbow slightly bent. Raise dumbbell in an arc to the starting position, exhaling in the process. Suggested repetitions: 8-12.

- **Alternate Dumbbell Shrug:** *to strengthen muscles in shoulders, upper back and neck.* Stand comfortably with dumbbells in each hand. Elevate shoulders as high as possible, rolling them first backward and then down to the starting position. On the second repetition, roll the shoulders forward and down. Alternate first backward and then forward. Exhale as you lower the shoulders. Suggested repetitions: 10 forward, 5 backward. Ø

- **One Arm Dumbbell Extension:** *to strengthen triceps (back of arm) and improve range of motion.* With a straight arm, lift a light weight overhead. Slowly lower it behind the back as far as is comfortable. Extend arm to original position. Inhale on the way down, exhale on the way up. Suggested repetitions: 8-12 on each arm. Ø

- **Dumbbell Calf Raise:** *to strengthen calf muscle and improve range of motion of ankle joint.* Stand with feet shoulder-width apart, weights in each hand, toes on a 2" x 4" block (preferred but not necessary). Raise up on toes lifting heels as high as possible. Slowly lower heels to starting position. Breath normally. Suggested repetitions: 5 with heels straight back, 5 with heels turned out, 5 with heels turned in.

- **Dumbbell Half Squats:** *to strengthen thigh muscles in front.* Stand with feet shoulder-width apart and w heels on a 2" x 4" block (not necessary, but preferred). Holding weights in each hand, slowly descend to a comfortable position where the tops of the thighs are about at a 45 degree angle to the floor. There is no benefit to a deeper squat. Inhale on the way down. Stand up slowly, keeping knees slightly bent. Exhale on the way up. Suggested repetitions: 10-12.

- **Sit up:** *to strengthen stomach muscles.* Lie on back, knees bent, feet on floor, placing your finger tips behind your ears. Curl torso to upright position and touch elbows to knees while exhaling. Curl down to starting position while inhaling. Suggested repetitions: 5.

Endurance

Endurance-building or aerobic exercises improve the functions of the heart, lungs, and blood vessels. Vital to fitness are a strong heart to pump blood to nourish billions of body cells, healthy lungs where the gases of cell metabolism are exchanged for oxygen and elastic blood vessels free of obstructions. Without a healthy level of endurance, you may feel tired, lack zest. You may also experience shortness of breath, rapid heartbeat or even nausea.

Activities to improve endurance include brisk walking, cycling, swimming, dancing, and jogging. Walking is actually one of the best all-around exercises. The massaging action the leg muscles exert on the veins as you walk improves the flow of blood back to the heart and also strengthens the leg muscles.

Walking for Fitness

The following walking program has been designed to help mid-life and older persons build and maintain cardiovascular endurance. Walking offers several advantages over other forms of exercise; it requires no previous instructions, it can be done almost anywhere, it can be done at almost anytime, it costs nothing and it has the lowest rate of injury of any form of exercise.

It takes a little longer to achieve conditioning results through walking than through more strenuous activities, but not much. One study showed, for example, that jogging a mile in 8 ½ minutes burns only 26 more calories than walking a mile in 12 minutes. Conditioning benefits from walking improve dramatically if you increase the pace to faster than 3 miles per hour (20-minute mile). In another study, participants burned an average of 66 calories per mile walking 3 miles per hour, but 124 calories per mile when they increased the pace to 5 miles per hour.

Choose a comfortable time of day to exercise, not too soon after eating and when the air temperature is not too high. Many people find it more enjoyable to exercise with others. Follow the program at the recommended rate but be careful not to overexert. Stop if you find yourself panting or feeling nauseous, if your breathing does not return to normal within ten minutes after exercising or if your sleeping is affected. If you feel uncomfortable progressing at the recommended rate, spend additional weeks at each level of exercise. For example, if you reach a comfortable limit in the fifth week of the program at 3 one-mile walks on alternate days, continue one-mile walks but increase the frequency to 5, 6, 7 or more walks weekly until you can move on to activity recommended for the sixth week.

How to Walk

A good walking workout is a matter of stepping up your pace, increasing your distance and walking more often. Here are some tips to help you get the most out of walking:

- Move at a steady clip, brisk enough to make your heart beat faster and cause you to breathe more deeply.

- Hold your head erect, back straight and abdomen flat. Toes should point straight ahead and arms swing at your sides.

- Land on your heel and roll forward to drive off of the ball of your foot. Walking only on the ball of the foot or walking flat-footed may cause soreness.

- Take long easy strides, but don't strain. When walking up hills or walking rapidly, lean forward slightly.

- Breathe deeply, with your mouth open if that's more comfortable.

What to Wear

Shoes that are comfortable, provide good support and don't cause blisters or calluses are the only special equipment necessary. They should have arch supports and should elevate the heel one-half to three-quarters of an inch above the sole. They should also have uppers made of materials that "breathe" such as leather or nylon mesh. Some examples are: training models of running shoes with thick soles, light trail or hiking boots or casual shoes with thick rubber or crepe rubber soles.

Wear lighter clothing than the temperature would ordinarily dictate because brisk walking generates a lot of body heat. In cold weather, wear several layers of light clothing. They trap body heat and are easy to shed if you get too warm. A woolen cap and mittens are important in very cold temperatures.

Endurance Exercises

Endurance: Level I

1st Week and 2nd Week:	3 sessions on alternate days—1/4 mile. Use good posture and proper walking techniques. Dress correctly.
3rd Week:	3 sessions on alternate days—1/2 mile. Gradually lengthen stride. Practice deep breathing each 220 yards.
4th Week:	3 sessions on alternate days—3/4 mile. Practice deep breathing each 220 yards.
5th Week:	3 sessions on alternate days—1 mile. Practice deep breathing each 220 yards.

Endurance: Level II

6th Week:	5 sessions—1 mile each. Practice forced breathing. Emphasize good posture.
7th Week:	5 sessions—1 mile each in 20 minutes.
8th Week:	5 sessions—1½ miles each in 30 minutes.
9th Week:	5 sessions—2 miles each in 40 minutes.
10th Week:	5 sessions—2 miles each in 40 minutes.

Endurance: Level III

11th Week	5 sessions—2½ miles each in 50 minutes.
12th Week:	5 sessions—3 miles each in 60 minutes.
13th Week:	5 sessions—3 miles each in 55 minutes.
14th Week:	5 sessions—3 miles each in 50 minutes.
15th Week:	5 sessions—2 miles each in 45 minutes.

Part Three

Exercise and Specific Medical Conditions

Chapter 14

Exercise and Your Arthritis

Understanding Arthritis

The word arthritis literally means joint inflammation ("arth" = joint; "itis" = inflammation). It refers to more than 100 different diseases. These diseases usually affect the joints and the tissues around the joints, such as muscles and tendons. Some of these diseases can also affect other parts of the body, including the skin and internal organs.

Nearly 40 million Americans have arthritis. These people face many challenges because of the disease. The good news is there are many ways to meet those challenges and lead a fulfilling life in spite of arthritis.

This chapter is for people who have arthritis and for their families and friends. It explains the importance of a regular exercise program so you can take an active role in learning how to control your arthritis as much as possible.

What Can Exercise Do for Me?

Some kind of exercise is good for almost everyone! For many years it was thought that people with arthritis should not exercise because it would damage their joints. Now doctors and therapists know that

Pub. no. 9704/6-95, Arthritis Foundation, 1995.

people with arthritis can improve their health and fitness through exercise without hurting their joints.

If you have arthritis, exercise is especially important. Exercise is beneficial because it can help:

- keep your joints moving; keep the muscles around your joints strong;

- keep bone and cartilage tissue strong and healthy;

- improve your ability to do daily activities; and

- improve your overall health and fitness, by:

  - giving you more energy;

  - helping you sleep better;

  - controlling your weight;

  - making your heart stronger;

  - making your bones and muscles stronger;

  - decreasing depression; and

  - improving your self-esteem and sense of well-being.

Along with medicine, rest and other parts of your treatment program, regular exercise can help keep your joints in working order so you can continue your daily activities. It also may help prevent further joint damage.

What Could Happen if I Don't Exercise?

If your joints hurt, you may not feel like exercising. However, if you don't exercise, your joints can become even more stiff and painful. Exercise is beneficial because it keeps your bones, muscles and joints healthy.

Because you have arthritis, it is important to keep your muscles as strong as possible. The stronger the muscles and tissue are around your joints, the better they will be able to support and protect those joints—even those that are weak and damaged from arthritis. If you don't exercise, your muscles become smaller and weaker, and your bones can become more brittle.

Many people with arthritis keep painful joints in a bent position because at first it's more comfortable. If your joints stay in one position for too long (without movement), you may lose your ability to straighten them out. If this happens, you may be unable to use those joints. Exercise helps keep your joints as flexible as possible, allowing you to continue to do your daily tasks as independently as possible.

Exercise can lift your spirits. If you're in pain, you may feel depressed. If you feel depressed, you may not feel like moving or exercising. And without exercise, you may feel more pain and depression. Research has shown that participating in a regular exercise program is a great way to feel better and move more comfortably.

Who Can Help Me Start an Exercise Program?

Two health professionals can help you plan a total fitness program. They can work with you to design a program that meets your specific needs.

Physical therapists can show you special exercises to help keep your bones and muscles strong.

Occupational therapists can show you how to do certain activities in ways that will not place extra stress on your joints. Occupational therapists also can provide you with splints or assistive devices if you need them.

Contact your doctor, local hospital, health clinic or Arthritis Foundation office for more information on how to reach these professionals.

Are There Any Risks in Exercising?

The most common risk is working your joints or muscles too much. This can happen if you exercise too long or too hard—especially when you're first beginning your exercise program. Most of these problems can be prevented by following the tips on pages 171–173.

Remember that exercise is only one part of your treatment program. Other parts of your program should include:

- proper diagnosis by a doctor;

- using your joints correctly;

- education about arthritis;

- conserving your energy;

- medication;

- eating right;

- rest/relaxation;

- splints (for some people); and

- using heat or cold treatments.

What Are the Main Types of Exercise?

People with arthritis often benefit from a balanced exercise program including different types of exercise. Three main types of exercise that should be included in your exercise program are range-of-motion (flexibility), strengthening and endurance exercises.

Range-of-Motion (Flexibility) Exercises

These exercises are beneficial because they reduce stiffness and help keep your joints flexible—something that can help you carry out your activities of daily living. The "range of motion" is the normal amount your joints can move in certain directions. Examples of range-of-motion (ROM) exercises are shown on pages 176–177 of this chapter. If your joints are very painful and swollen, move them gently through their range of motion.

Health Tip

Try to move your joints through their full range of motion every day. Daily activities such as housework, climbing stairs, dressing, bathing, cooking, lifting or bending **do not** move your joints through their full range of motion. Daily activities should **not** replace range-of-motion exercises.

Strengthening Exercises

These exercises are beneficial because they help maintain or increase muscle strength. Strong muscles help keep your joints stable and more comfortable. Two common strengthening exercises for people with arthritis are isometric and isotonic exercises.

Isometric Exercises

In these exercises, you tighten your muscles but don't move your joints. This helps build your muscles without moving painful joints. Examples of isometric exercises are quadriceps sets, in which you tighten the large muscle at the front of your thigh, or gluteal sets, in which you tighten the muscles in your buttocks. The illustration below shows another example of an isometric exercise.

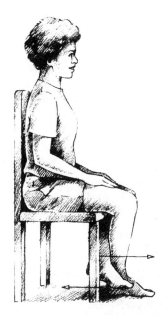

This exercise strengthens the muscles that bend and straighten your knee. Sit in a straight-backed chair and cross your ankles. Your legs can be almost straight, or you can bend your knees as much as you like. Push forward with your back leg and press backward with your front leg. Exert pressure evenly so that your legs do not move. Hold and count out loud for 10 seconds. Repeat. Change leg positions.

Isotonic Exercises

In these exercises, you move your joints to strengthen muscles. Isotonic exercises seem like ROM exercises, but they become strengthening exercises by increasing the speed at which they are done, increasing the number of exercises that are done, or adding light weight to the exercise being done (one to two pounds). Water exercises can help strengthen muscles because water is a form of both assistance and resistance. Changing the position in which you do exercises also can help strengthen muscles. For example, you encounter more resistance when you try to raise your arms from a sitting position than when you try to raise your arms from a lying-down position.

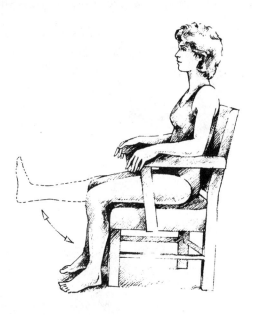

This exercise strengthens your thigh muscle. Sit in a chair with both feet on the floor and spread slightly apart. Raise one foot until your leg is as straight as you can make it. Hold and count out loud for five seconds. Gently lower your foot to the floor. Relax. Repeat with your other leg.

Strengthening exercises must be carefully designed for people with arthritis. Knowing which muscle needs to be strengthened and how to perform the exercise without overstressing the joints are key elements in a successful program. Your physical therapist, occupational therapist and/or doctor can provide appropriate recommendations.

Endurance Exercises

Endurance exercises are beneficial because they strengthen your heart. They make your lungs more efficient and give you more stamina so you can work longer without tiring as quickly. Endurance exercises also help you sleep better, control your weight and lift your spirits.

Some of the most beneficial endurance exercises for people with arthritis are walking, water exercise and using a stationary bicycle.

Walking

Walking is better for people with arthritis than running because it puts less stress on your joints. It requires no special skills and is inexpensive.

However, you will need a good pair of supportive walking shoes. You can walk almost any time and anywhere. If you have severe hip, knee, ankle or foot problems, talk to your doctor; walking may not be for you.

The Talk Test

A quick test to see if you are exercising at a moderate pace is called the Talk Test. When you are exercising, you should be able to talk easily and not be out of breath. If you are exercising so hard that you can't talk normally, you may need to slow down.

Water Exercise

Swimming and exercise in warm water are especially good for stiff, sore joints. Warm water helps relax your muscles and decrease pain. The water should be between 83 and 90 degrees. Water helps support your body so there is less stress on your hips, knees and spine. You can do warm-water exercises while standing in shoulder- or chest-height water or while sitting in shallow water. In deeper water, use an inflatable tube or floatation vest or belt to keep you afloat while you exercise.

Health Tip

Gradually build up your endurance exercises to 20 to 30 minutes per day, at least three times per week. Endurance exercises should be only one part of your total exercise program. **Do not** substitute endurance exercises for the therapeutic exercises your health-care team recommends.

Bicycling

Bicycling, especially on an indoor, stationary bicycle, is a good way to improve your fitness without putting too much stress on your hips, knees and feet. Adjust the seat height so that your knee straightens when the pedal is at the lowest point. When you begin, do not pedal faster than 15 to 20 miles per hour, or 60 revolutions per minute. Add resistance only after you have warmed up for five minutes. Don't add so much resistance that you have trouble pedaling. Exercising on a stationary bicycle should be started slowly, using limited or no resistance if you have knee problems.

How Should I Start?

If you haven't been exercising on a regular basis or have pain, stiffness or weakness that interrupts your daily activities, start your fitness program with flexibility and strengthening exercises.

Once you feel comfortable doing these exercises, gradually include endurance exercises as well. You can begin by exercising five minutes, three times a day, to get a total of 15 minutes for that day. Over a period of time, try extending the endurance part of your exercise program to get a total of 20 to 30 minutes for the day, at least three times per week.

When Should I Exercise?

Try exercising at different times of the day until you decide what is best for you. Some people find that doing morning ROM exercises helps them loosen up for the day's activities; others find that gentle ROM exercises before bed makes them less stiff in the morning. Each person is different. You may find it helpful to do a few short sessions of ROM exercises during different times of the day. A good guideline is to exercise during the time of the day when you are feeling less pain and stiffness and when you have adequate time to do them.

Don't do strenuous exercises just after you eat or just before you go to bed. Wait at least two hours after a meal.

Exercise on a regular basis. Try to do range-of-motion exercises daily and strengthening and endurance exercises every other day. If you miss a day, pick up again where you left off. If you miss several days, you may need to start again at a lower level.

Tips for Better Exercise

Before Exercise

Massage or Apply Heat Treatments

Massage the stiff or sore areas or apply heat treatments to the area you will be exercising. Heat relaxes your joints and muscles and helps relieve pain. Cold also reduces pain and swelling for some people.

There are many ways you can apply heat or cold. Some methods you may want to try are:

- Take a warm (not hot) shower before you exercise.

- Apply a heating pad or hot pack to the sore area.

- Sit in a warm whirlpool.

- Wrap a bag of ice or frozen vegetables in a towel and place it on the sore area.

Be sure to apply the heat or cold correctly. Heat treatments should feel soothing and comfortable, not hot. Apply for about 20 minutes. Use cold for 10 to 15 minutes at a time For more information on the correct use of heat or cold, contact your local chapter of the Arthritis Foundation for a copy of the booklet *Managing Your Pain.*

Warm Up First

Do gentle range-of-motion and strengthening exercises at least 10 to 15 minutes before more vigorous endurance-type exercise. Begin your activity at a slow pace and gradually work to a faster pace. Taking the time to warm-up before exercising will help you prevent injuries.

Wear Comfortable Clothes and Shoes

Your clothes should be loose and comfortable for easy movement. Layering your clothes will help you adapt to changes in temperature and activity level. Your shoes should provide good support, and the soles should be made from non-slip, shock-absorbent material. Wearing shock-absorbent insoles also can make your exercise more comfortable.

During Exercise

Don't Hurry

Exercise at a comfortable, steady pace that allows you to speak without running out of breath (see the Talk Test on page 169). Exercising at this pace gives your muscles time to relax between each repetition. For range of motion and flexibility, it is better to do each exercise slowly and completely rather than to do many repetitions at a fast pace. You can gradually increase the number of repetitions as you get into shape.

Breathe While you Exercise

Don't hold your breath. Breathe out as you do the exercise and breathe in as you relax between repetitions. Counting out loud during the exercise will help you breathe deeply and regularly.

Be Alert for "Warning Signs"

Stop exercising right away if you have chest tightness or severe shortness of breath or feel dizzy, faint or sick to your stomach. If these symptoms occur, contact your doctor immediately. If you develop muscle pain or a cramp, gently rub and stretch the muscle. When the pain is gone, continue exercising with slow, easy movements. You may need to change position or the way you are doing the exercise.

Know Your Body's Signals

During the first few weeks of your exercise program, you may notice that your heart beats faster, you breathe faster and your muscles feel tense when you exercise. You may feel more tired at night, but awake feeling refreshed in the morning. These are normal reactions to exercise that mean your body is adapting to your new activities and getting into shape.

Don't Do Too Much Too Fast

Building endurance should be a gradual process spread out over several weeks. You'll know you have done too much if you have joint or muscle pain that continues for two hours after exercising or if your pain or fatigue is worse the next day. Next time, decrease the number of times you do each exercise, or do them more gently. If this doesn't help, ask your therapist about changing the exercise. A good general rule to remember is to stop exercising if you start having sharp pain or more pain than usual. Pain is your warning signal that something is wrong.

After Exercise

Cool Down

After exercising, cool down for five to 10 minutes. This helps you cool off, lets your heart slow down and helps your muscles relax. To cool down, simply do your exercise activity at a slower pace, such as walking slowly. Also try gentle stretching to avoid stiff or sore muscles the next day.

How Do I Keep Going?

Keep a positive attitude about yourself and your exercise program. Remember that exercise can help reduce pain and help you keep up with most of your daily activities. But also remember that there will be days when you won't feel like doing as much. On these days, do a little less exercise.

The keys to keeping up with your program are:

- Make exercise a regular part of your day.

- Stay in the habit by doing at least some exercise even on those days when you aren't motivated. Make some effort, because interrupting the routine can decrease the benefits you get from exercise.

- Listen to your body's signals. Know when to cut back or change your exercise.

We all can find many reasons not to exercise. Listed below are some common problems you may experience and ways to overcome them.

"I haven't exercised in so long. What if I can't do it?" It's normal to feel hesitant about something you haven't done for a while. To overcome such feelings, try not to think of exercise as competition with

173

others. Instead, focus on your own abilities, and do what you can. Think positively. Each accomplishment, no matter how small, will help reinforce your confidence and self-esteem.

"I'm out of shape. It will take too long to see results." Often long-term problems can be addressed and managed by setting goals. These same steps can be applied to your exercise program:

- Decide what you want to accomplish (your long-term goal). Determine the steps to accomplish this goal. List your options, then choose one or two you would like to work on.

- Make short-term plans to help reach the options you have chosen. These plans identify specific actions that you can realistically expect to accomplish within a short time, such as a week. These actions should be something that you want to do, that you feel you can do, and that contribute to your long-term goal. Make an exercise contract with yourself: Write down what you are going to do, how much you will do, when you will do it and how often you will do it. Post your contract where you will see it every day.

- Carry out your plan. Record your progress and any problems you have. Also, get your family and friends to provide feedback on how you are doing.

- Check the results of your short-term plans at the end of each week.

- Modify your plans if something doesn't seem to be working. If you continue having problems, ask others for assistance.

"It hurts." It's normal to have some pain or soreness when you begin an exercise program. Always remember to warm up beforehand and to cool down afterwards to help relax your muscles and reduce the pain. Also, remember that exercising to build strong muscles and joints often reduces the pain of arthritis.

Try to move your joints gently by yourself. If you need help, ask a therapist who is trained to help people with arthritis. The therapist also can train your friends or family members to help you.

On those days when your joints are more painful and swollen, cut back on the number of exercises you do. Do not do vigorous exercises. If you notice a big change in what you are able to do, talk to your doctor or therapist about it. If just one or two joints are swollen or painful, you can adapt your exercises to put less stress on those joints. For example, if your knee flares up, switch to water exercises or use a stationary bicycle without resistance instead of walking.

"My arthritis is acting up." If you are having a flare, don't skip your exercises entirely. While rest will help settle down a flare, too much rest can be harmful. To do absolutely nothing leads to stiff and weak muscles. A balance between rest and activity is necessary, especially when you have a flare. Get plenty of rest, but also do range-of-motion exercises. They will help maintain joint mobility. As the flare settles down, continue doing your range-of-motion exercises, but also begin some strengthening exercises.

"I don't have enough time." Follow an exercise schedule. Several short exercise periods are just as good as one long period. Making time for exercise should not be a burden. Think of your exercise time as special time for yourself. Use this time to think about other creative goals for yourself.

"It's boring." Do exercises you enjoy. Ask your therapist about new exercises that can add variety to your program. Listen to your favorite music while exercising. Exercise with friends or family members. If you walk or bicycle, go to the park or another pleasant area.

"The weather's bad." If you usually exercise with a group and can't get to your class, do your exercises at home. If you swim or walk, have a backup plan for indoor exercises when the weather is bad. For example, walk around a shopping mall if it's too cold or hot to walk outside.

"I don't like to exercise alone." Ask friends or family members to exercise with you, or join an exercise class. Another option is to use one of the Arthritis Foundation's exercise videotapes to get the feeling of a group experience.

"It's too much work." Maybe you're being too ambitious about your exercise program. Maybe you're trying to do too much. Relax! Enjoy the good feelings while you exercise and afterward. Join an exercise group. Exercising for fun is the best way to keep it up.

"I lose interest and forget about it." If you're having trouble sticking to your program, think about the things that can affect your attitude. Why did you want to start the program? Are these reasons still important? Keep a record of what you do and at the end of each day, check off the exercises you did.

"My joints are not bothering me anymore." Exercise probably has a lot to do with this. Instead of stopping, try some different exercises or activities that will vary your program.

Range-Of-Motion Exercises

The exercises outlined below will help keep your joints moving. Follow these tips to get the most benefit:

- Set reasonable goals.

- Find a buddy who is willing to exercise with you.

- Do these exercises once or twice per day.

- Do each exercise three to 10 times.

- Move slowly. Do not bounce.

- Breathe while you exercise. Count out loud.

- Stop exercising if you have severe pain. Don't overdo it.

- Check with your doctor before beginning any exercise program. The Arthritis Foundation is not responsible for any injury incurred while doing these exercises.

Knee And Hip

Lie on your back with one knee bent and the other as straight as possible. Bend the knee of the straight leg. Use your hands to pull your knee to your chest. Push the leg into the air and then lower it to the floor. Repeat, using the other leg. If you feel pain in your knee, do not kick it into the air. Just lower it to the floor.

Hip

(This exercise is not recommended for people who have had total hip replacements, who have low back problems or who have osteoporosis.) Lie on your back with your legs straight and about six inches apart. Point your toes up. Slide one leg out to the side and return. Try to keep your toes pointing up. Slide your leg only. Do not lift it. Repeat with your other leg. (This exercise also can be done from a standing position.)

Shoulder

Lie on your back. Raise one arm over your head, keeping your elbows straight. Keep your arm close to your ear. Return your arm slowly to your side. Repeat with your other arm. (This exercise also can be done from a standing position.)

Hip And Knee

Lie on your bask with your legs as straight as possible, about six inches apart. Keep your toes pointed up. Roll your hips and knees in and out, keeping your knees straight. To further strengthen knees, while lying with both legs out straight, attempt to push one knee down against the floor. Tighten the muscle on the front of the thigh. Hold this tightening for a slow count of five. Relax. Repeat with the other knee.

Fingers

Open your hand, with fingers straight and spread apart. Bend all the finger joints except the knuckles. Touch the top of your palm with your fingertips. Reach your thumb across your palm until it touches the second joint of your little finger. Stretch your thumb out and repeat.

Chapter 15

Being a Sport With Exercise-Induced Asthma

By Ruth Papazian

You wouldn't call Nicholas, 16, a jock. He harbors no dreams of Olympic glory, has no intention of trying out for a school sports team, and has faked more injuries to get out of gym class than even he can count. His hobbies run more to the creative and intellectual—playing bass guitar in a garage band and fooling around on his computer.

But Nicholas (who asked that his last name not be used) didn't always avoid sports. At one time, he was an avid basketball player. But all that changed about four years ago.

"We were supposed to run a mile in gym, and about halfway through, I started coughing, wheezing and felt nauseous. I told the teacher I couldn't go on, but he said that he didn't like quitters. I tried to finish, but I couldn't," he recalls. Nicholas went to the doctor and found out he had exercise-induced asthma.

"My friends stopped inviting me to play B-ball or soccer after school because they were afraid that I would have an attack in the middle of a game. Some of the kids called me 'wheeze boy'," Nicholas says. "After a while, I decided they were right, so even though I loved sports, I gave up on all physical activities."

Asthma is a lung disease that is either inherited or may develop as a severe allergic reaction to pollen, viruses, dust, cigarette smoke, and other "triggers" (but not everyone with allergies develops asthma

FDA Consumer: January/February, 1994

and not every asthmatic has allergies). Exercise-induced asthma (EIA) is a common form of asthma. It occurs only when a person exercises. People who have chronic asthma, on the other hand, can develop symptoms whenever they are exposed to a trigger.

About 80 to 90 percent of people who have chronic asthma also have EIA. But you can have EIA even if you don't have chronic asthma. Nicholas is among the 35 to 40 percent of people with seasonal allergies who have EIA, and his symptoms are always worse during the spring and fall when gym classes are held outdoors.

How an EIA Attack Happens

During an asthma attack, the bronchial airways (the large and small tubes that bring air into the lungs) become partly blocked. A trigger, such as pollen, causes immune system cells in the lungs to release histamine and other chemicals. These chemicals cause the lining of the airways to swell, making them narrower. At the same time, tiny rubberband-like muscles wrapped around the outside of the bronchi (the two large tubes that branch out from the windpipe into the lungs) tighten in what is known as "bronchospasm." Completing the process, mucus cells in the airways produce secretions that plug up the works even more.

In about half of chronic asthmatics, the initial attack (known as "early response") is followed by a delayed reaction ("late response"). This delayed reaction happens because lung inflammation makes the airways and lungs extremely sensitive to irritation. Some asthma specialists believe that EIA differs from chronic asthma because exercise-induced bronchospasm (another name for EIA) does not cause lung inflammation, so there is no late response.

With asthma, the problem isn't getting air into the lungs, but exhaling air out through the obstructed airways. (People who don't have asthma can get an idea of what an asthma attack feels like by taking a breath and holding it for a second, then trying to take another breath without exhaling first.)

Cold, dry air is believed to trigger EIA. So, exercising outdoors in the winter or breathing through your mouth during heavy exertion is likely to set off an attack. (Breathing through your nose warms and moistens the air before it reaches the lungs.) EIA symptoms typically occur after three to eight minutes of strenuous activity, and can last 20 to 30 minutes. They can range from mild to severe, and include coughing, wheezing, tightness or pain in the chest, shortness of breath, and reduced stamina.

EIA Need Not Bench You

"Many people who have EIA don't know it because they blame their symptoms on being out of shape," notes John Weiler, M.D., a professor in the department of internal medicine at the University of Iowa Hospitals and Clinics in Iowa City. Others may experience symptoms only when they push themselves to the "max" or exercise outdoors when air quality is poor.

But if you're susceptible to it, EIA can affect you, regardless of your fitness level or athletic ability. In fact, according to various studies, 10 to 12 percent of athletes have EIA. At the 1984 summer Olympics in Los Angeles, 67 of the 597 members of the American team had EIA; among them, they won 41 medals.

Obviously, EIA need not limit participation or success in vigorous activities. Today it can be medically managed and its effects minimized.

"In the past, doctors discouraged people with asthma from exerting themselves to avoid triggering an attack. But the current thinking is that it is important for asthmatics to engage in regular exercise to condition and strengthen their lungs," says Stanley Szefler, M.D., director of clinical pharmacology at the National Jewish Center for Immunology and Respiratory Medicine in Denver.

Swimming in an indoor pool may be the ideal exercise for asthmatics because the warm, humid air keeps the airways from drying and cooling. However, "with proper management, virtually no sport is off-limits," says Szefler.

Proper management of EIA, Szefler says, includes monitoring air flow with a peak-flow meter, avoiding allergic triggers, and using medication before exercise.

Asthma symptoms can change a lot. They are often worse at night than during the day. They may be worse in the winter or during "allergy seasons" when pollen counts are high. The new National Heart, Lung, and Blood Institute guidelines recommend that people 5 years or older who have moderate to severe asthma use a peak-flow meter twice a day (morning and evening).

A peak-flow meter measures how fast you blow air out of your lungs. When a person blows into the device—which looks something like a kazoo—a slide indicates the force of the exhaled air. The farther the slide is pushed, the greater the peak flow.

181

"Peak-flow meters can help asthmatics monitor their symptoms so attacks can be better anticipated," explains Michael Gluck, D.Sc., chief of FDA's anesthesiology and respiratory devices branch.

Once a doctor determines normal peak flow, a treatment approach can be tailored just for you. For instance, your doctor may instruct you to take more medicine than usual if your peak flow drops a certain amount, say 70 percent of normal, or to get medical help right away if it falls to 30 percent of normal.

"In the past, a vague sense of not feeling well was the only indication a person had that an asthma attack was imminent. By that time, it was often too late to head off the attack," says Gluck. "Peak-flow meters give you...a much earlier indication of an oncoming attack."

"Drugs that relax the muscle spasm in the walls of the bronchial tubes to open them are often the first line of treatment in preventing EIA," says Tunde Otulana, M.D., a medical reviewer in FDA's oncology and pulmonary drugs division. Such drugs are called bronchodilators. They are typically prescribed in aerosol (inhalant) form. They are sprayed into the mouth and breathed directly into the lungs. Doctors recommend using the medication from five minutes to an hour before exercise. If breathing problems develop during exercise, you may need to take another dose. The most common side effect of bronchodilators is feeling jittery, says Otulana.

Cromolyn sodium is often prescribed to treat athletes who have EIA. This drug, which is also an inhalant, prevents the lining of the airways from swelling in response to cold air or allergic triggers, explains Otulana, and must be taken on a regular basis for the treatment of asthma. Cromolyn sodium can be used up to 15 minutes before engaging in physical activity.

Cromolyn has few side effects, according to Otulana. "The most common complaint is that it leaves an unpleasant taste in the mouth for a few seconds. Some people may experience coughing due to dryness and throat irritation and, in rare instances, patients have become nauseated."

In addition to bronchodilators and cromolyn, which are used primarily to head off an attack of EIA, the National Heart, Lung, and Blood Institute treatment guidelines recommend the use of inhaled corticosteroids for patients with moderate to severe chronic asthma. "Instead of using a 'rescue' approach to treat episodes of breathlessness, doctors are now focusing on the big picture and using a preventive approach to treat airway inflammation, which is the underlying cause of asthma," says Szefler.

"Corticosteroids work by reducing swelling in the bronchial tubes and by enhancing the action of bronchodilators. They are meant to be used as preventive medication, usually on an ongoing basis," says Otulana.

Corticosteroid inhalants can occasionally cause throat irritation and thrush (a fungal infection in the mouth), says Otulana. (He advises gargling with warm water after using the inhaler to help avoid both side effects.) Prolonged use of very high doses may increase the risk of the same type of health problems associated with the drug in pill form: high blood pressure, diabetes, and softening of the bones.

"It is very difficult to recognize EIA, especially when exercise is the only trigger for asthma," says Weiler. "If you can't keep up with the other kids, can't seem to be able to 'get into shape' no matter how much you exercise, or experience problems after exercise that your classmates don't, EIA may be to blame."

Today, Nicholas carries a bronchodilator with him and uses cromolyn 20 minutes before gym class. Although he still dislikes exercise, he doesn't cut gym now that he can keep up with the other kids. "If I premedicate, I have no problems," he says. "Asthma can be a setback, but it doesn't have to be—if you learn how to deal with it."

Tips on Coping With EIA

- Start with a 15-minute warm-up to allow the lungs to adjust to the increased demand for oxygen.

- In cold weather, cover your mouth and nose with a scarf to help warm the air before it gets to the lungs.

- Avoid triggers that may cause or worsen EIA (for example, don't exercise outdoors when pollen counts are high).

- End with a 15-minute cool-down rather than stopping abruptly.

- Follow your doctor's instructions about using medication before or after exercise. If you're on a team, let your coach know about your doctor's instructions.

- If you have symptoms, use a bronchodilator right away. Remember, cromolyn and corticosteroids are not recommended during an asthma attack because they do not immediately open the airways.

Ruth Papazian is a health and medical writer in the Bronx, N.Y.

Chapter 16

Exercise and Diabetes

Chapter Contents

Section 16.1

Starting to Exercise

Source: American Diabetes Association. *Diabetes Day-By-Day*, No. 8, 1996. Used by permission.

The journey of a thousand leagues starts from where your feet stand. You may have heard the proverb. Exercise is like that. It all boils down to single steps you take each day It can be as simple and as difficult as starting any journey. There's no question, taking that first step can be hard. Maybe you've never exercised. Maybe you used to but stopped. Maybe you've just been diagnosed with diabetes and feel like you'll never be fit again. We've all got plenty of reasons not to exercise. We're

- too old,

- too fat,

- too weak,

- too sick,

- too busy,

- too tired.

What we need to remember is that it's never too late. With few exceptions, even if you're disabled or injured you can still improve your level of fitness. Once you get going, you'll be amazed how quickly your excuses fade.

Too old? Join a class with others in your age group. There are seniors' mall walking clubs, water exercise classes, senior stretch programs, even chair aerobics classes. Check your local YMCA, YWCA, or county recreation program. Nothing in your area? Start your own program with a partner, such as a relative or friend.

Too fat? If you feel too awkward or embarrassed to exercise, join the club. Most people feel slightly silly when they start out. Exercise is not just for skinny minnies. In fact, once you get going, look around. Few regular exercisers have perfect physiques. Most fitness buffs will respect your efforts and root for your success. If you're trying to lose weight, even a modest amount of regular physical activity can help.

Too weak? Regular physical activity will help you have more strength and energy for daily tasks.

Too sick? Of course, you can't exercise when you're ill or when your blood glucose levels are out of control. But once you are feeling better, regular physical activity will help you stay well. If you stick with it, you may even find you don't get sick as much and may need less medication.

Too busy? You don't have to spend hours exercising to see a health benefit. Depending on your fitness level, you may need to start with as little as 10 minutes of walking three times a week. If you really want to make a change, you can find ways to get more activity into your daily routines. Park farther away from the entrances at the mall. Plan an after-dinner walk with someone you want to talk to. Ride a stationary bike while you watch the morning or evening news.

Too tired? Believe it or not, regular physical activity will give you more energy. Toning your muscles and conditioning your heart, lungs, and blood vessels will better equip you to handle the work and stress of daily life.

Lots of people think of exercise programs the way they think of diets. They plan to get in shape for a certain event. Or they join an exercise class hoping it will help them lose 5 or 10 pounds. But physical activity and healthful eating are habits we need to stay with over the long haul. That doesn't mean doing the same exercise or eating the same meals forever. You may enjoy trying new forms of physical activity, in the same way new recipes are fun. Or you may find an activity that works for you and stay with it.

The First Step

The first step to fitness is a visit to the doctor. Before you begin any exercise program, get a thorough medical exam. The exam should check:

- blood pressure,
- blood fat levels,
- glycohemoglobin and current blood glucose level,

187

- health of heart and circulatory system,
- body composition (fat versus lean),
- eyes,
- feet.

Your doctor should help determine your level of fitness. You need to know what types of exercise or exercise programs are good choices for you. Some complications of diabetes make certain types of physical activity bad choices. The benefits of an exercise program need to outweigh the risks.

If possible, get an exercise prescription. This is an exercise plan that takes into account your current level of fitness, special health concerns, and your diabetes treatment plan. Your health-care providers are your best resources.

Set Goals

Goals help give shape to your exercise plan. They give you something specific to work toward. Reaching a goal marks your success. Setting new goals keeps you going. Start out by asking yourself why you plan to exercise. Do you want to

- feel better?
- move easier?
- lose weight?
- get stronger?
- have more energy?
- reduce stress?
- stay fit while learning to live with diabetes?
- reduce your risk of diabetes complications such as heart disease?
- get your doctor or partner to stop nagging you?

Once you know why you plan to exercise, talk with your doctor about realistic ways to reach your goal. With your doctor or exercise specialist, you can plan an exercise routine with your goal in mind.

Your program will need to take into account your diabetes management routine. Your doctor and diabetes educator can help you plan

- the best times to exercise,

- when to test your blood glucose levels and what your test results mean in terms of exercise,

- how to avoid problems with low blood glucose levels,

- how to inspect your feet before and after exercise,

- other specific health concerns.

Here's how this might work. Suppose you have non-insulin-dependent (type II) diabetes and are overweight. You work in an office and drive to work. You don't have an exercise plan. Your doctor says that if you lose some weight and start to exercise, you may be able to improve your blood glucose control. After your physical exam and an exercise stress test, the doctor says you can start a walking program.

Your health goal: to lose 10 pounds.

Your fitness goal: to stay with a regular walking program for 3 months, building up to 20 minutes of walking three times a week.

Current fitness level: couch potato.

Now you need to break your fitness goal down into smaller steps. Make your goals realistic, measurable, and achievable. Your long-term goal is to walk for 30 minutes three times a week. Your short-term goal is to walk 10 minutes without stopping three times a week for a month.

Write your goal down. Keep a log, or diary, of your exercise. You can buy a special notebook, write on your calendar, or make a note in your blood glucose record book. You might also want to jot down how you feel while exercising, or any problems you have. This gives you something to look over when you're ready to make changes.

When your goal period is up, look at your log. Were there good days and bad? Did you start feeling different? As you set your new goal, use your log to decide on changes. Do you need to reduce your level of physical activity? Or are you ready to move up a notch? Discuss changes with your health-care team. Be sure to reward yourself when you reach a goal.

Knowing that physical activity is something you'll do for the rest of your life can help. You can take the long view. If your first attempt doesn't work, try again. Do something different. Join a class or a mall walkers club. Think about what you enjoy doing and find a fitness activity that matches. Do you like to exercise to music? To TV? Alone

189

or with friends? Outdoors or indoors? There are so many choices, you can find something to enjoy.

Fringe Benefits

You know that regular physical activity is good for your health. It also brings fringe benefits such as:

- looking better,
- meeting new friends,
- escaping from the daily grind,
- learning new skills, and
- reducing stress.

Still, after you've been exercising for a while, you'll no doubt go through a spell where your motivation slips. Anyone who has a long-term exercise program has "off" days, times when he or she just doesn't want to stick with it. Or you may have a setback due to illness or injury. When it happens to you, don't mistake it for failure. Give yourself a break. Call an exercise buddy. Review your exercise log. Read an inspirational book. Try a new activity. Join a class. Celebrate your successes. Treat yourself to something new to wear when you exercise—a new T-shirt, even new shoes. Before you know it, your exercise slump will be over.

Reprinted with permission from American Diabetes Association, Inc., Copyright © 1996, The American Diabetes Association, Inc. The American Diabetes Association has many publications to help you live better with diabetes. For more information or to order, call the American Diabetes Association at 1-800-DIABETES.

Section 16.2

20 Steps To Safe Exercise

Source: American Diabetes Association. *Diabetes Day-byDay,* No. 9, 1996. Used by permission.

Exercise can improve your health and your outlook on life. Because you have diabetes, however, it pays to be doubly careful not to injure yourself or upset your diabetes control. You'll want to follow the basic guidelines that everyone who exercises needs to follow. And you'll want to add some extra safety steps that take your diabetes into account. These 20 steps to safe exercise will help you deal with both these types of needs.

1. Get a thorough medical exam before you start. Your doctor should check your

- blood pressure
- blood fat levels
- glycated hemoglobin levels
- health of heart and circulatory system
- body composition (fat versus lean)
- vision
- feet

2. Choose exercises that fit your health. Talk to your health-care team about what types of exercise are best for you. Diabetes can cause health problems, such as eye or nerve disease, that make certain types of exercise poor choices. For example, if you have lost feeling in your feet, swimming may be better than walking. If you have trouble seeing or have frequent low blood glucose reactions, you may need to exercise indoors or with a friend. Your health-care team can help, you choose fitness goals tailored to your health.

3. Take it easy. Slow and steady wins the race. Trying to do too much too soon can leave you discouraged or even injured.

One way to pace yourself is to count your heart rate and make sure it stays below a certain level. Another is to rate how difficult exercise feels and avoid too much huffing and puffing. Your health-care team can teach you how to avoid pushing yourself too hard.

Step up your workout as you become more fit. Gradually increase how long and how hard you exercise. For instance, you may start out walking for just 5 or 10 minutes. Over many weeks, you may build up to 25 or 30 minutes. You and your health-care team should adjust your plans for exercise, meals, and medications as you get in shape.

4. Warm up and stretch when you start exercising. Warm up with a low-impact exercise like walking. This gets your heart and muscles prepared to work. After you are warmed up, you may want to stretch gently. Stretching helps keep muscles and joints flexible. Tight muscles and joints are more prone to injury.

5. End your workout with a cool-down. Slow down gradually, until your breathing becomes more normal. For example, if you've been jogging, walk for 5 minutes to cool down. When your breathing is back to normal, start your stretching, routine. Some people prefer to stretch at the end of their workout, when muscles are warm and can stretch more easily.

6. Drink plenty of liquids. Sweating means you're losing fluid. It's important to drink to replace fluids lost in sweat. Water is almost always the best choice. If you are exercising for a long time, you may want the extra calories in a drink that contains carbohydrate. Choose drinks that are no more than 10% carbohydrate.

7. Watch the temperature. Avoid exercising when it's too hot or cold. During the summer months, do not exercise when it's hot or humid or when air quality is poor. Instead, exercise indoors where it's air conditioned. In the winter, move your workout indoors when you feel it's too cold, especially if the wind-chill is 15°F or lower.

8. Wear clothes that are right for the weather and your sport. It won't help to wear heavy clothes in the warm weather. Sweating more won't help you lose fat, just water weight. (In fact, it's unhealthy. You'll just increase your risk or overheating.)

In the summer, wear lightweight, light-colored clothes. Be sure to use sunscreen and a hat. In winter, dress in layers. Polypropylene, silk, or thin, fine wool make a good first layer. These materials help lift sweat from your body and prevent chafing. Your outer layer should be made of material that can "breathe" and let sweat escape. Be sure to protect your feet, hands, and head from the cold.

Use the safety gear that goes with your sport. If you're cycling, wear a helmet. If you're playing racquetball, wear eye protection.

9. Remember your feet. Wear the right shoes for your sport. This means basketball shoes to play basketball, walking shoes for walking, aerobics shoes for aerobics, etc. Replace shoes when they begin to wear out. Always put on clean, smooth-fitting socks. Check your feet after exercise. Look for blisters, warm areas, or redness. If you do see problems, call your doctor.

10. Watch for low blood glucose. If you take insulin or oral diabetes medicine, you may have low blood glucose levels during and after exercise. In fact, you may get low blood glucose 12 or more hours after a workout. People who have non-insulin-dependent (type II) diabetes controlled by diet and exercise usually don't have problems with low blood glucose.

Glucose fuels your muscles during exercise. At the same time, exercise helps pep up insulin's action. Both things lower your blood glucose level. Through careful planning, you and your doctor will learn to adjust your treatment to avoid low blood glucose levels caused by exercise.

11. Test your blood glucose before you exercise. If you take insulin or diabetes pills, self-monitoring of blood glucose is the key to avoiding low blood glucose levels.

It's best to test your blood glucose twice before exercise. Test 30 minutes before, and again just before you begin. This tells you whether your blood glucose level is stable or dropping. If it is dropping, you may need an extra snack.

12. Be ready to test during exercise. This is especially important if you try a new activity or sport. A test can help you predict how this sport will affect your blood glucose levels.

You may also want to test if you will be exercising for more than an hour. Generally, you'll want to test every 30 minutes. If your blood glucose starts to fall, stop and have a snack.

13. Test again after exercise. Exercise—especially long, hard workouts—can lower your blood glucose for hours after you've stopped. This happens because workouts draw on your body's supply of glu-

193

cose, stored in your muscles and liver as glycogen. Later, your body rebuilds its stores of glycogen by taking glucose from the blood. For as long as 24 hours, your body needs the glucose you get from meals to fill up your glycogen stores. Your health-care team can suggest at what times you should do extra tests to avoid low blood glucose.

14. Use your testing results to learn how exercise affects your body. Exercise makes insulin work harder. Your blood glucose may drop more than usual when you take your normal insulin dose. Exercise can make insulin go to work faster, too.

On the other hand, long, hard exercise sessions can sometimes raise your blood glucose, especially if it was very high before you started. Hard exercise can signal your liver to start breaking down glycogen into glucose. Hard exercise means whatever is difficult for you. It could he just walking a mile faster than usual or pedaling your bike hard up a steep hill.

If you take insulin or diabetes pills to control your blood glucose levels, you need to plan your exercise and diabetes care to avoid levels too low or too high.

15. Time your exercise according to your meals and insulin. Generally, you want to exercise after you have eaten. The food will help keep your blood glucose from becoming too low. It's best to exercise 1 to 3 hours after a meal. You'll also want to avoid exercising when your insulin is peaking (at its strongest). Avoiding your insulin's peak times will help you avoid low blood sugar. Your doctor may suggest that you try decreasing the insulin dose that will be working while you exercise.

16. Eat before exercise. Because exercise lowers your blood glucose, you may need larger meals or extra snacks before exercise. Ask your health-care team for tips. If your blood glucose level is between 150 and 250 mg/dl before exercise, you probably won't need a snack. But check your blood glucose during exercise to be sure. If your blood glucose is less than 100 mg/dl, your health-care team may advise you to eat half a sandwich or a piece of fruit before you exercise.

If you are exercising for an hour or more, you may need to eat a snack every 30 minutes to 1 hour. You may also need extra snacks after long exercise to build back your energy stores.

17. Be prepared to treat low blood glucose. Always carry juice, regular (nondiet) soft drink, glucose gel, raisins, or another fast-acting source of sugar. If you feel a reaction coming on, stop and treat it right away.

18. Know when not to exercise. If your fasting blood glucose is more than 300 mg/dl, no matter what type of diabetes you have, it is in poor control. Don't exercise before you bring your glucose levels back down or before checking with your health-care team.

19. Know when to test for ketones. If you have insulin-dependent (type I) diabetes and your blood glucose tests are 250 mg/dl before exercise, stop and test your urine for ketones. If you test positive for moderate or large amounts of ketones, do not exercise. Ketones are a sign that your insulin level is too low. Exercise could cause the body to make more ketones.

Ketones add acid to the blood. When too many ketones are produced, they disrupt your body's chemical balance. This can be dangerous. Wait until your urine tests show negative or trace ketone levels to return to exercise.

20. Update your exercise plan regularly. If you take insulin or diabetes pills, be sure to talk to your doctor about exercise and your blood glucose levels. Ask your doctor to tailor exercise guidelines to meet your individual needs. Once you get going in a regular exercise program, you may find that you need less insulin or lower doses of diabetes pills. Your doctor may also be able to leach you how to change your own insulin dose on days when you plan a different exercise routine.

Exercise with diabetes does demand a few extra safety steps. You'll find that once you're into regular exercise, these will become a part of your routine. And you'll find the rewards of exercise well worth a little extra effort.

Chapter 17

Exercise and Your Heart: A Guide to Physical Activity

Do We Get Enough Exercise from Our Daily Activities?

Most Americans get little vigorous exercise at work or during leisure hours. Today, only a few jobs require vigorous physical activity. People usually ride in cars or buses and watch TV during their free time rather than be physically active. Activities like golfing and bowling provide people with some benefit. But they do not provide the same benefits as regular, more vigorous exercise.

Evidence suggests that even low- to moderate-intensity activities can have both short- and long-term benefits. If done daily, they help lower your risk of heart disease. Such activities include pleasure walking, stair climbing, gardening, yardwork, moderate to heavy housework, dancing and home exercise. More vigorous exercise can help improve fitness of the heart and lungs, which can provide even more consistent benefits for lowering heart disease risk.

Today, many people are rediscovering the benefits of regular, vigorous exercise—activities like swimming, brisk walking, running, or jumping rope. These kinds of activities are sometimes called "aerobic"—meaning the body uses oxygen to produce the energy needed for the activity. Aerobic exercises can condition your heart and lungs if performed at the proper intensity for at least 30 minutes, 3-4 times a week.

NIH Pub. No. 93-1677

197

But you don't have to train like a marathon runner to become more physically fit! Any activity that gets you moving around, even it it's done for just a few minutes each day, is better than none at all. For inactive people, the trick is to get started. One great way is to take a walk for 10-15 minutes during your lunch break. Other ideas in this pamphlet will help you get moving and living a more active life.

What Are the Benefits of Regular Physical Activity?

These are the benefits often experienced by people who get regular physical activity.

Feeling Better

Regular physical activity—

- gives you more energy
- helps in coping with stress
- improves your self-image
- increases resistance to fatigue
- helps counter anxiety and depression
- helps you to relax and feel less tense
- improves the ability to fall asleep quickly and sleep well
- provides an easy way to share an activity with friends or family and an opportunity to meet new friends

Looking Better

Regular physical activity—

- tones your muscles
- burns off calories to help lose extra pounds or helps you stay at your desirable weight
- helps control your appetite

You need to burn off 3,500 calories more than you take in to lose 1 pound. If you want to lose weight, regular physical activity can help you in either of two ways.

First, you can eat your usual amount of calories, but be more active. For example: A 200-pound person who keeps on eating the same amount of calories, but decides to walk briskly each day for 1½ miles will lose about 14 pounds in 1 year. Or second, you can eat fewer calories and be more active. This is an even better way to lose weight.

About three-fourths of the energy you burn every day comes from what your body uses for its basic needs, such as sleeping, breathing, digesting food and reclining. A person burns up only a small amount of calories with daily activities such as sitting. Any physical activity in addition to what you normally do will burn up extra calories.

The average calories spent per hour by a 150-pound person are listed below. (A lighter person burns fewer calories; a heavier person burns more.) Since exact calorie figures are not available for most activities, the figures below are averaged from several sources and show the relative vigor of the activities.

Activity	Calories burned
Bicycling 6 mph	240 cals./hr.
Bicycling 12 mph	410 cals./hr.
Cross-country skiing	700 cals./hr.
Jogging 5 1/2 mph	740 cals./hr.
Jogging 7 mph	920 cals./hr.
Jumping rope	750 cals./hr.
Running in place	650 cals./hr.
Running 10 mph	1280 cals./hr.
Swimming 25 yds/min.	275 cals./hr.
Swimming 50 yds/min.	500 cals./hr.
Tennis-singles	400 cals./hr.
Walking 2 mph	240 cals./hr.
Walking 3 mph	320 cals./hr.
Walking 4 1/2 mph	440 cals./hr.

The calories spent in a particular activity vary in proportion to one's body weight. For example, a 100-pound person burns 1/3 fewer calories, so you would multiply the number of calories by 0.7. For a 200-pound person, multiply by 1.3.

Working harder or faster for a given activity will only slightly increase the calories spent. A better way to burn up more calories is to increase the time spent on your activity.

Working Better

Regular physical activity—

- helps you to be more productive at work
- increases your capacity for physical work
- builds stamina for other physical activities
- increases muscle strength
- helps your heart and lungs work more efficiently

Consider the benefits of a well-conditioned heart:

In 1 minute with 45 to 50 beats, the heart of a well-conditioned person pumps the same amount of blood as an inactive person's heart pumps in 70 to 75 beats. Compared to the well-conditioned heart, the average heart pumps up to 36,000 more times per day, 13 million more times per year.

Feeling, looking, and working better—all these benefits from regular physical activity can help you enjoy your life more fully.

Can Physical Activity Reduce my Chances of Getting a Heart Attack?

Yes! Various studies have shown that physical inactivity is a risk factor for heart disease. Overall, the results show heart disease is almost twice as likely to develop in inactive people than in those who are more active. Regular physical activity (even mild to moderate exercise) can help reduce your risk of heart disease. In fact, burning calories through physical activity may help you lose weight or stay at your desirable weight—which also helps lower your risk of heart disease. The best exercises to strengthen your heart and lungs are the aerobic ones like brisk walking, jogging, cycling and swimming.

Coronary artery disease is the major cause of heart disease and heart attack in America. It develops when fatty deposits build up on the inner walls of the blood vessels feeding the heart (coronary arteries). Eventually one or more of the major coronary arteries may become blocked—either by the buildup of deposits or by a blood clot forming in the artery's narrowed passageway. The result is a heart attack.

We know that there are several factors that can increase your risk for developing coronary artery disease—and thus the chances for a heart attack. Fortunately, many of these risk factors can be reduced or eliminated.

The Risk Factors for Heart Disease that You Can Do Something About Are:

Cigarette Smoking, High Blood Pressure, High Blood Cholesterol, Physical Inactivity and Obesity. The more risk factors you have, the greater your risk for heart disease and heart attack.

Cigarette Smoking. Heavy smokers are two to four times more likely to have a heart attack than nonsmokers. The heart attack death rate among all smokers is 70 percent greater than among nonsmokers. People who are active regularly are more likely to cut down or stop cigarette smoking.

High Blood Pressure. The higher your blood pressure, the greater your risk of developing heart disease or stroke. A blood pressure of 140/90 mmHg (millimeters of mercury) or greater is generally classified as high blood pressure. Regular physical activity, even of moderate intensity, can help reduce high blood pressure in some people. This type of activity may also help prevent high blood pressure.

High Blood Cholesterol. A blood cholesterol level of 240 mg/dl (milligrams per deciliter) or above is high and increases your risk of heart disease. A total blood cholesterol of under 200 mg/dl is desirable and usually puts you at a lower risk of heart disease. Cholesterol in the blood is transported by different types of particles. One of these particles is a protein called high density lipoprotein or HDL. HDL has been called "good" cholesterol because research has shown that high levels of HDL are linked with a lower risk of coronary artery disease. Regular moderate-to-vigorous physical activity is linked with increased HDL levels.

Physical Inactivity. The lack of physical activity increases your risk for developing heart disease. Even persons who have had a heart attack can increase their chances of survival if they change their habits to include regular physical activity. It can help control blood lipids, diabetes and obesity as well as help to lower blood pressure. Also, physical activity of the right intensity, frequency and duration can increase the fitness of your heart and lungs—which may help protect you against heart disease even if you have other risk factors.

Obesity. Excess weight may increase your risk of developing high blood pressure, high blood cholesterol and diabetes. Regular physical activity can help you maintain your desirable body weight. People at their desirable weight are less likely to develop diabetes. And, exercise may also decrease a diabetic person's need for insulin.

Remember that even if you are active, you should not ignore other risk factors. Reduce or eliminate any risk factors you can to lower your chances of having a heart attack.

Tips for your heart's health:

- Stay physically active.
- Stop smoking and avoid other people's smoke if possible.
- Control high blood pressure and high blood cholesterol.
- Cut down on total fats, saturated fats, cholesterol and salt in your diet.
- Reduce weight if overweight.

Are There Any Risks in Exercising?

Muscles and Joints

The most common risk in exercising is injury to the muscles and joints. This usually happens from exercising too hard or for too long—particularly if a person has been inactive for some time. However, most of these injuries can be prevented or easily treated as explained in "Effective ways to avoid injuries" on page 215.

Heat Exhaustion and Heat Stroke

If precautions are not taken during hot, humid days, heat exhaustion or heat stroke can occur—although they are fairly rare. Heat stroke is the more serious of the two. Their symptoms are similar:

Heat exhaustion	Heat stroke
dizziness	dizziness
headache	headache
nausea	nausea
confusion	thirst
body temperature below normal	muscle cramps
	sweating stops
	high body temperature

The last two symptoms of heat stroke are important to know. If the body temperature becomes dangerously high, it can be a serious problem.

Both heat exhaustion and heat stroke can be avoided if you drink enough liquids to replace those lost during exercise. And be sure to take the other important precautions listed on page 216 in the section on avoiding injuries.

Heart Problems

In some cases, people have died while exercising. Most of these deaths are caused by overexertion in people who already had heart conditions. In people under age 30, these heart conditions are usually congenital heart defects (heart defects present at birth). In people over age 40, the heart condition is usually coronary artery disease (the buildup of deposits of fats in the heart's blood vessels). Many of these deaths have been preceded by warning signs such as chest pain, lightheadedness, fainting and extreme breathlessness. These are symptoms that should not be ignored and should be brought to the attention of a doctor immediately.

Some of the deaths that occur during exercise are not caused by the physical effort itself. Death can occur at any time and during any kind of activity—eating, sleeping, sitting. This does not necessarily mean that a particular activity caused the death—only that the two events happened at the same time.

No research studies have shown that physically active people are more likely to have sudden, fatal heart attacks than inactive people. In fact, a number of studies have shown a reduced risk of sudden death for people who are physically active.

Exercising too hard is not beneficial for anyone, however, and is especially strenuous for out-of-shape, middle-aged and older persons.

It is very important for these people to follow a gradual and sound exercise program.

If you consider the time your body may have been out of shape, it is only natural that it will take time to get it back into good condition. A gradual approach will help you maximize your benefits and minimize your risks.

Comparing the Benefits and the Risks

Should you begin a regular exercise program? Consider the ways physical activity can benefit you and weigh them against the possible risks.

Potential Benefits

- more energy and capacity for work and leisure activities
- greater resistance to stress, anxiety and fatigue, and a better outlook on life
- increased stamina, strength and flexibility
- improved efficiency of the heart and lungs
- loss of extra pounds or body fat
- help in staying at desirable weight
- reduced risk of heart attack

Potential Risks

- muscle or joint injuries
- heat exhaustion or heat stroke on hot days (rare)
- aggravation of existing or hidden heart problems

Should I Consult a Doctor Before I Start an Exercise Program?

Most people do not need to see a doctor before they start since a gradual, sensible exercise program will have minimal health risks. However, some people should seek medical advice. Use the following checklist to find out if you should consult a doctor before you start or significantly increase your physical activity.*

Mark those items that apply to you:

❏ Your doctor said you have a heart condition and recommended only medically supervised physical activity.

❏ During or right after you exercise, you frequently have pains or pressure in the left or mid-chest area, left neck, shoulder or arm.

❏ You have developed chest pain within the last month.

❏ You tend to lose consciousness or fall over due to dizziness.

❏ You feel extremely breathless after mild exertion.

❏ Your doctor recommended you take medicine for your blood pressure or a heart condition.

❏ Your doctor said you have bone or joint problems that could be made worse by the proposed physical activity.

❏ You have a medical condition or other physical reason not mentioned here which might need special attention in an exercise program. (For example, insulin-dependent diabetes.)

❏ You are middle-aged or older, have not been physically active, and plan a relatively vigorous exercise program.

If you've checked one or more items, see your doctor before you start. If you've checked no items, you can start on a gradual, sensible program of increased activity tailored to your needs. If you feel any of the physical symptoms listed above when you start your exercise program, contact your doctor right away.

* This checklist has been developed from several sources, particularly the Physical Activity Readiness Questionnaire, British Columbia Ministry of Health, Department of National Health and Welfare, Canada (revised 1992).

What if I've Had a Heart Attack?

Regular, brisk physical activity can help reduce your risk of having another heart attack. People who include regular physical activity in their lives after a heart attack improve their chances of survival. Regular exercise can also improve the quality of your life—how you feel and look. It can help you do more than before without pain (angina) or shortness of breath.

If you've had a heart attack, consult your doctor to be sure you are following a safe and effective exercise program. Your doctor's guidance is very important because it could help prevent heart pain and / or further damage from overexertion.

Five Common Myths About Exercise

Myth 1. Exercising makes you tired.

As they become more physically fit, most people feel physical activity gives them even more energy than before. Regular, moderate-to-brisk exercise can also help you reduce fatigue and manage stress.

Myth 2. Exercising takes too much time.

It only takes a few minutes a day to become more physically active. To condition your heart and lungs, regular exercise does not have to take more than about 30 to 60 minutes, three or four times a week. If you don't have 30 minutes in your schedule for an exercise break, try to find two 15-minute periods or even three 10-minute periods. Once you discover how much you enjoy these exercise breaks, you may want to make them a habit! Then physical activity becomes a natural part of your life.

Myth 3. All exercises give you the same benefits.

All physical activities can give you enjoyment. Low-intensity activities—if performed daily—also can have some long-term health benefits and lower your risk of heart disease. But only regular, brisk and sustained exercises such as brisk walking, jogging or swimming improve the efficiency of your heart and lungs and burn off substantial extra calories. Other activities may give you other benefits such as increased flexibility or muscle strength, depending on the type of activity.

Myth 4. The older you are, the less exercise you need.

We tend to become less active with age, and therefore need to make sure we are getting enough physical activity. In general, middle-aged and older people benefit from regular physical activity just as young people do. Age need not be a limitation. In fact, regular physical activity in older persons increases their capacity to perform activities of daily living. What is important, no matter what your age, is tailoring the activity program to your own fitness level.

Myth 5. You have to be athletic to exercise.

Most physical activities do not require any special athletic skills. In fact, many people who found school sports difficult have discovered that these other activities are easy to do and enjoy. A perfect example is walking—an activity that requires no special talent. athletic ability or equipment.

How Do Different Activities Help My Heart and Lungs?

Some types of activity will improve the condition of your heart and lungs if they are brisk, sustained and regular. Low-intensity activities do not condition the heart and lungs much. But they can have other long-term health benefits.

The columns below describe three types of activities and how they affect your heart.

Column A—These vigorous exercises are especially helpful when done regularly. To condition your heart and lungs, the AHA recommends that you do them for at least 30 minutes, three or four times a week, at more than 50 percent of your exercise capacity. (See page 23 on target heart rate zone.) Other health experts suggest a shorter period for higher-intensity activities. These exercises can also burn up more calories than those that are not so vigorous.

Column B—These activities are moderately vigorous but still excellent choices. When done briskly for 30 minutes or longer, three or four times a week, they can also condition your heart and lungs.

Column C—These activities are not vigorous or sustained. They still have benefits—they can be enjoyable, improve coordination and muscle tone, relieve tension, and also help burn up some calories.

These and other low-intensity activities—like gardening, yardwork, housework, dancing and home exercise—can help lower your risk of heart disease if done daily.

A **Do condition heart and lungs**	B **Can condition heart and lungs**	C **Do not condition much**
Aerobic Dancing	Downhill Skiing	Badminton
Bicycling	Basketball	Baseball
Cross-Country Skiing	Field Hockey	Bowling
Hiking (uphill)	Calisthenics	Croquet
Ice Hockey	Handball	Football
Jogging	Racquetball	Gardening
Jumping Rope	Soccer	Golf (on foot or by cart)
Rowing	Squash	Housework
Running in Place	Tennis (singles)	Ping-Pong
Stair-climbing	Volleyball	Shuffleboard
Stationary Cycling	Walking Moderately	Social Dancing
Swimming		Softball
Walking Briskly		Walking Leisurely

The Key to Success

How Do I Begin?

The key to a successful program is choosing an activity (or activities) that you will enjoy. Even moderate levels of activity have important health benefits. Here are some questions that can help you choose the right kind of activity for you:

1. How physically fit are you?

If you've been inactive for a while, you may want to start with walking or swimming at a comfortable pace. Beginning with less strenuous activities will allow you to become more fit without straining your body. Once you are in better shape, you can gradually change to a more vigorous activity if you wish.

2. How old are you?

If you are over 40 and have not been active, avoid very strenuous programs such as jogging when you're first starting out. For the first few months, build up the length and intensity of your activity gradually. Walking and swimming are especially good forms of exercise for all ages.

3. What benefits do you want from exercising?

If you want the benefits of exercise that condition your heart and lungs, check the activities in columns A and B on page 208. These activities—as well as those listed in column C—also give you other benefits as described in this booklet.

4. Do you like to exercise alone or with other people?

Do you like individual activities such as swimming, team sports such as soccer, or two-person activities such as racquetball? How about an aerobics class or ballroom dancing? Companionship can help you get started and keep going. If you would like to exercise with someone else, can you find a partner easily and quickly? If not, choose another activity until you can find a partner.

5. Do you prefer to exercise outdoors or in your home?

Outdoor activities offer variety in scenery and weather. Indoor activities offer shelter from the weather and can offer the convenience of exercising at home as with stationary cycling. Some activities such as bench stepping, running in place or jumping rope can be done indoors or outdoors. If your activity can be seriously affected by weather, consider choosing a second, alternate activity. Then you can switch activities and still stay on your regular schedule.

6. How much money are you willing to spend for sports equipment or facilities?

Many activities require little or no equipment. For example, brisk walking only requires a comfortable pair of walking shoes. Also, many communities offer free or inexpensive recreation facilities and physical activity classes.

209

7. When can you best fit the activity into your schedule?

Do you feel more like being active in the morning, afternoon, or evening? Consider moving other activities around. Schedule your activity as a regular part of your routine. Remember that exercise sessions are spread out over the week and needn't take more than about 10 to 15 minutes at a time.

By choosing activities you like, you will be more likely to keep doing them regularly and enjoying the many benefits of physical activity.

How Do I Pace Myself?

Build up slowly. If you've been inactive for a long while, remember it will take time to get into shape. Start with low- to moderate-level activities for at least several minutes each day. See the sample walking program on page 218, for example. You can slowly increase your time or pace as you become more fit. And you will feel more fit after a few weeks than when you first started.

How Hard Should I Exercise?

It's important to exercise at a comfortable pace. For example, when jogging or walking briskly you should be able to keep up a conversation comfortably. If you do not feel normal again within 10 minutes of stopping exercise, you are pushing yourself too much.

Also, if you have difficulty breathing, experience faintness or prolonged weakness during or after exercising, you are exercising too hard. Simply cut back.

If your goal is to improve the fitness of your heart and lungs, you can find out how hard to exercise by keeping track of your heart rate. Your maximum heart rate is the fastest your heart can beat. Exercise above 75 percent of your maximum heart rate may be too strenuous unless you are in excellent physical condition. Exercise below 50 percent gives your heart and lungs little conditioning.

Therefore, the best activity level is 50 to 75 percent of this maximum rate. This 50-75 percent range is called your target heart rate zone.

When you begin your exercise program, aim for the lower part of your target zone (50 percent) during the first few months. As you get into better shape, gradually build up to the higher part of your target zone (75 percent). After 6 months or more of regular exercise, you can exercise at up to 85 percent of your maximum heart rate—if you wish. However, you do not have to exercise that hard to stay in good condition.

To find your target zone, look for the age category closest to your age in the table below and read the line across. For example, if you are 30, your target zone is 95 to 142 beats per minute. If you are 43, the closest age on the chart is 45; the target zone is 88 to 131 beats per minute.

Age	Target HR Zone 50-75%	Average Maximum Heart Rate 100%
20 years	100-150 beats per min.	200
25 years	98-146 beats per min.	195
30 years	95-142 beats per min.	190
35 years	93-138 beats per min.	185
40 years	90-135 beats per min.	180
45 years	88-131 beats per min.	175
50 years	85-127 beats per min.	170
55 years	83-123 beats per min.	165
60 years	80-120 beats per min.	160
65 years	78-116 beats per min.	155
70 years	75-113 beats per min.	150

Your maximum heart rate is approximately 220 minus your age. However, the above figures are averages and should be used as general guidelines.

Note: A few high blood pressure medicines lower the maximum heart rate and thus the target zone rate. If you are taking high blood pressure medications, call your physician to find out if your exercise program needs to be adjusted.

To see if you are within your target heart rate zone, take your pulse immediately after you stop exercising.

1.   When you stop exercising, quickly place the tips of your first two fingers lightly over one of the blood vessels on your neck (carotid arteries) located to the left or right of your Adam's apple. Another convenient pulse spot is the inside of your wrist just below the base of your thumb.

2.   Count your pulse for 10 seconds and multiply by six.

3. If your pulse falls within your target zone, you're doing fine. If it is below your target zone, exercise a little harder next time. And if you're above your target zone, exercise a little easier. Don't try to exercise at your maximum heart rate—that's working too hard.

4. Once you're exercising within your target zone, you should check your pulse at least once each week during the first 3 months and periodically after that.

A special tip: Some people find that exercising within their target zone seems too strenuous. If you start out lower, that's okay, too. You will find that with time you'll become more comfortable exercising and can increase to your target zone at your own rate.

How Long Should I Exercise?

That depends on your age, your level of physical fitness, and the level of intensity of your exercise. If you are inactive now, you might begin slowly with a 10-15 minute walk or other short session, three times a week. As you become more fit, you can do longer sessions or short sessions more often.

If you're active already and your goal is to condition your heart and lungs, try for a minimum of 30 minutes at your target heart rate zone. Each exercise session should include:

Warm up 5 minutes

Begin exercising slowly to give your body a chance to limber up and get ready for more vigorous exercise. Start at a medium pace and gradually increase it by the end of the 5-minute warm-up period.

Note: With especially vigorous activities such as jumping rope, jogging or stationary cycling, warm up for 5-10 minutes by jumping rope or jogging slowly, warming up to your target zone. It is often a good idea to do stretching exercises after your warm-up period and after your exercise period. Many of these stretching exercises can be found in books on sports medicine and running. Below are three stretches you can use in your warm-up period and after your cool-down period. Each of these exercises help stretch different parts of your body. Do stretching exercises slowly and steadily, and **don't bounce** when you stretch.

- **Wall push:** Stand about 1½ feet away from the wall. Then lean forward pushing against the wall, keeping heels flat. Count to 10 (or 20 for a longer stretch), then rest. Repeat one to two times.

- **Palm touch:** Stand with your knees slightly bent. Then bend from the waist and try to touch your palms to the floor. Count to 10 or 20, then rest. Repeat one to two times. If you have lower back problems, do this exercise with your legs crossed.

- **Toe touch:** Place your right leg level on a stair, chair, or other object. With your other leg slightly bent, lean forward and slowly try to touch your right toe with right hand. Hold and count to 10 or 20, then repeat with left hand. Do not bounce. Then switch legs and repeat with each hand. Repeat entire exercise one to two times.

Exercising within your target zone 30-40 minutes

Build up your exercising time gradually over the weeks ahead until you reach your goal of 30-60 minutes. Once you get in shape, your exercising will last from 30 to 60 minutes depending on the type of exercise you are doing and how briskly you do it. For example—for a given amount of time, jogging requires more energy than a brisk walk. Jogging will thus take less time than walking to achieve the same conditioning effect. For two examples of how to build up to the goal of 30-60 minutes, see "Two Sample Exercise Programs" beginning on page 218.

Cool down 5 minutes

After exercising within your target zone, slow down gradually. For example, swim more slowly or change to a more leisurely stroke. You can also cool down by changing to a less vigorous exercise, such as changing from running to walking. This allows your body to relax gradually. Abrupt stopping can cause dizziness. If you have been running, walking briskly, or jumping rope, repeat your stretching and limbering exercises to loosen up your muscles.

213

How Often Should I Exercise?

If you are exercising in your target zone, exercise at least three or four times per week (every other day). If you are starting with less intense exercise, you should try to do at least something every day.

Exercising regularly is one of the most important aspects of your exercise program. If you don't exercise at least three times a week, you won't experience as many of the benefits of regular physical activity as you could or make as much progress. Try to spread your exercise sessions throughout the week to maximize the benefits. An every-other-day schedule is recommended and may work well for you.

What if I Miss a Few Sessions?

Whenever you miss a few sessions (more than a week), you may need to resume exercising at a lower level than before.

If you miss a few sessions because of a temporary, minor illness such as a cold, wait until you feel normal before you resume exercising. If you have a minor injury, wait until the pain disappears. When you resume exercising, start at one-half to two-thirds your normal level, depending on the number of days you missed and how you feel while exercising.

Whatever the reasons for missing sessions, don't worry about the missed days. Just get back into your routine and think about the progress you will be making toward your exercise goal.

Is There a Top Limit to Exercising?

That depends on the benefits you are seeking.

Anything beyond 60 minutes daily of a vigorous or moderately vigorous activity, such as those in columns A and B on page 208, will result in little added conditioning of your heart and lungs. And it may increase your risk of injury.

If you want to lose extra pounds or control your present weight, there is no upper limit in that the longer you exercise, the more calories you burn off. But remember that the most effective weight loss program includes cutting down on calories in addition to exercise.

Remember: How you exercise is just as important as the kind of activity you do. Your activity should be brisk, sustained and regular— but you can do it in gradual steps. Common sense and your body will tell you when you are exercising too long or too hard. Don't push your-self to the point where exercise stops being enjoyable.

Effective Ways to Avoid Injuries

The most powerful medicine for injuries is prevention. Here are some effective ways to avoid injuries:

1. Build up your level of activity gradually over the weeks to come.

- Try not to set your goals too high—otherwise you will be tempted to push yourself too far too quickly.

- For activities such as jogging, walking briskly and jumping rope, limber up gently and slowly before and after exercising.

- For other activities, build up slowly to your target zone, and cool down slowly afterwards.

2. Listen to your body for early warning pains.

- Exercising too much can cause injuries to joints, feet, ankles and legs. So don't make the mistake of exercising beyond early warning pains in these areas or more serious injuries may result. Fortunately, minor muscle and joint injuries can be readily treated by rest and aspirin.

3. Be aware of possible signs of heart problems such as:

- Pain or pressure in the left or mid-chest area, left neck, shoulder or arm during or just after exercising. (Vigorous exercise may cause a side stitch while exercising—a pain be-low your bottom ribs—which is not the result of a heart problem.)

- Sudden lightheadedness, cold sweat, pallor or fainting.

Ignoring these signals and continuing to exercise may lead to se-rious heart problems. Should any of these signs occur, stop exercis-ing and call your doctor.

215

4. For outdoor activities, take appropriate precautions under special weather conditions.

On hot, humid days:

- Exercise during the cooler and/or less humid parts of the day such as early morning or early evening after the sun has gone down.

- Exercise less than normal for a week until you become adapted to the heat.

- Drink lots of fluids, particularly water—before, during and after exercising. Usually, you do not need extra salt because you get enough salt in your diet. (And a well-conditioned body is better able to conserve salt so that most of the sweat is water.) However, if you exercise very vigorously for an extended time in the heat (for example, running a marathon), it's a good idea to increase your salt intake a little.

- Watch out for signs of heat stroke—feeling dizzy, weak, lightheaded, and/or excessively tired; sweating stops; or body temperature becomes dangerously high.

- Wear a minimum of light, loose-fitting clothing.

- Avoid rubberized or plastic suits, sweatshirts, and sweat pants. Such clothing will not actually help you lose weight any faster by making you sweat more. The weight you lose in fluids by sweating will be quickly replaced as soon as you begin drinking fluids again. This type of clothing can also cause dangerously high temperatures, possibly resulting in heat stroke.

On cold days:

- Wear one layer less of clothing than you would wear if you were outside but not exercising. It's also better to wear several layers of clothing rather than one heavy layer. You can always remove a layer if you get too warm.

- Use old mittens, gloves, or cotton socks to protect your hands.

- Wear a hat, since up to 40 percent of your body's heat is lost through your neck and head.

On rainy, icy or snowy days:

- Be aware of reduced visibility (for yourself and for drivers) and reduced traction on pathways.

5. *Other handy tips are:*

- If you've eaten a meal, avoid strenuous exercise for at least 2 hours. If you exercise vigorously first, wait about 20 minutes before eating.

- Use proper equipment such as goggles to protect your eyes for handball or racquetball, or good shoes with adequate cushioning in the soles for running or walking.

- Hard or uneven surfaces such as cement or rough fields are more likely to cause injuries. Soft, even surfaces such as a level grass field, a dirt path, or a track for running are better for your feet and joints.

- If you run or jog, land on your heels rather than the balls of your feet. This will minimize the strain on your feet and lower legs.

- Joggers or walkers should also watch for cars and wear light-colored clothes with a reflecting band during darkness so that drivers can see you. Remember, drivers don't see you as well as you see their cars. Face oncoming traffic and do not assume that drivers will notice you on the roadway.

- If you bicycle, you can help prevent injuries by always wearing a helmet and using lights and wheel-mounted reflectors at night. Also, ride in the direction of traffic and try to avoid busy streets.

- Check your shopping malls. Many malls are open early and late for people who do not wish to exercise alone in the dark. They also make it possible to be active in bad weather and to avoid summer heat, winter cold or allergy seasons.

Two Sample Activity Programs

There are many ways to begin an activity program. Below are two examples—a walking and a jogging program. These activities are easy ways for most people to get regular exercise because they do not require special facilities or equipment other than good, comfortable shoes.

If walking or jogging does not meet your needs, look for other exercise programs in pamphlets and books on aerobic exercise and sports medicine. Check out the programs and facilities of your local park and recreation department or community recreation centers. Many programs have adapted facilities for the disabled and for seniors.

If you find a particular week's pattern tiring, repeat it before going on to the next pattern. You do not have to complete the walking program in 12 weeks or the jogging program in 15 weeks.

A new AHA brochure called 'Walking. . .Natural Fun, Natural Fitness" has a walking readiness questionnaire and a one-mile fitness test. You can ask your local American Heart Association for a copy.

A sample walking program

	Warm up	Target zone exercising	Cool down	Total time
Week 1				
Session A	Walk 5 min.	Then walk briskly 5 min.	Then walk more slowly 5 min.	15 min.
Session B	Repeat above pattern			
Session C	Repeat above pattern			

Continue with at least three exercise sessions during each week of the program.

	Warm up	Target zone exercising	Cool down	Total time
Week 2	Walk 5 min.	Walk briskly 7 min.	Walk 5 min.	17 min.
Week 3	Walk 5 min.	Walk briskly 9 min.	Walk 5 min.	19 min.

	Warm up	Target zone exercising	Cool down	Total time
Week 4	Walk 5 min.	Walk briskly 11 min.	Walk 5 min.	21 min.
Week 5	Walk 5 min.	Walk briskly 13 min.	Walk 5 min.	23 min.
Week 6	Walk 5 min.	Walk briskly 15 min.	Walk 5 min.	25 min.
Week 7	Walk 5 min.	Walk briskly 18 min.	Walk 5 min.	28 min.
Week 8	Walk 5 min.	Walk briskly 20 min.	Walk 5 min.	30 min.
Week 9	Walk 5 min.	Walk briskly 23 min.	Walk 5 min.	33 min.
Week 10	Walk 5 min.	Walk briskly 26 min.	Walk 5 min.	36 min.
Week 11	Walk 5 min.	Walk briskly 28 min.	Walk 5 min.	38 min.
Week 12	Walk 5 min.	Walk briskly 30 min.	Walk 5 min.	40 min.

Week 13 on:

Check your pulse periodically to see if you are exercising within your target zone. As you become more fit, try exercising within the upper range of your target zone. Gradually increase your brisk walking time to 30 to 60 minutes, three or four times a week. Remember that your goal is to get the benefits you are seeking and enjoy your activity.

A sample jogging program

If you are over 40 and have not been active, you should not begin with a program as strenuous as jogging. Begin with the walking program instead. After completing the walking program, you can start with week 3 of the jogging program below.

	Warm up	Target zone exercising	Cool down	Total time
Week 1				
Session A	Walk 5 min., then stretch and limber up	Then walk 10 min. Try not to stop	Then walk more slowly 3 min. and stretch 2 min.	20 min.

Session B Repeat above pattern

Session C Repeat above pattern

Continue with at least three exercise sessions during each week of the program.

	Warm up	Target zone exercising	Cool down	Total time
Week 2	Walk 5 min., then stretch and limber up	Walk 5 min., jog 1 min., walk 5 min., jog 1 min.	Walk 3 min., stretch 2 min.	22 min.
Week 3	Walk 5 min., then stretch and limber up	Walk 5 min., jog 3 min., walk 5 min., jog 3 min.	Walk 3 min., stretch 2 min.	26 min.
Week 4	Walk 5 min., then stretch and limber up	Walk 4 min., jog 5 min., walk 4 min., jog 5 min.	Walk 3 min., stretch 2 min.	28 min.
Week 5	Walk 5 min., then stretch and limber up	Walk 4 min., jog 5 min., walk 4 min., jog 5 min.	Walk 3 min., stretch 2 min.	28 min.

	Warm up	Target zone exercising	Cool down	Total time
Week 6	Walk 5 min., then stretch and limber up	Walk 4 min., jog 6 min., walk 4 min., jog 6 min.	Walk 3 min., stretch 2 min.	30 min.
Week 7	Walk 5 min., then stretch and limber up	Walk 4 min., jog 7 min., walk 4 min., jog 7 min.	Walk 3 min., stretch 2 min.	32 min.
Week 8	Walk 5 min., then stretch and limber up	Walk 4 min., jog 8 min., walk 4 min., jog 8 min.	Walk 3 min., stretch 2 min.	34 min.
Week 9	Walk 5 min., then stretch and limber up	Walk 4 min., jog 9 min., walk 4 min.; jog 9 min.	Walk 3 min., stretch 2 min.	36 min.
Week 10	Walk 5 min., then stretch and limber up	Walk 4 min., jog 13 min.	Walk 3 min., stretch 2 min.	27 min.
Week 11	Walk 5 min., then stretch and limber up	Walk 4 min., jog 15 min.	Walk 3 min., stretch 2 min.	29 min.
Week 12	Walk 5 min., then stretch and limber up	Walk 4 min., jog 17 min.	Walk 3 min., stretch 2 min.	31 min.
Week 13	Walk 5 min., then stretch and limber up	Walk 2 min., jog slowly 2 min., jog 17 min.	Walk 3 min., stretch 2 min.	31 min.

A sample jogging program (cont.)

	Warm up	Target zone exercising	Cool down	Total time
Week 14	Walk 5 min., then stretch and limber up	Walk 1 min., jog slowly 3 min., jog 17 min.	Walk 3 min., stretch 2 min.	31 min.
Week 15	Walk 5 min., then stretch and limber up	Jog slowly 3 min., jog 17 min.	Walk 3 min., stretch 2 min.	30 min.

Week 16 on:

Check your pulse periodically to see if you are exercising within your target zone. As you become more fit, try exercising within the upper range of your target zone. Gradually increase your jogging time from 20 to 30 minutes (or more, up to 60 minutes), three or four times a week. Remember that your goal is to get the benefits you are seeking and enjoy your activity.

The exercise patterns for both of the sample activity programs are suggested guidelines. Listen to your body and build up less quickly, if needed.

How Do I Keep Going?

Here are some tips to help you stay physically active:

1. Set your sights on short-term as well as long-term goals. For example, if your long-term goal is to walk 1 mile, then your short-term goal can be to walk the first quarter mile. Or if your long-term goal is to lose 10 pounds, then focus on the immediate goal of losing the first two or three pounds. With short-term goals you will be less likely to push yourself too hard or too long. Also, think back to where you started. When you compare it to where you are now, you will see the progress you've made.

2. Discuss your program and goals with your family or friends. Their encouragement and understanding are important

sources of support that can help you keep going. Your friends and family might even join in.

3.   If you're having trouble sticking to your regular activity program, use the questions on pages 208–210 to think through the kinds of things that can affect your exercise enjoyment.

4.   What were your original reasons for starting an activity program? Do these reasons still apply or are others more important? If you are feeling bored or aren't enjoying a particular activity, consider trying another one.

By continuing to be active regularly, you'll be building a good health habit with benefits you can enjoy throughout your life.

How Can I Become More Active Throughout My Day?

To become more physically active throughout your day, take advantage of any opportunity to get up and move around. Here are some examples:

*   Use the stairs—up and down—instead of the elevator. Start with one flight of stairs and gradually build up to more.

*   Park a few blocks from the office or store and walk the rest of the way. Or if you ride on public transportation, get off a stop or two before and walk a few blocks.

*   Take an activity break—get up and stretch, walk around and give your muscles and mind a chance to relax.

*   Instead of eating that extra snack, take a brisk stroll around the neighborhood.

*   Do housework, such as vacuuming, at a more brisk pace.

*   Mow your own lawn.

*   Carry your own groceries.

*   Go dancing instead of seeing a movie.

*   Take a walk after dinner instead of watching TV.

If you have a family, encourage them to take part in an exercise program and recreational activities they can either share with you or do on their own. It is best to build healthy habits when children

223

are young. When parents are active, children are more likely to be active and stay active after they become adults.

Whatever your age, moderate physical activity can become a good health habit with lifelong benefits.

A prescription for your health:

> Feel better
> Look better
> Work better
> Live an active life!

For more information about heart health, contact:

- National Heart, Lung, and Blood Institute Education Programs Information Center P. O. Box 30105 Bethesda, Maryland 20824-0105, or

- Your local American Heart Association or call 1-800-AHA-USA1 (1-800-242-8721)

Chapter 18

Living Actively Following Hip Replacement

Each year, hip replacement surgery relieves pain and improves mobility for virtually all of the 120,000 patients who undergo the procedure. Although most patients are in their 60s and 70s, hip replacement is appropriate for any adult with severe hip pain and limited ability to walk—from those in their 80s to athletes as young as Bo Jackson, the baseball and football player who received an implant at age 29. Entertainer Liza Minnelli had a hip replacement last winter at age 49. While implant recipients must "retire" from certain activities, many more can be resumed or started for the first time—and there's widespread agreement about which ones are safe.

Even under the best of circumstances, however, hip implants may slowly wear out or loosen, and eventually need to be replaced because of the possibility of failure (a sudden, painful event that can cause serious injury). For this reason, implant recipients should be followed regularly. Many patients don't receive such monitoring for two reasons: First, data from long-term follow-up studies have only recently become available; second, insurance coverage is often limited to a few months following surgery. To address this shortcoming, the National Institutes of Health (NIH) recently issued a consensus statement stressing the importance of lifetime care for all hip replacement patients.

The Johns Hopkins Medical Letter, August, 1995.

What Activities Are Safe?

Hip replacement nearly always provides dramatic pain relief and major improvements in walking speed, stride, and the ability to climb stairs. But with a growing number of people receiving implants before age 60, and the increased emphasis on the benefits of exercise throughout life, improved function has become an important goal.

Today, only a few high-risk activities are forbidden, and implant recipients can participate in many low- and non-impact activities. Most surgeons urge their patients to remain active because of the healthful benefits of exercise. According to a study in the Mayo Clinic Proceedings, more than three-quarters of the surgeons who performed 1,015 hip replacements at the Mayo Clinic in 1993 recommended sailing, swimming, scuba diving, cycling, golfing, and bowling for their patients.

Other activities the surgeons sometimes recommended include speed walking, tennis, volleyball, ice skating, hiking, backpacking, cross-country skiing, and ballet. More than three-quarters of the surgeons said they advised against running, football, baseball, basketball, hockey, soccer, handball, racquetball, water skiing, and karate.

The specific activities recommended for an individual patient depend on general health, fitness, motivation, and familiarity with the activity. Exercise must be undertaken sensibly because the implant doesn't contain nerve fibers and can't produce injury-warning sensations (i.e. pain) the way a normal hip can. As a result, some recipients may be inclined to work out too hard for too long, which can accelerate wear and premature failure of the implant.

Physical therapy and exercise can help condition patients for the activities they wish to pursue, and special footwear can provide extra cushioning and support. Ms. Minnelli has been able to include some dance routines in her performances, while Mr. Jackson has permanently retired from playing baseball and football.

Causes Of Implant Failure

Each step a hip replacement patient takes causes thousands of very small particles to be released from the plastic lining of the prosthesis because of the pressure placed on the joint. These particles stimulate certain cells to boost production of proteins known as cytokines. The cytokines switch on other cells that slowly erode the hip bone around the implant and gradually weaken it, in a process known as osteolysis. Osteolysis has no external symptoms and occurs at variable rates. Eventually, it may loosen the implant enough to make it fail unless a second procedure is performed. Usually, only the weakened portion of the device needs to be replaced.

Although most implants don't fail for at least a decade (and may last up to 25 years), the NIH recommends regular x-rays from the start because failure may occur without any obvious warning signs. A safe schedule for most patients, according to Dr. Lee Riley, Johns Hopkins Distinguished Service Professor of Orthopedic Surgery, includes an exam and x-ray every 12 to 18 months for life.

Choosing the Best Procedure

The type of implant you receive depends mostly on the quality and density of your bone. All implants contain a ball attached to a stem, which is inserted into the thigh bone, and a socket that must be fixed to the pelvis at the other end. This can be accomplished with or without cement. In the latter approach, the ends of the implant are coated with a porous material and tightly fitted into place; the porous material encourages new bone growth, which fuses with the device and provides additional reinforcement.

Often, however, the stem of the implant is cemented to the thighbone, and the socket is secured without cement (a "hybrid" hip). Sometimes screws or other hardware are used as additional anchors. If your bones are strong enough, a prosthesis without cement is usually preferred.

Chapter 19

Exercise and Pregnancy

Chapter Contents

Section 19.1

A Little Exercise Goes A Long Way

Source: *Parents Magazine*, July, 1994

For most of her life, Kathy Ryan was what she calls "a born-and-bred couch potato." When it came to exercise, she sighs, "the mind was willing, but the flesh was weak."

Then Kathy, who is 30, became pregnant. One day in her third month, she noticed a pregnancy exercise program near her home in Mount Vernon, New York. Much to her amazement, Kathy found herself signing up. "It went totally against my grain," she says. "Maybe it was a pregnancy craving."

Feeling dubious, Kathy went to her first class. "When I came home," she says, "the first thing I said to my husband was, 'Get the dog and let's go for a walk!' I felt energized."

As Kathy discovered, pregnancy can be a catalyst for beginning an exercise program. The rewards are many: Along with providing a burst of energy like the one that Kathy experienced, exercise can help alleviate many of pregnancy's unpleasant side effects, including swelling, insomnia, backache, constipation, shortness of breath, and depression according to experts. And while exercise probably won't make your labor shorter or less painful, it will give you more stamina and better muscle tone, both of which can make labor more bearable.

If you are still not convinced that it's worth getting off the couch, try thinking of pregnancy as a nine-month marathon, as some experts suggest. "Pregnancy really is an endurance test," says Paula Bernstein, M.D., attending physician at Cedars-Sinai Medical Center, in Los Angeles. Bernstein also stresses that giving birth is the hardest work that most women will ever do. Being fit will help you meet the physical challenges of both pregnancy and birth; it will also help you get back into shape more easily after you deliver.

The cardiovascular benefits of exercise are especially helpful during the 267-odd days of pregnancy, when your heart must pump about 30 percent more blood than usual. By promoting better circulation, regular exercise reduces the likelihood of swelling in the feet and legs and may help lessen the severity of varicose veins, if they develop.

Give Your Spirits A Boost

There are also many psychological benefits to being in shape at a time when you may be feeling as if your body is out of control. "Many pregnant women never had to worry about their weight before, and when they see their bodies getting bigger, it can be unsettling," says Bet Stapleton, founder of Perinatal Fitness of Westchester, a pre- and postnatal exercise program in New York. Exercise can also help tone the extra pounds of pregnancy.

Before you begin or continue a fitness program, however, you must consult with your doctor to be sure that you do not have a medical condition that would rule out exercising now. (See "Safety Checklist," on page 233.)

Women who are fitness buffs and whose pregnancies are progressing normally can usually continue many of the activities that they enjoyed before. Tennis and jogging, for example, when done in moderation, are often acceptable. Some sports, of course, are out now: Water-skiing and downhill skiing, for example, could both result in a bad fall that might hurt you or your baby. Scuba diving is also inadvisable (your baby needs a steady supply of oxygen), as are contact sports (you could be hit in the stomach or knocked down).

Moderation Is The Key

Avid exercisers need to resist the temptation to overdo their workouts. "A lot of women come in thinking that they'll exercise just as they did before, and we really have to encourage them to pace themselves," says Nancy Kramer, who teaches in the Motherwell Maternity Health and Fitness Program at Lenox Hill Hospital, in New York City. Moderating your exercise routine is especially important during the third trimester, when you must be extra sensitive to signs of overexertion.

If you did not exercise regularly before and are now inspired to get in shape, what type of exercise is best for you? Much depends on your level of activity and fitness before you became pregnant—plus some common sense. Ideally you should ease into a moderate, low-intensity exercise program—say, three times a week—that will get you into better shape and put you on the road to a fitness routine after you give birth.

"The type of exercise you do should be enjoyable in addition to being safe—otherwise you are less likely to stick with it " explains

Sheldon H. Cherry, M.D., clinical professor of obstetrics and gynecology at the Mount Sinai School of Medicine, in New York City. The safest pregnancy exercises are noncompetitive and non-weight-bearing and involve smooth, nonjarring movements. At the top of the list is swimming, which offers the most support for your body. If you do not know how to swim—pregnancy is not the time to learn a new sport—you may want to look into water-aerobics classes for pregnant women. Check your local Y to see if it offers such classes. Almost as beneficial as swimming is cycling—stationary cycling is especially good during pregnancy because there is less risk of falling.

One exercise that does not require any previous experience and is easily accessible to nearly everyone is walking. "Going for a brisk, 15-minute walk three times a week is a good way of getting aerobic exercise," says Cherry.

Classes Have Many Pluses

Another good choice for beginners is a low-impact-aerobics class tailored to pregnant women. Many women like the structure of an organized class, as well as exercising in a group in which everyone else is as large as they are. Pregnancy classes concentrate on your special needs, such as strengthening abdominal muscles and improving posture. They also offer individualized attention as to how—and how hard—you should do the exercises.

These classes can also become a support group in which you can network about baby-sitters, grouse about heartburn, and often forge lasting friendships. Kramer says that she was continually amazed last winter that even during the biggest snowstorms in New York, her pregnant students never failed to show up excited for class.

You may also want to investigate exercise videos, which are cheaper than classes and let you work out at odd hours—a real boon after you give birth.

A pregnancy exercise video was successful in getting Cathy Boyce on the fitness track. Cathy, who lives in Orlando, says that she became "soft and overweight" after the birth of her first child. Too busy to make time for exercise, she felt that "I wasn't doing anything for me." When Cathy became pregnant again, a friend convinced her to try an exercise tape. Cathy began doing the routine three days a week and also started taking long walks on weekends. Not only did she feel better physically, but she was also delighted to be making time for herself. Now, two years later, Cathy gets up at 5:00 AM to exercise before her daughter, Delaney, wakes up .

Cathy Clarke, of the Bronx, New York, began to exercise for the first time when she was three months pregnant, largely on the advice of her midwife. Somewhat to her surprise, she has continued to work out in a postpartum class. She believes that being fit, besides making her feel good, has helped her cope with the strenuous demands of motherhood.

"I have found that mothering is as much a physical job as it is a mental and emotional one," she says, pointing to her energetic son, Joseph, who at 8 months already weighs 20 pounds.

Safety Checklist

Who should not exercise:

The American College of Obstetricians and Gynecologists says that the following risk factors preclude exercise during pregnancy:

- Pregnancy-induced hypertension;

- Ruptured membranes before term;

- Incompetent cervix;

- Persistent second-or third-trimester bleeding;

- Premature labor during your previous or current pregnancy;

- Slow fetal growth;

- Other conditions, including heart and lung disease, may also eliminate exercise as an option; they should be evaluated by your doctor.

Rules to follow while exercising:

- Always warm up before exercising and cool down afterward, because your joints are more susceptible to injury during pregnancy.

- Drink lots of liquids to replace fluids lost through perspiration.

- Avoid jarring motions or rapid changes of direction that could throw you off balance.

- Don't get overheated or exercise when it's very hot or humid.

- Keep your pulse below 140 beats per minute.

- After the first trimester, don't do any exercise on your back.

- Wear athletic shoes and a support bra.

- Stop as soon as you start feeling fatigued.

Danger signs during exercise:

If you experience any of these symptoms, stop exercising and consult your doctor:

- Shortness of breath;

- Bleeding or fluid from the vagina;

- Abdominal pain;

- Dizziness, numbness, nausea, or tingling.

Section 19.2

Say Bye-Bye To Baby Fat

Eating For Two Doesn't Mean You Have To Look Like It After Delivery

Source: *Prevention,* Feb., 1996

Motherhood may mean some sacrifices, but one of them doesn't have to be your figure. That little black prepregnancy dress can become a little black postpregnancy dress. And it doesn't require mortgaging all of life after pregnancy to your aerobics instructor.

That's because recovering your figure isn't something to think about later, when the baby's born. Recent research suggests that the way you put on pregnancy weight as well as when may determine whether you drop weight after birth or whether your skirts will still be snug months later.

The Right Way To Eat For Two

While you may want to emerge from your pregnancy looking more like a swan than an elephant, the first and most important thing to remember is that you are going to gain weight. A healthy, growing baby alone will pack on about 7 ½ pounds. And then, of course, there's the placenta, the amniotic fluid and all the other vital components of pregnancy that you don't want to get stingy with at dinnertime. Additionally, about 25 percent of that weight is going to be fat. And this, too, is very necessary for the health of mother and child. In other words, you never want to try to reign in calorie intake to your prepregnancy levels.

But you shouldn't let pregnancy be an excuse to go wild on calories, either. Yes, you're eating for two, but the other person you're eating for is a baby, not a 200-pound truck driver.

A woman of normal weight should gain approximately 25 to 35 pounds over nine months (28 to 40 pounds for those women who are prone to be underweight, only 15 to 25 pounds for the overweight). And, according to one study over one-third of women who gain more than these recommended amounts are still toting around an extra 9 pounds a year after delivery.

Now, a prescribed nine-month gain of 25 to 35 pounds may seem like your nonstop passport to chocolate-bar city, but the reality is that it only translates into an extra 300 calories per day. That's equivalent to, say, an additional 3½ cups of skim milk or six Oreos. It's not equivalent to an extra bag of chips, a bucket of dip and an avocado, rum-raisin ice cream and pastrami sandwich.

But the difference between 300 calories of milk and 300 cookie calories is a big one as far as you and your baby's health are concerned. "The main area where you're clearly eating for two is when it comes to nutrients," says Barbara Abrams, R.D., D.P.H., professor of public health and epidemiology at the University of California, Berkeley. "You need more iron, more calcium, B vitamins and zinc—in some cases as much as 100 percent more during pregnancy."

Three and a half cups of skim milk can provide you with the necessary 300 calories and valuable calcium, vitamin D and protein. But 300 calories of cookies provides you with...300 calories, not much more. "While the average pregnant woman answers she can have the milk and the cookies, that's just not true if her prenatal weight gain is higher than expected," Dr. Abrams says. "The decision to be made is milk or cookies."

And the decision is simple. In a nutshell, the secret to eating for two during pregnancy and still ending up looking like one after delivery is to eat a little more—and a lot smarter. By always choosing nutritionally dense calories over empty ones, you can maximize benefits without having to pack on more weight than you actually need. You'll also want to watch a natural tendency to grab calorie-laden "craving" foods. You and your baby don't need the extra calories, and your body will tuck away the fat stores it requires quite nicely without your help. Again, stick to foods that pack the most nutritional wallop for the least amount of calories.

Finally, watch for hidden calories in your beverages. "I had a patient mysteriously gaining much more weight than we could explain," recalls Dr. Abrams. "One day in my office she pulled out a large container of orange juice. It turned out she was drinking several a day."

While plenty of liquids are a must during pregnancy due to increased blood volume and the possibility of dehydration four 8-ounce glasses of OJ pack a whopping 450 calories. If it's vitamin C and flavor you're wanting, try mixing equal portions of fruit juice and water for the nutrition you need without the calories you don't need. But if it's merely a matter of thirst, no-cal water alone is the hands-down choice. Check with your doctor concerning prenatal supplements. If your diet is shipshape, you may not need them. But according to Mona Shangold, M.D., gynecologist in Philadelphia and author of *Complete Sports Medicine Book for Women* (Simon & Schuster, 1992), "most women should begin taking prenatal vitamin-and-mineral supplements prior to conception." In many cases they can be an excellent safeguard against vitamin and mineral deficiencies.

The Right Timing

When you put on the pounds may be just as important to the future of your waistline after pregnancy as how many you put on. Researchers have found that women who gained the most weight during the first trimester retained more weight after their pregnancies (*International Journal of Obesity*, August 1994).

While everyone's pregnancy runs a unique course, women on average should gain only about three to six pounds in the first trimester. After that, about a pound a week is recommended. Unlike the first trimester, weight gain in the second and third trimesters appears to be crucial for a baby's normal development.

The big problem is that you may be only into your second month ... and you're *hungry now!* Keeping in mind that this is more a mental perception than any "I want more food, Mommy" message from your baby, there are a couple ways to deal with the hunger.

First, split up your meals. Instead of eating three big meals a day, make it six smaller ones. It'll seem like you're eating more, but in reality you'll still be consuming only as much as you were before. Second, hit the water cooler. Water fills you up for free. No calories, and there's the added benefit of protecting yourself from possible dehydration during your pregnancy.

Workouts Tame The Gain

If you thought your delicate condition was going to excuse you from exercising, forget it. Next to not smoking and avoiding alcohol and other harmful drugs, exercise is one of the most important things you can do. It's not only a wonderful thing for the health of you and your baby but for the shape of your figure, as well, says James F. Clapp III, M.D., professor of reproductive biology at Case Western Reserve University, Cleveland.

Dr. Clapp found that women who exercised at least three times a week for a minimum of 30 minutes throughout pregnancy gained an average of seven pounds less than women who didn't exercise. And part of that weight savings was in the fat department (*Medicine and Science in Sports and Exercise*, February 1995).

If you're a regular exerciser, you can continue—with your doctor's O.K. and a few modifications. Even if you don't work out now, you can take up a low-intensity program as long as your doctor approves. Here are a few guidelines to ensure a safe workout:

- If you have been working out, maintain your usual level of activity—don't increase it.

- Exercise at least three times a week.

- Drink plenty of water to prevent overheating and dehydration.

- Never exercise to exhaustion.

- Choose exercises like stationary cycling, walking, swimming and weight training with light or three- to five-pound hand weights.

- Avoid any activities with a risk of falling or trauma to the abdomen.

- As pregnancy progresses and your center of gravity shifts, be careful of activities requiring balance.

- If the additional weight is presenting a difficulty, switch to non-weightbearing exercises, such as swimming or stationary cycling.

- Stop exercising immediately and go to see your doctor right away if you experience any pain or bleeding or if your water breaks.

Postdelivery Body Slimmers

You've done everything right and delivered a healthy, beautiful baby. But you've still got quite a few unwanted pounds hanging around afterward.

Here's how to kiss them bye-bye:

Move that body. As soon as you feel up to exercising, go for it. Now, that doesn't mean a 4-mile-per-hour walk or an hour-long aerobics class. Start out with an easy walk, 15 or 20 minutes, and slowly increase the intensity over the next several weeks. Enlist family members to watch the baby while you exercise. Other options are a hired baby-sitter or a health club with child care.

Strollers specially designed for walking or jogging may make it easy to bring your baby along on workouts. Until the baby has good head control at about four months, roll up blankets for head support and stick to smooth terrain, says Mark Widome, M.D., professor of pediatrics at Penn State College of Medicine, Hershey. Even as baby gets older, avoid speeds and terrains that may cause his head to shake.

Curb overeating. Even though breast-feeding burns an extra 500 calories or more a day, weight loss may plateau if you're eating too much, says Kathryn Dewey, Ph.D., professor of nutrition at the University of California, Davis. She theorizes that prolactin, the milk-inducing hormone, may increase appetite during the first few months.

The idea is to eat roughly what you've been eating throughout pregnancy.

Get out of the house. Being home all day, especially for working women, means easy access to the refrigerator. In fact, one study found that the earlier women went back to work, the more weight they lost. Researchers suspect that the working mothers had less access to food. We're not telling you to give up maternity leave. Instead, try joining a mother's group. (Check with your pediatrician or local hospital for a group in your area.)

Try the milk diet. Research has found that moms who breastfed their babies for more than six months lost about 10 pounds during the first year, while those who fed them formula lost a little more than five (*American Journal of Clinical Nutrition,* August 1993).

Evaluate your birth-control method. Keep in mind that some birth-control drugs containing estrogen and/or progesterone may make weight loss tougher. Although they haven't been tested in postpartum women, birth-control pills and injections have been shown to cause weight gain in some women. To reduce the risk, ask for the lowest effective does or opt for a nondrug method of birth control.

Where Does Pregnancy Weight Go?

Location	Avg. Weight (in pounds)	When It's Usually Lost
Fetus	7.5	at birth
Placenta	1.5	at birth
Amniotic fluid	2.0	at birth
Uterus	2.0	3 weeks postpartum
Breasts	1.0	*
Blood	3.0	3-6 weeks postpartum
Water	3.5	3-6 weeks postpartum
Fat	7.5	*

(*) Variable and partly dependent on whether you breastfeed your baby or not.

Abs Toners During Pregnancy

Shaping up adbominal muscles after pregnancy can be a real workout. For the best chance at a flat belly afterward, tone and tighten them before and during pregnancy. Crunches, or partial sit-ups, are the ab exercise of choice. But after the first trimester, you're not supposed to lie on your back, so we asked Julie Tupler, R.N., certified childbirth educator, personal trainer and owner of Maternal Fitness, in New York City, for some "upright" exercises to keep your abs in shape.

Pelvic Tilt

Start by standing with your feet about shoulder-width apart, knees bent and your back flat. Pull your abdominals in as you tuck your buttocks under. Hold for 5 seconds, then release. The movement is similar to pressing your lower back against the floor if you were lying down. Repeat the exercise while you're on your hands and knees. Remember to start with a flat back and work only your lower back. Do 10 tilts in each position.

Tupler Technique

Sitting cross-legged on the floor, support your back against a wall. Think of your abdomen as a sideways elevator: first floor-abdomen relaxed; fifth floor-belly button "touches" the spine. Begin by inhaling and expanding your belly. As you exhale, pull your belly button back to the third floor. This is your starting position. Now pull the belly button to the fifth floor. Hold for 2 seconds and release to third floor. Repeat 10 times. (Count out loud to ensure that your keep breathing.) Your back shouldn't move. Do 5 sets a day.

Chapter 20

Exercise and Mental Health

Chapter Contents

Section 20.1

Physical Fitness & Mental Health

Source: DHHS Pulication No. (ADM) 84-1364, 1984.

*By Ruth Kay in consultation with mental
health and recreation specialists.*

- *Do you feel physically and mentally fit, or are you out of
  shape and out of sorts?*

- *Is your weight under control and are you feeling good, or are
  the scales going up and your spirits down?*

These are questions that relate to mind and body. How you react
to them may tell you something about your physical and emotional
health. If you feel physically fit, chances are you also feel mentally
fit. You feel good about yourself and the world around you. You're confident about today and. Look forward to tomorrow. Your physical fitness has a direct bearing on how you look at life.

What follows are some ideas about keeping in shape, reasons why
you should, and some suggestions about physical activities for special groups of people.

Exercise, Health, and Fitness

Exercise is a key factor in keeping fit—physically and mentally.
There is a positive relationship between exercise, health, and fitness.
Regular, sensibly vigorous physical activity, for example, is a valuable
tool in preventing or controlling obesity, and heart, lung, and circulatory system diseases. Inactivity, on the other hand, can actually
contribute to the risk of developing these ailments. But Dr. Kenneth
H. Cooper of the Aerobic Center in Dallas believes that most people
continue to exercise because of the psychological effects—not because
"their resting heart rate decreases, their oxygen consumption increases,
their work capacity goes up, but . . . because they feel better."

Making sure that you have a sensible balance of physical activity
suitable to your age and capability is a good way to stay mentally
healthy. Mental health experts say that appropriate exercise can help
relieve emotional stress—anger, tension, hostility, and aggression. It

242

also helps some people sleep longer and better. Others find exercise helps them feel more alert and energetic.

Research shows that exercise can help in the prevention and treatment of mild depression. For some, exercise is an effective antidepressant because it gives them a sense of mastery and self-control. Since women are twice as likely as men to suffer from this mental health problem, it's helpful for them to know that exercise is one way to deal with depression.

Be Sensible

Before you start out on a new program of vigorous physical activity, it's a good idea to get a medical evaluation, especially if—

* you're over 40 and haven't been exercising regularly, or

* you have medical problems, or

* you haven't had a physical checkup in a while.

Ask your physician to help you tailor exercise or physical activities that are right for you and appropriate for physical fitness. Keep an open and receptive mind about this. A trial of different workouts and time schedules may be necessary to help determine what's best for your needs. Build your program gradually, using particular caution if you've been inactive for a long time.

If you think you'd enjoy the discipline of a class, you might consider the structured physical fitness programs offered by the community recreation departments/centers, schools, or the local "Y". Commercial health clubs and spas also offer exercise programs with a variety of rates and apparatus. You don't, however, need expensive equipment, special clothes, shoes, or a gym in order to keep fit. Your own home or the community playground could be the ideal place for you to work out.

Keeping in Shape

To be effective, exercise needs to be rhythmic, regular, reasonably vigorous, and continuous for 20 minutes or more at least three times a week, preferably every other day. If you save it all for the weekend, you may overexert yourself and do more harm than good. For muscle strength, flexibility, endurance, and weight control you can choose from a variety of physical activities including tennis, dancing, racquetball, swimming, backpacking, jogging, running, walking, calisthenics, cycling, or cross-country skiing. These are but some of the fun ways to keep fit.

Physical activities include more than formally programmed exercise. Climbing stairs, for instance, will provide some aerobic activity, stimulating to the heart and lungs. Gardening can be good stretching, pulling, and bending exercise, and it's great for working off anxieties. Think of other ways to get your share of physical activity. You might ride your bike instead of a bus whenever it's practical. A light lunch and a long walk are a good alternative to a heavy noonday meal and a short drive in a car. It makes good sense to exert muscle and energy for physical fitness, and you'll put more zip into your life if you do.

Children

Physical fitness activities begin with play early in life, starting with arm and leg movements in infancy. As children grow, they need the guidance of parents, teachers, coaches, recreation directors and physicians in selecting individual and team play activities for physical and emotional development. Besides helping to build physical fitness and a sense of physical power, play is a child's outlet for expressing joy, frustration, anger, and pride. Group play and sports encourage growth in emotional stability and maturity and offer that good feeling of "belonging." The ability to win or lose gracefully and to take pride in the success of others are added values learned through these activities which also provide lessons in honesty, cooperation, teamwork, tolerance, and consideration for others.

Parents and teachers know that when students are in good health, they get better grades in school, gaining in self-esteem and self-confidence. It's one more reason for schools to provide physical fitness programs for all students—kindergarten through high school and college. Schools and parents need to take an active interest and, where possible, work together in creating physical education programs in which all students, whatever their capabilities or special needs, can take part. Physical fitness training programs help students understand the relationships of exercise, diet, rest and relaxation to all aspects of health. Well-planned physical education programs can help children establish lifetime patterns of wholesome and rewarding physical activities.

Adults

The recreation and exercise activities of many adults are often the reflections of favorite play activities they enjoyed during their school experiences or growing-up years. Now, as adults, they still need to release physical energy and emotional stress. They can do it constructively and within social limits through exercise—from cooperative adventures in nature to strenuous sports. These are ways to keep body and mind young and give balance to life. Physical activities like tennis, golf, and bowling offer opportunities for sharing the joy of doing things with others. Conversely, running, walking, or cycling can be done alone, with the freedom to think solitary thoughts and compete with no one but oneself. Both group and independent activities are good for physical fitness. Let your emotional needs, as well as time and circumstance, help you choose activity that's also good for your mental health.

Interest in physical fitness often increases with age, even though the incidence of chronic illness also increases. Some older adults, 60-years-of-age or more, spend more time exercising than people in their 40s and 50s, often because they're not as involved with growing families and have more time for themselves. Popular physical activities for the over-60 adults include walking, golfing, swimming, calisthenics, and even jogging, if their doctor approves. The elderly who are active, interested, and involved in a variety of physically and mentally stimulating activities add meaning and purpose to their own lives—not to mention the lives of their families. Keeping physically and mentally Fit will help maintain a good self-image and prevent premature dependence on others.

People with Special Needs

Through carefully planned physical fitness programs, disabled or handicapped persons can be encouraged to develop and sustain abilities necessary for self-care tasks. For some, this gives them the ability to be independent and self-sufficient at home rather than being dependent and needing institutional care. Patients confined to beds or wheelchairs often need special mobility exercises to increase and maintain their muscular endurance, strength, motor flexibility, and cardiac output for maximum physical capabilities.

Physicians and health-care providers need to be sensitive to the emotional as well as the physical needs of their patients and make appropriate provisions for physical activity programs and the environment in which they take place. Physical fitness activities can relieve weariness and boredom. They can effect a change in outlook—helping fear and depression give way to confidence and peace of mind. Appropriately adapted physical training for disabled persons can also help them better understand and appreciate their own abilities. Physical activities can help improve attitudes about themselves and others. They also offer challenges in responding to successes and failures, and allow opportunity for self-evaluation as well as self-satisfaction. Comprehensive physical fitness programs for the handicapped can help pave the way to happier, more successful, useful lives.

Physical fitness programs are also important for psychiatric patients. Recreational activities, particularly with small groups, help to promote relaxation, cooperation, self-expression, and creativity. Dancing to music is a good example of an effective recreational activity for these patients. Physical activities also provide experiences that test exposure to reality and permit those patients who are withdrawn and who have regressed to become involved socially. Fitness training for depressed patients can promote improvement in mood states and self-concept as well as help maintain or develop physical health.

For the mentally retarded, many or whom also suffer from physical handicaps, physical recreation provides opportunity to develop a positive self-image and improve intellectual functioning. Recreation is a means of relaxation and enjoyment and provides a necessary break in daily routines. Sports and games suitably chosen for the retarded help bolster their social, emotional, and physical well-being.

To respond to the special needs of the mentally retarded, the Joseph P. Kennedy, Jr. Foundation, Washington, DC, created Special Olympics. It is an international program of year-round sports training and athletic competition for mentally retarded people, 8-years-of-age or older, and promotes the philosophy that competing and winning are secondary to experiencing and participating. Write to Special Olympics, Inc., 1701 K Street, N.W., Washington, DC 20006, if you want more information about the program.

An Old Truth

The benefits of physical activity or exercise were recognized a long time ago. In ancient Greece, home of the original Olympic Games, the physician Hippocrates, known as the "Father of Medicine," believed exercise to be a person's best friend. Since then many others have shared his belief, as does modern-day society.

And why not? Exercise helps one achieve what everyone hopes for, a sense of well-being—physically fit and mentally healthy.

References

Duffy, Tony, and Paul Wade. *Winning Women: The Changing Image of Women in Sports*. New York: Times Books, 1983.

Fixx, James F. *Jim Fixx's Second Book of Running*. New York: Random House, Inc., 1980.

Frankel, Lawrence J., and Betty Byrd Richard. *Be Alive as Long as You Live: The Older Person's Complete Guide to Exercise for Joyful Living*. New York: Lippincott and Crowell, 1980.

Fuenning, Samuel I., Kenneth D. Rose, Fred D. Strider, Wesley Sime, eds. *Physical Fitness and Mental Health: Proceedings of the Research Seminar on Physical Fitness and Mental Health*. Lincoln, Nebraska: University of Nebraska Foundation, 1981.

Gilmore, C.P. *Exercising for Fitness*. Alexandria, Virginia: Library of Health/Time-Life Books, 1981.

Section 20.2

The Psychological Benefits of Exercise

Source: *American Health,* June, 1995.

By Susan Chollar

Sarah Cain loves to run. Most days after work she makes her way along the trails that cut through the redwood forest near her home, leaping over roots that snake across the tree-lined path. And when winter's failing light darkens the forest, she pounds the streets of the small towns that edge California's Monterey Bay. Forty-five miles each week, more than 2,000 miles a year. Year in and year out.

The 35-year-old agricultural research technician likes what exercise does for her body. It keeps her fit, muscular and slim. But she loves what it does for her mind. "It keeps me from being depressed and calms me down," she says. "I get a warm, glowing feeling after I run. It takes the edge off."

Although many people are lured to exercise for its well-known cardiovascular benefits or because it makes them look good, a growing number are working up a sweat for the psychological benefits. Exercise can't transform an aggressive, type A personality into a calm type B, but scientists now know that even moderate activity—say, a brisk walk at lunchtime—can lift spirits or dispel tension. And therapists are increasingly prescribing exercise to help their patients cope with more long-term psychological ailments such as anxiety and clinical depression.

A study at the University of Western Australia in Perth, for instance, compared college students in an aerobic dance class with a sedentary group. After their workouts, the dancers scored significantly higher on self-esteem tests than the nonexercisers.

Regular physical activity also improves alertness and energy. Corwyn Mosiman, a 40-year-old optometrist in Watsonville, Calif., works out during his lunch break four times a week for an hour and a half. "If I don't do it, I get tired in the afternoon," he says. "Exercise gives me a burst of energy that gets me through the day."

Another study at Brooklyn College in New York City found that students enrolled in a swimming class reported having more vigor after spending 30 to 60 minutes in the pool. They also had significantly lower levels of depression, tension and anger. And in a 15-week study at Loma Linda (Calif.) University, a group of overweight, formerly sedentary women reported significantly higher energy levels than controls after walking for 45 minutes, five times a week. "They loved it," says exercise scientist and study author David Nieman. "They kept telling us how great they felt—that they wanted to keep going."

Exercise also improves mood. "The effects are most obvious immediately after a workout and can last for several hours," say psychologist Thomas Plante at Santa Clara (Calif.) University. Even more important, long-term exercisers seem to possess an overall sense of well-being that extends into other areas of their lives. Dr. Nieman found that after six weeks, the walkers in his study were significantly less stressed than the sedentary women.

"Exercise gives me a better outlook," says Tim Landeck, a 34-year-old teacher in Watsonville, Calif., who turns to kayaking and trail-biking when the pressures of work and taking care of his two small children get him down. "Afterward, I feel more jazzed up about what I'm doing."

There's even evidence that exercise helps the creative juices flow. In studies at New York City's Baruch College, exercise psychologist Joan Gondola found that college students who ran regularly or took aerobic dance classes scored significantly higher on a standard psychological test of creativity than students who hadn't exercised. Dr. Gondola says that during her own workouts, she frequently slips into an almost trancelike state where feelings and intuition prevail over more structured thoughts. She calls it her "Aha!" state because creative solutions to nagging problems often pop into her head during those times.

Long-term exercise may also help head off the decline in mental skills, including slowed reaction time and loss of short-term memory, that often accompanies aging. Psychologists Alan Hartley and Louise Clarkson-Smith of Scripps College in Claremont, Calif., studied 300 men and women 55 and over who were either sedentary or active. The exercisers, who had run the equivalent of six mile-a-day for many years scored higher on tests of reaction time, working memory and nonverbal reasoning than did their sedentary counterparts. "By becoming active when you're young, and staying active," says Dr. Hartley, "you're guarding against the mental deterioration that can occur with age and inactivity." (There's no evidence, however, that exercise improves mental skills among the young or middle-aged or that it boosts IQ at any point in life.)

The impact of exercise on cognitive skills in the elderly may be due to superior cardiovascular fitness, which assures adequate blood flow and oxygen transport to the brain and may slow the cell death that accompanies normal aging. The alertness and vigor many people report immediately following exercise may also be linked to increased blood flow to the brain. But exercise also triggers the release of several key neurotransmitters, including epinephrine and norepinephrine, that are known to boost alertness.

Alternatively, exercise's calming effects may be due to the rise in body temperature brought on by a vigorous workout. The core temperature of the average jogger, for instance, rises to over 100°, which produces a brief tranquilizing effect not unlike a lazy soak in a hot tub.

Exercise also reduces tension by desensitizing the body to stress. A vigorous workout stimulates the body to pump out the so-called stress hormones, such as cortisol and epinephrine, that prepare your heart, lungs and muscles for "fight or flight." But regular workouts train the body to react less intensely to stress, leaving exercisers better able to cope with anxiety-provoking events.

Another reason to work up a sweat: Exercise acts as nature's form of Prozac, boosting brain levels of norepinephrine, dopamine and serotonin, three neurotransmitters that elevate mood. Studies have shown that depressed people often have abnormally low levels of these chemicals. Most common antidepressants work by correcting this imbalance, and to some extent, exercise also does.

In fact, exercise may be just as effective as more traditional therapies when it comes to treating psychological ills. In a study of 74 depressed men and women at the University of Wisconsin in Madison, psychologist Marjorie Klein compared the effects of two 45-minute running sessions a week with both meditation and group therapy. After 12 weeks, Dr. Klein found that exercise was just as effective in alleviating depression, and that all three approaches reduced anxiety and tension.

What of the proverbial runner's high, the intense pleasure reported by many exercisers during a long, grueling workout? Beta-endorphins (one of a group of opioids that act within the central nervous system to reduce feelings of pain and induce euphoria) have long been credited with these good feelings. When 13 runners at the University of New Mexico in Albuquerque were given an endorphin-blocking drug before a strenuous 28.5-mile mountain race, their performance wasn't affected, but their moods were: Twelve of the 13 runners reported that they didn't get their usual psychological rush during the second half of the race.

Yet some scientists are skeptical of the endorphin high. "It's not exactly what a scientist would consider a tight story," says neuroscientist Huda Akil at the University of Michigan in Ann Arbor. Some studies show that beta-endorphins increase in the bloodstream during strenuous exercise, but whether they also increase within the brain is unclear. For one thing, endorphins are barred from receptors in the brain's pleasure center by the blood-brain barrier, a biochemical surveillance system that protects the blood supply to the brain. "The high many athletes describe," says Emory University neuropharmacologist Michael Owens, "may not be an opiate-induced euphoria but rather a deep sense of relaxation and well-being."

It' s also possible that rhythmic exercise such as swimming or cycling may induce a meditative state that brings deep relaxation. Or a session at the gym may simply provide a time-out from unpleasant thoughts and emotions. That may explain why even a slow walk can banish a bad mood. "In some ways, then, exercise may not be much different from a hobby, meditation or prayer," says Santa Clara's Dr. Plante.

Whatever the mechanism, therapists are increasingly tapping into the prescriptive powers of exercise to help troubled patients. "I don't need to worry about the why," says Concord, N.H.-based sports psychologist Kate Hays, who became hooked on exercise 14 years ago during a time of personal crisis. "After a run I come home energized and better able to cope," says Dr. Hays, 51, who now runs three to five miles five times a week, and swims half a mile twice a week. "It made me feel wonderful then, and it still does."

Sarah Cain also discovered the therapeutic power of aerobic exercise in her early 20s, when she was suffering from depression. Now whenever she' s anxious or blue, Cain laces up her running shoes and hits the trail. "Back then, I didn't have the discipline to make myself exercise when I was depressed," she says. "Now I do. I know better than to just sit there flopping around the house."

How to Get the Exercise High

Looking for more than bulging biceps from your workout? If the promise of a more positive psychological state appeals to you, here's how to maximize the emotional benefits of exercise.

Find the right fit. Although virtually any physical activity can lift your mood, some types are more effective than others. Sports that are noncompetitive, repetitive (such as swimming laps or riding a stationary bike) and predictable (such as a run to the end of a familiar trail and back), offer the most consistent mental payoff. Pursuits that encourage deep rhythmic breathing such as yoga and tai chi help induce relaxation as well.

Set realistic goals. Don't vow to run 10 miles a day, every day; you'll set yourself up for failure. If you're out of shape, try a low-intensity activity such as walking 30 to 45 minutes, three or four times a week. Not only does it give you a psychological boost, but it's also cheap and easy to stick with.

Don't get derailed by excuses. Make things easier for yourself by setting aside time for exercise in advance, just as you would for any important appointment, and have your gear packed and ready to go. "Keep in mind that the days you feel least energetic and eager to exercise are exactly when you need it the most," says exercise specialist Bonnie Berger at the University of Wyoming in Laramie.

Don't push too hard. If you overdo it in the gym, your mood may actually suffer rather than improve. For the best results, beginners should keep their pulse at around 65% of their maximum heart rate (to calculate that number, subtract your age from 220 and multiply by .65) and limit the aerobic part of the workout to 30 minutes. As you become fitter, you may need to increase the intensity or duration of your sessions to maintain a sense of well-being.

Stick with it. Even novices will be able to reap the most immediate psychological benefits of exercise: the boost in mood most people experience an hour or two after a workout. To attain more lasting improvements in psychological well-being, however, you'll need to keep at it consistently for at least 10 weeks.

Addicted to Exercise?

We've all seen them: the Lycra-clad woman who takes three back-to-back step classes a day; the impossibly thin neighbor who never misses a morning run, even when he's got the flu; the friend who constantly begs off dinner in favor of a date with the stair climber. Hard as it may be for most of us to believe, certain people become so dependent on the physical and psychological benefits of exercise that their quest for a fix literally controls their lives.

Gwen Townsend (not her real name) first joined a gym to control her weight. Almost before she knew it, the 28-year-old New York City public relations executive was hooked. She worked out six or seven days a week for two-hour stretches, moving from the stair climber to the stationary bike to the treadmill, then finishing off with 45 minutes of strength training. Townsend exercised when she was sick or injured, ignoring a painful knee condition that was exacerbated by her grueling sessions. She cut corners at the office and turned down social invitations to keep her nightly date with the gym. "It was a huge release for me," she says. "When I had a tough day at work or if I was upset, getting into that exercise groove could really clear my mind. I had to force myself to take a day off. And when something came up to prevent me from going to the gym, it really flipped me out."

How can you tell whether you're an exercise junkie? Psychologist Connie Chan at the University of Massachusetts in Boston says that if you must work out daily in spite of illness or injury to maintain a sense of emotional well-being, your habit isn't healthy. More warning signs: You organize your life around exercise; you feel irritable, guilty or tense when you lay off for a few days; or you experience serious depression, insomnia or loss of interest in life when you're forced to quit for more than a week.

Why some people become addicted to exercise still isn't clear. There may be a physiological component involving endorphins or other pleasure-producing chemicals, Dr. Chan says. But she also suspects that many exercise junkies strive for perfection in the gym because they feel they've failed in other areas of their life. In one study at the University of Arizona, researchers found parallels between the personalities of compulsive mole runners and anorexic women. Both had unrealistically high expectations of themselves, an unusual ability to deny pain and higher levels of repressed anger.

"It's all about control," says Townsend, who struggled with bulimia in college and who, after seeing a nutritionist and making other positive changes in her life, feels as though she finally has her eating and exercise habits in check. "With both compulsive exercise and compulsive eating," she says, "you're trying to control something you can never fully control—your body."

Susan Chollar is an Aptos, Calif.-based writer specializing in science and health.

Part Four

Specific Activities

Chapter 21

Aerobics Gets Real

By Mary Duffy and Maura Rhodes

Ten years ago, many women donned form-fitting leotards and pranced and puffed their way through an hour-long aerobics class for the express purpose of looking good in said garment. Spurred by vanity and a diehard crash-dieting mentality, dance exercisers faced the music and the mirror in hopes of sweating off—fast—what flab they couldn't diet off. Despite talk of target heart rate and increased endurance, most aerobic dancers exercise primarily to get slimmer—not healthier.

A funny thing happened on the way to thinner thighs, however. The more people exercised (and this goes for runners, cyclists, swimmers, and walkers), the better they felt between workouts. the rush of energy they experienced right after class never entirely died out, but simmered gently: They discovered they had more stamina to get through intense work days and chore-packed weekends. They found they were able to measure their progress not only by the number of push-ups they could do, but by how many grocery bags they could lug. And with every extra crunch they performed, the easier it was to lift a toddler without straining the back. Lunch-hour aerobicizers metamorphosed into weekend warriors who ventured onto tennis courts, or into canoes, or onto the sides of mountains undaunted. As a result,

Source: *Women's Sports & Fitness.* November/December, 1993. Used by permission.

for many aficionados of aerobic dance, the aesthetic payoffs took a backseat to the pragmatic.

Now this switch in motive is contributing to a slow but sure switch in the mode and mood of exercise classes. "It's been a gradual evolution of awareness away from the emphasis on how we look to how we feel," says New York fitness instructor Molly Fox, whose 14 years in the business have afforded her the opportunity to watch it progress.

"People now realize there are enormous benefits to fitness other than a skinny waist and firm thighs," agrees Peter Francis, Ph.D., professor of physical education at San Diego State University and biomechanics consultant for the U.S. Olympic Committee. "They know that exercise builds a relative immunity to heart disease, for example, and that they can improve their body composition to some extent rather than just lose pounds." Adds Kari Anderson, owner of Seattle's Pro-Robics Conditioning clubs, "I hear fewer women talking about how much they weigh."

Instead, the fitness shoptalk of the '90s is peppered with terms like functional strength," "protective exercise," and "joint integrity," and women are less obsessed with looking great for next month's high school reunion than with felling greater for decades to come. To accommodate these goals, there's a movement toward exercise that mimics what the body is called upon to do on a day-to-day basis. "Look at how humans move in daily life. We're always stopping and starting, picking things up, putting things down, rushing here, rushing there. We're constantly changing our pace." asserts Keli Roberts, an instructor and trainer at L.A.'s Martin Henry Studio, who also has two new videos in the offing. The integration of interval training (in which the pace is purposely varied throughout a workout) and cross-training into fitness classes reflects this desire to make exercise more "real."

As to the reasons for motivation, Fox points out that crunches have become important for reasons beyond honing a washboard belly. "People realize that just about everything they do involves the abs and lower back."

"Before people wanted to strengthen their stomach muscles to get rid of a spare tire," agrees Roberts. "Now they want to stabilize themselves."

What's more, according to Roberts, aerobics class classics are being replaced by moves that reflect real-life movements, thereby using muscles the way they're meant to be used. For example, leg lifts performed while lying on one's side make little sense because people rarely recline on their sides in daily life. These moves are making way for lunges and squats, which use the leg muscles in ways they're needed. The irony is that these particular exercises were once thought to be unsafe, at least for people with bad knees; now they're considered therapeutic. In fact, many modern movements are taken from physical therapy, which is designed to bring an injured body back into the realm of normal and natural function. Step Reebok's Gin Miller originated the idea of step training after rehabilitating an injured knee by stepping on and off of a porch step.

Likewise, lateral exercise such as the side-to-side motion of sliding is fast becoming commonplace in exercise classes. This "plane" of movement, pretty much ignored until now, works the abductor and adductor muscles (of the outer and inner thighs, respectively) and helps stabilize joints. There are umpteen advantages to lateral strength: It aids ease of movement in many sports and allows you to neatly negotiate a patch of ice on the jogging trail, for example. In addition, lateral strength is protective, stabilizing the quads to help the knees to track properly and strengthening muscles and tendons around the ankle to prevent sprains.

Injury among instructors and exercisers has much to do with the current changes in aerobic classes. Early on, most teachers were professional dancers (or at least had a dance background), working part-time to improve their cash flow. In many cases, they led their classes in front of a mirror, their backs to the chorus line of amateur dancers, performing as much as teaching. Little was known about the toll all that leaping and jumping had on the body until people started getting hurt. The resulting high rate of injury was unfortunate, but is was an eye-opener. "I got injuries early in my career," says Leslie Howes, owner of Crosy Street Gym in New York City. "But getting hurt affected my teaching dramatically, forcing me to replace some dance movements with more natural moves that are less stressful and more fluid."

Injuries have also led to an increasingly high level of professionalism among instructors. Those who attended the earliest meetings of IDEA: The Association for Fitness Professionals, asked naive questions, according to Francis, who lectured at the very first IDEA convention in 1972. "The questions have gradually grown more sophisticated," he says, adding that his seminars on biomechanics drew several hundred attendees at the last IDEA convention.

The word "natural" is key to the changes that are afoot in fitness classes these days. The pace is less frenetic, and "going for the burn" is passé. "They're looking for a class complete with everything they'll need to help them do what they really want to do—hike on weekends, take long bike rides," says Howes.

"Exercise has to be convenient, practical, and enjoyable. People have lives and they just can't devote all their time to getting a nice body. If they want to have it all, they have to be moderate in what they do," adds Karen Voight, owner of Voight Fitness and Dance in Los Angeles.

And women expect staying in shape to help them get through the rigors of daily life. Anderson finds it especially rewarding to hear her students say being fit makes them better parents because they're more limber and able to keep up with their physically active kids.

What it all boils down to is a more holistic approach to exercise. The concern is not just how strong, toned, and well-developed certain muscles are, but how well all the major muscle groups work together as a team. Squats and lunges that are becoming mainstays of legwork are compound moves that teach various muscle groups in the legs to work well together, producing smoother movements, according to Howes. Because it is important not to overdevelop a single muscle, form is also essential—making sure the knee is over the foot and paying attention to where the head is in relation to the knee.

The current change in exercise classes is a sign of the times, according to Francis, "A lot of people subscribe to the idea that quality of life is important, and that goes hand-in-hand with a more thoughtful and reasonable rationale for everything we do—including exercise."

Maura Rhodes is a New York-based writer who specializes in health and fitness.

Chapter 22

Cross-Country Skiing

A Wonderful Winter Workout

By David H. Jelley

The first snowfall of the season doesn't have to mean an end to your physical exercise program. On the contrary, it signals the beginning of the winter sports season. As North America's fastest growing winter sport, cross-country skiing has seen astronomical growth over the past two decades. Commonly known as Nordic skiing, its origins can be traced back to ancient Scandinavian hunters. Today more than 6 million men, women, and children are cross-country skiers, compared with only 50,000 in 1970. Much of the enthusiasm stems from people's desire to get outdoors and enjoy nature.

Increased awareness of health and fitness have also played a part in the popularity of cross-country skiing. Regular exercise offers benefits to most people, and for many who have diabetes, physical fitness is an important part of a healthy lifestyle. A good exercise program may help you maintain ideal body weight, improve blood sugar control, lower insulin requirements, and perhaps improve your cardiovascular system.

First, before you start skiing, consult with your doctor, a diabetes specialist, or an exercise specialist trained in diabetes care. Although exercise can help many people stay healthy, people with diabetes who have eye disease, nerve damage, or other complications can be harmed by exercise. Your doctor can determine whether cross-country skiing

Diabetes Forecast: January, 1992. Used by Permission. (See editor's note at end of chapter.)

can meet your needs. Your doctor and health-care team also can advise you about the intensity, frequency, and duration right from the start.

Nordic skiing is excellent for all-round strength conditioning, and sports medicine experts rate it better than any other sport when it comes to cardiovascular benefits. Almost every muscle in the body is used in cross-country skiing, but the joint and ligament stress is minimal compared with most other aerobic activities.

Cross-country skiing is often readily accessible and relatively inexpensive. There are no age limits or gender-specific requirements, and few physical barriers—if you can walk, you can probably ski. But before you begin, you may need some tips to get started smoothly on the trail.

Getting Started

Recreational cross-country skiing is not hard to do. One way to describe it is that you apply a slightly bent-over shuffling style to walking while wearing skis. Although simply getting moving on skis is easy, feeling comfortable with these skinny boards strapped to your feet as you move across slippery packed snow is more difficult.

To help ensure a successful start in your new sport, take a lesson the first time you go out. The fundamental skills you learn in an introductory lesson will enable you to ski safely and efficiently. Your instructor can offer practical advice on how to hold your poles correctly, how to dress, how to fall safely on tricky downhills, and, because skis have no brakes, how to stop. An instructor also can answer any questions you may have regarding equipment.

Last, taking a lesson can make your introduction to Nordic skiing more enjoyable because the better you ski, the more fun you'll have.

Where To Ski?

You can ski anyplace where there is 6 inches of snow on the ground—your local park, nearby fields, or perhaps your own backyard. In some cities, such as Minneapolis and Toronto, you can tour zoos on your skis. You may find cross-country touring centers that have marked, preset trails called groomed trails. The snow on these trails usually is packed by machines into narrow tracks so your skis glide more easily than they do on ungroomed trails with deep snow and obstacles.

Organized touring centers frequently offer warming huts, rental equipment, and formal instruction, as well as free advice on everything from waxing skis to wearing knickers. The main disadvantage of these centers is that they have trail fees ranging from $5 to $15 dollars a day. This is still a bargain in comparison to downhill resorts which charge three to four times as much for daily lift tickets.

Equipment

Renting your ski gear is usually your best bet the first few times you go. One of the first decisions you'll have to make is choosing your skis.

Nordic skiers traditionally have used waxable skis, which require a "sticky" wax under the center of the ski for traction. When applied correctly, waxed skis provide the fastest, smoothest ride around. Waxing can be a hassle, however, because it is sometimes necessary to wax your skis several times during an outing.

Today there are waxless models that have scales on the bottom to provide one-way traction without wax. Waxless skis are convenient and provide relatively good performance for a diversity of conditions.

In addition to waxable and waxless varieties, there are four or five kinds of skis, boots, bindings, and poles corresponding to the different kinds of cross-country skiing: touring, light touring, skating or racing, mountaineering, and children's.

Touring skis are wide and stable, making them easier to control for beginners and off-trail skiers. Light touring skis weigh less and are thinner than touring skis for fast skiing on machine-set tracks, and the lightest of these are used for racing. Mountaineering skis are wider skis with metal edges and are designed for trips into the backcountry or anywhere with rugged terrain and steep slopes. These skis are better for downhill turns, providing extra security on icy trails. The heaviest and most expensive skis are those made exclusively for downhill ski areas.

Most people opt for touring or light-touring gear to start because of its versatility. It can be used on groomed tracks or on wilderness trails. A decent introductory package that includes skis, bindings, boots, and poles can be bought for less than $150.

That To Wear?

Dressing for cross-country skiing can be as high tech as a one-piece lycra racing suit or as down-to-earth as knickers and a turtleneck sweater. The goal is to stay warm and dry, which is not always easy when you alternate exercising and rest periods over a snow-covered course.

Factors to consider are weather, such as the temperature, the chance of precipitation, and the windchill factor, along with how fast and hard you can ski. Most beginners overdress. This is not a major problem if you remember the first rule of dressing for any outdoor activity where conditions may vary—layer your clothing.

The first layer next to the skin should be a non-moisture-absorbing layer. Polypropylene underwear is a good choice because the fabric does not retain moisture, so heated perspiration passes through to the next layer and away from your skin.

The next, or middle, layer should serve as insulation to hold warm air close to the body. A light wool or synthetic turtleneck and knickers are good choices. For colder weather, the middle layer can be heavier, such as a wool shirt, a fleece or pile jacket, or a down vest.

The outer layer should be a shell that is wind- and water-resistant. The best fabrics are those that repel water yet are "breathable," allowing perspiration to evaporate. The value of layering clothes in this fashion is that you can remove or add layers as needed to adjust to the weather and your level of comfort.

Although cotton clothing is comfortable, you should avoid it because cotton absorbs and holds water. Wool and newer synthetics such as polypropylene, fiberpile, and fleece stay warm even when wet. Knickers are a good idea because they can reduce the chafing that comes from the legs of your long pants rubbing together.

Don't hesitate to remove layers if you start to feel too warm. Waiting until you are soaked with perspiration defeats the purpose of layering. You can always put the outer layers back on if you get chilled.

It's also handy to always have a hat with you. Up to 70 percent of the body heat that escapes from your body is lost through the skin of your head and neck. If that doesn't convince you to bring a hat, note that the face and ears are the parts of your body most susceptible to frostbite. You can lose another 15 percent of your body heat from your hands and feet.

Conditioning

Although being in good physical condition is not a prerequisite, it's a definite advantage when it comes to your first time out on skis. Those who walk, run, or do other aerobic exercises regularly should have no problem moving along the trail. However, if you're not in good shape, you should begin slowly, using Nordic skiing as a way to improve fitness.

On the other hand, if you plan to ski more challenging terrain, longer distances, or more often than once or twice a season, some specific preseason conditioning is well worth the effort. Even the best skier's technique falls apart when fatigue sets in, and it's not much fun to be exhausted at your turn-around point and then have to limp home.

Cross-country skiing is touted as one of the best sports for all-around physical conditioning because it is such a well-balanced exercise. As a power sport, Nordic skiing builds muscular strength and endurance. A good stride is the result of a strong kick and a forceful push with your poles. The kick-and-glide action utilizes virtually all of the various muscles of the legs and buttocks and also exercises the abdominal muscles.

As an endurance activity, cross-country skiing is better than almost any other sport for improving aerobic fitness. The arms, shoulders, back, and abdomen are worked by using the poles. Because your muscles need more oxygen during aerobic exercise, your rib, abdominal, and shoulder muscles also get a workout as you breathe faster and more deeply.

If you're convinced of the benefits of cross-country skiing, how can you prepare for the season? As with other sports, skiing is muscle-specific. The more closely you mimic the muscle movements of actual cross-country skiing, the better prepared you will be when you hit the trail.

Roller skiing duplicates the total movement of cross-country skiing better than any other off-season exercise. Roller skis are made of wood or aluminum and have hard rubber tires about 5 inches in diameter. They are about three feet long and can use any boot-and-binding combination. A ratchet mechanism in the hubs of the front wheel allows the ski to roll forward but prevents it from sliding backward, thus simulating a kick-and-glide action. At a cost of $125 to $175 for the skis alone, they are designed for the more serious skier.

The next-best form of training is a stationary cross-country skiing machine. The best of these has a flywheel and a one-way clutch mechanism to provide a continuous motion, closely mimicking the real thing. Good machines can cost more than $500, but they are also frequently available in health clubs. And you may also want to try using in-line roller skates, which are skates with wheels that are all in a line rather than side-by-side in pairs.

The easiest and most accessible ways of getting fit before you go out skiing, however, are walking and running. Also, weight training can add needed strength in certain muscle groups. A carefully planned weight-training program will not only help build muscle power but, more important for skiing, muscle endurance.

Diabetes Management

As with any other form of exercise, it is important to manage your diabetes in cross-country skiing. The first step, of course, is to confer with your doctor or health-care team about your physical condition, as well as about how skiing will affect your diet and blood sugar levels.

Getting your doctor's advice is particularly important because some common guidelines for athletes without diabetes who are preparing for prolonged physical activity may not be right for you. For instance, carbohydrate-loading, a practice that some athletes use to build up their carbohydrates before an event, can affect your blood sugar levels. Knowing how your body may react will help you plan your outing, particularly if you expect to ski for several hours.

Guidelines for people with diabetes that hold true for other sports are also good for cross-country skiing. Ski with a partner in case you need help and keep some fast-acting sugars on hand. As for where to inject your insulin, the abdomen is usually a sensible spot. Because skiing uses most muscle groups in the lower and upper body, insulin injected there may get to the important muscles sooner.

Watch Out For Cold Temperatures

When participating in outdoor winter sports, it's important to pay attention to the air temperature and the windchill. Extreme cold can cause what are known as cold injuries. Frostbite and hypothermia are the two most common types of cold injuries.

Frostbite is the medical term for the freezing of skin tissue caused by decreased peripheral blood circulation combined with cold, wind, or wetness. The ears and face are the most commonly affected areas of skin. When the windchill factor falls below -10°F, cover your head and face to avoid serious frostbite.

Changes in the color of your skin are good indicators of the severity of frostbite. A change from pink or dark-colored skin to white indicates superficial frostbite. Warming the area with your hands or going indoors to a heated area usually will take care of this kind of frostbite. The appearance of a dull gray spot on the skin along with numbness are signs Of more severe frostbite, and you should see a doctor as soon as possible. In the meantime, keep dry and covered with protective clothing, but don't actively rewarm the area.

Hypothermia refers to a lowered core-body temperature, and it can be caused by wearing the wrong clothing and by a combination of exhaustion and wetness. Most cases of hypothermia occur in air temperatures between 30° and 50° F. Wind and moisture are the biggest culprits. The presence of moisture, in sweat, is one reason why it's important that the layer of clothing next to your skin draws sweat away from your body.

Hypothermia produces both mental and physical symptoms. A person may appear very fatigued while denying fatigue, or maybe incoherent and irrational. Other symptoms are shivering, slurred speech, clumsiness, apathy, and drowsiness.

Many of these symptoms are common in hypoglycemia as well, so a person with diabetes who has these symptoms should be given food in the form of fast-acting sugars, then taken to a warm place and given dry clothing to wear.

If someone has hypothermia but is still rational, it is important to act quickly. If his or her core-body temperature is above 92°F, rewarming with extra heat, shelter, or covering is a safe response. But if the body-core temperature is lower than 92, or if the person falls unconscious, it is usually better to postpone rewarming until you can get him or her to a hospital or medical center.

Although these warnings and guidelines may seem intimidating, try not to let them get you down. As with most other activities and exercise programs, knowing some basic guidelines about safety and cross-country skiing will help you enjoy the sport from the beginning and for a longer time.

A new world of exercise and fun awaits you with the next snowfall. By following a few simple guidelines and being well-prepared, you can make cross-country skiing a healthy part of your wintertime lifestyle.

David H. Jelley, MD, is a fellow in Pediatric Endocrinology and Diabetes at the University of Colorado Health Sciences Center and the Barbara Davis Center for Childhood Diabetes.

[*Editor's Note:* Because exercise is an important part of managing the symptoms of diabetes, the American Diabetes Association devotes a considerable amount of its resources to providing information regarding physical fitness activities. Much of this material represents some of the best introductory information to various physical activities available, and is therefore included in this section as a useful reference for all readers.]

Reprinted with permission from American Diabetes Association, Inc., Copyright © 1992, The American Diabetes Association, Inc. The American Diabetes Association has many publications to help you live better with diabetes. For more information or to order, call the American Diabetes Association at 1-800-DIABETES.

Chapter 23

Cycling

Chapter Contents

Section 23.1

Fitness Cycling

Source: Charmichael, Chris, and Edmund R. Burke. *Fitness Cycling*. Champaign, IL: Human Kinetics, 1994. "Assessing Your Cycling Fitness" on pp. 282-285 from J. Henderson. *Jog, Run, Race*. Mountain View, CA: Anderson World, 1978. Used by permission.

Cycling for Fitness

Experts have long recognized bicycling as one of the best forms of aerobic exercise. Almost anyone of any age can cycle for fitness, and anyone in good health can become a proficient rider with practice. Thanks to the efficiency of the bicycle, cycling is an excellent way to build cardiorespiratory and muscular fitness. One of the beauties of bicycling is that you can strengthen your body and your spirits simultaneously. Fun and fitness building go hand in hand.

Even more encouraging is the diversity of the people on bicycles. Those of all ages are working out, racing, or just having a good time. No matter how differently they use their bicycles, riders from the professional cyclist to the weekend tourist have two things in common: they are getting satisfaction from their activity, and they are getting a good workout and burning calories. Everyone who cycles regularly can achieve health and fitness benefits.

A Sport for Everyone

Cycling ranks among the most popular of sporting activities in the United States. The total number of cyclists who exercise regularly is estimated at more than 50 million by the Bicycle Institute of America. The Sporting Goods Manufacturing Association tells us that over 5 million Americans cycle more than 100 days a year. Adults make up 54% of this population, and children under the age of 16 make up 44%. Among adults, 55% of cyclists are women and 45% are men.

One of today's most popular home equipment exercise items is a stationary bicycle—more than 3 million are bought every year. Like many people, you probably do some of your exercising at home. Stationary indoor cycling is an excellent complement to your outdoor cycling.

Benefits of Cycling

Bicycling is an excellent way to exercise 20 to 60 minutes a day, 3 to 5 days a week for achieving good health and fitness. Cycling is as effective as walking and running for toning the large muscles of the lower body. It provides the needed aerobic boost to the cardiovascular system but with less stress on your joints.

Aerobic exercise researchers say that cycling is as good as running and swimming for attaining fitness. Sports medicine specialists prescribe cycling because it causes less wear and tear on the joints and muscles than jogging. They often advise older adults and people with joint problems to choose cycling as their primary exercise.

Let's look specifically at how cycling can improve each fitness component: cardiovascular fitness, body composition, flexibility, and muscular endurance and strength.

Cardiovascular Fitness

Cycling is one of the best activities for improving cardiovascular fitness. Cardiovascular fitness is measured in terms of aerobic capacity, which is the ability to do large-muscle, whole-body exercise of moderate to high intensity over extended periods of time. Cycling works primarily the muscles of the legs, hips, and buttocks, and the upper body is used during hill climbing. It increases the oxidative capacity of these muscles, thereby improving the body's ability to do extended work.

By engaging in regular vigorous cycling that improves aerobic capacity, you can reduce the risk of heart disease. This kind of activity, called aerobic exercise, helps your heart get stronger.

Body Composition

Aerobic cycling several times a week is a fun and fast way to burn fat and calories and increase lean weight. Your body can be divided into two basic components: lean weight (muscle, bone, internal organs) and fat weight. For good health and fitness, you should try to maintain a proper ratio of one to the other. By assessing your body composition, it is possible to determine if you are underweight, muscular, or overweight.

Estimates of body composition are easily determined by measuring skinfolds with calipers. This gives a percentage of body fat, which means that out of a total body weight a certain percentage is estimated to be stored fat. Therefore, if your percentage of fat is 23, the remaining 87% is lean body mass. You should try to maintain body fat below 20% if you are male and below 25% if you are female.

Controlling what you eat (caloric intake) combined with regular aerobic exercise (caloric output) is an ideal way to maintain a balance in body composition. Cycling works all of the major muscle groups of the lower body and can produce a lean, muscular look. Table 1.2 lists the calories burned while cycling at various speeds.

Table 1.2 Calories Burned During Cycling

Cycling speed (mph)	Calories per mile
10	26
15	31
20	38
25	47
30	59

Flexibility

Flexibility is the ability to move muscles and joints through their full range of motion. Being flexible turns sports like cycling into lifetime activities that can make a real difference in long-term health.

Cycling has very little effect on improving your flexibility. Your goal is to supplement your cycling to avoid what some riders call "cycling rigor mortis"—joint stiffness and gradual loss of muscle elasticity caused by excessive saddle time. Suggestions on how to incorporate stretches into your cycling fitness program for improved performance and for improved overall health are provided at the end of this section.

Muscular Endurance and Strength

Muscular fitness includes both endurance (how many times or how long you can lift or hold an object) and strength (how much weight you can lift). Many activities in your daily life such as lifting grocery bags and walking up several flights of stairs require some degree of muscular fitness.

Cycling enhances muscular strength and endurance, especially for the muscles of the lower body. Figure 1.1 shows how cycling affects the muscles.

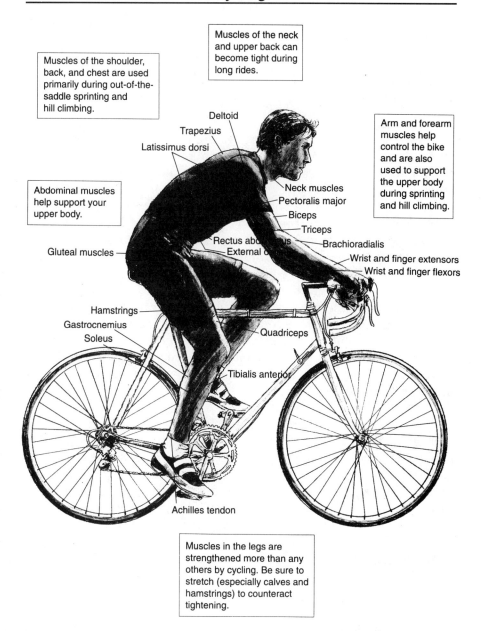

Muscles of the neck and upper back can become tight during long rides.

Muscles of the shoulder, back, and chest are used primarily during out-of-the-saddle sprinting and hill climbing.

Arm and forearm muscles help control the bike and are also used to support the upper body during sprinting and hill climbing.

Abdominal muscles help support your upper body.

Deltoid
Trapezius
Latissimus dorsi
Neck muscles
Pectoralis major
Biceps
Triceps
Rectus abdominus
Brachioradialis
External oblique
Wrist and finger extensors
Wrist and finger flexors
Gluteal muscles
Hamstrings
Gastrocnemius
Soleus
Quadriceps
Tibialis anterior
Achilles tendon

Muscles in the legs are strengthened more than any others by cycling. Be sure to stretch (especially calves and hamstrings) to counteract tightening.

Figure 1.1 Muscles used in cycling.

273

For example, a regimen of sprint cycling and riding up hills can strengthen the muscles of the back and shoulders more effectively than some weight-lifting programs. Generally, long-distance, lower-intensity cycling can improve your muscular endurance.

Comparing Cycling's Fitness Benefits

How do the fitness benefits of cycling compare to the benefits of other activities you may want to undertake? How much do you need to cycle to receive the same benefits from cycling as you would from other fitness activities? Let's compare the aerobic training effect of cycling to that of running and swimming. If you cycle 5 miles in less than 20 minutes, that is comparable to running 1 mile in less than 8 minutes and swimming 600 yards in less than 15 minutes.

Cycling is comparable to running, aerobics, and swimming in cardiovascular training, and equal to many activities for maintaining body weight, muscular endurance, and strength.

In addition to the physical benefits of regular aerobic cycling, you can also help increase your sense of well-being and enjoy a more productive and happier life. Kenneth Cooper, author of *Aerobics,* described exercise as "a means of putting more years in your life and more life in your years." As research has shown, even small improvements in fitness—like those achieved through cycling—can substantially reduce the risk of disease.

So don't underestimate the value of getting out and pedaling a bicycle 3 to 5 times a week. Combine a little cycling with other positive lifestyle changes and you have the recipe for better health.

Best of all, cycling is a lifetime activity that can be enjoyed in many different ways. If you are young and full of energy you may want to race, or ride 25 miles in under an hour. If the weather's bad and you want to be fit, you may choose a stationary bike workout.

Getting Equipped to Cycle

You can still hop on the old 10-speed in your worn pair of tennis shoes, denim shorts, and cotton shirt, but you'll be a lot more comfortable—and therefore more willing to ride—if you invest a little time and money in choosing the right bike and clothing. This section will help you make the right selections.

These days you have many choices to make. Do you want a road bike, a mountain bike, or a hybrid? Do you want a basic stationary bike or a sophisticated exercise bike with all the bells and whistles? What cycling wardrobe will you select from the vast array of form-fitting synthetics? What shoes are best for the various forms of cycling?

Choosing a Bike

You probably already own a bike. But if you don't, or if you're planning to upgrade, the following sections will help you determine what type of bike is best for you. In searching for a bike, start by deciding what type of riding you want to do. Your local bike shop can provide a focus, but only after you give them the big picture.

Road Bikes

If you plan to stay strictly on the streets, pick a road bike—its light weight, drop bars, and skinny tires are best suited to pounding the pavement over the long haul. Today's road bikes have 14 to 16 speeds, a variety of shifting systems, and weigh about as much as the saddle on your old English racer.

Though mountain bikes account for the lion's share of the bike business these days, a road bike with a 27-inch or a 700c wheel is probably the best all-around fitness machine. The drop-style handlebars give you better aerodynamics and more hand positions—which can help you avoid fatigue and discomfort on long rides—than the straight bars of a mountain bike. The road bike's light weight and narrow tires mean less rolling resistance than a fat-tired mountain bike, but also a less forgiving ride, especially on pavement or dirt roads. Although the gearing range of a road bike is narrower than that of a mountain bike, with a larger "big gear" and a less-accommodating low gear, you don't need the extensive low-gear range a mountain bike offers unless you're planning a loaded-panniers tour of the Rocky Mountains. You will, however, welcome the road bike's bigger gears on long descents

The biggest drawbacks to buying a road bike are price and choice. Road bikes account for a much smaller share of the market than mountain bikes, so they generally cost more and offer fewer models to choose from.

Mountain Bikes

If you expect to ride mostly off-road, pick a mountain bike. You'll be in good company—6 of every 10 bikes sold in the United States are mountain bikes. With their broad range of gearing and fat, low-pressure tires, mountain bikes are great for pedaling up and down dirt roads and trails. Although they are designed for off-road use, their upright riding style and 26-inch wheels—reminiscent of the old beach cruisers and paperboy bikes from which they are descended—have made them a hit with newcomers to cycling and street riders who find them ideal for pedaling through the urban wilderness.

If you choose a mountain bike, you'll get fewer flats, thanks to the wide, heavy tires, and you'll stop faster, courtesy of the motorcycle-style cantilever brakes. But you'll also find the upright position, extra weight, and beefy rubber a hindrance on long rides.

There's a wide variety of mountain bikes, ranging from inexpensive steel bikes to top-dollar titanium trail tamers with front and rear suspension

Hybrids

If you plan to ride both road and trail but don't want to buy two bikes, you might consider buying a hybrid—a bike designed for both road and off-road riding. The hybrid bike is a legitimate choice for riders who want a little dirt (or a little asphalt) in their cycling diets. The tires are wider than road bike tires but narrower than mountain bike tires, and they are often on road-sized (27-inch or 700c) wheels. Although you can use a hybrid on road or trail, its straight bars and upright position aren't really suited for prolonged road rides, and its bigger wheels and narrower tires put technical trails out of reach for most riders. Still, many people who want a taste of both cycling worlds find them an acceptable compromise.

Buying a Bike

Even if you think you've found the bike of your dreams, don't buy it without taking it for a test ride. What you find to be minor annoyances in a 15-minute ride can become major headaches on longer rides. So, save yourself some money and aggravation by test riding a few bikes before buying one. After a number of test rides, one or two bikes will feel right to you.

Follow these two rules of thumb:

1. Stand astride your test bike and measure the distance between the top tube and your crotch. You need 1 inch of clear-

ance over the top tube for a road bike or hybrid, and 2 or more inches for a mountain bike.

2. While in the riding position, the handlebars and stem should block your view of the front wheel's hub.

If you are undecided about two frame sizes, it's usually best to choose the smaller size. It is critical for both safety and comfort to have the right size frame when cycling.

Accessories and Gear

Once you've found a bike to ride you may think you're done shopping, but we suggest you purchase a few items to make your cycling a lot safer and more comfortable.

Helmets

Your second major purchase should be a helmet meeting Snell, ANSI, or ASTM standards. Unlike their heavy, hard-shelled predecessors, today's lightweight expanded-polystyrene helmets weigh less than a half pound, provide ventilation to keep your head cool, and cost as little as $3—a small cost for the valuable protection they provide.

Some helmets blend internal plastic mesh with a Lycra cover; others employ a lightweight, hard-shell coating. All are designed to distribute and thus minimize the force of an impact. Make sure the salesperson shows you how to get a proper fit—a loose helmet is almost as bad as none at all. Most come in three standard sizes—small, medium, and large—and rely on removable pads to provide the custom fit each head requires. Never wear a helmet once it's been damaged in a spill. Many manufacturers will provide a replacement at little or no cost.

Padded Shorts

Next on your list of cycling accessories is a pair of good-quality cycling shorts. You'll find the smooth padding provided by the synthetic chamois liner much more comfortable than the seam running down the center of your old pair of cutoffs. These nylon-and-Lycra garments have a high back, designed to fit a body that's leaned over on a bike, and their length keeps your thighs from rubbing on the saddle. Elastic on the lower leg helps keep them from riding up while you're riding along. Some shorts designed for off-road riding even have hip and thigh pads to offer protection in the event of a spill.

Prices vary depending on quality, but you can expect to pay between $25 and $75. Consider buying at least two pairs, so you can wear one while the other is in the wash—riding in dirty shorts can lead to unpleasant bacterial invasions called saddle sores that are every bit as unpleasant as they sound. One way to minimize the likelihood of these eruptions is to rub the liner with vitamin A & D ointment, which also helps keep both real and synthetic chamois soft and pliable. Another is to wash occasionally with an antibacterial soap, such as Betadine. A third strategy is to remove your shorts as soon as possible after a ride.

Gloves

Your third purchase should be a pair of fingerless cycling gloves. These pad your hands where they contact the handlebars, a welcome buffer against some of the bumpy roads you're sure to encounter, and because your fingers aren't covered you retain the delicate control needed on shifting and brake levers. They also absorb sweat, giving you a better grip on the bars, and will protect your palms in the event of a spill, when your natural reaction will be to throw your hands out to catch yourself. It's much easier—and a good deal less painful—to buy a new pair of gloves than to wait for your palms to recover from a severe case of road rash. Expect to pay $15 to $30 for good gloves, and keep an eye out for a design that has a terrycloth thumb—it's handy for wiping the sweat away on a hot day.

Shoes

Finally, buy yourself a pair of cycling shoes. You may think running shoes are an acceptable compromise, but this is one purchase where half-stepping just won't do. The sole of a running shoe is too springy for cycling because it's intended to protect the foot as it pounds the ground. Cycling shoes, which make limited contact with the ground, have stiffer soles that help transmit power to the pedals—indeed, some models can be quite uncomfortable to walk in, even for a short distance.

In general, shoes fall into three categories—touring, racing, and off-road riding. Touring shoes resemble running shoes but have stiffer soles and rudimentary integrated cleats for gripping the pedal; you'll be able to do some walking in these, but don't plan any long hikes. Expect to pay $40 to $60.

Racing, or "cleated," shoes are more efficient for riding but almost useless for walking. Their soles are inflexible and equipped with removable, adjustable cleats designed to work either with standard pedals with toe clips and straps or with clipless pedals that incorporate a binding system similar to that used with skis. With the greater specialization comes a higher price—$60 to $140 and up. If you decide on this type of shoe, make sure your shop helps fit you and your new shoes to your pedals. Although some clipless systems provide a degree of "float" for the foot during the pedal stroke, poorly set-up cleats can lead to knee injuries.

Off-road shoes, which tend to look more like low-top hiking boots, have more rugged soles and some flexibility in the toebox, since they come in contact with the earth more often than their on-road counterparts. Versions are available both for standard and clipless pedals; some shoes can be used with either system. Because many off-road shoes are used for racing as well as riding, they run a little more expensive than touring shoes—$50 to $100 and up. And the caveat about cleat setup applies here, too.

Touring shoes are best for indoor cycling if they are used with toe clips and straps. Toe clips will help keep the ball of your foot centered over the pedals and should be an addition to your stationary bicycle.

Shoes will be one of the most important purchases you make, so take your time picking them out. If you find the choices too confusing, tell your salesperson what kind of riding you plan to do and let her or him fit you with the proper shoe for the job.

Other Essentials

You're going to get thirsty, so add two water bottle cages and water bottles (about $15 for all four items). And you're going to have flats, so pick out a frame pump ($20 and up) and a saddle bag ($10 and up). Fill the last item with tire irons ($2 and up), a patch kit ($2), and at least one spare tube ($5 and up). If you've never fixed a flat, ask the salesperson or a friend to show you how. A handlebar computer ($30 and up) can chart your road to fitness by logging elapsed time, distance, speed, and other information.

For indoor cycling, various accessories are also essential. Don't even consider indoor cycling without a fan. If you don't believe us, just try cycling for 30 minutes on your indoor bike in the summer or spring.

279

You'll work up such a sweat that you will probably not finish the work-out. For effective cooling, you need to use something as large as a window fan ($30). Many cyclists consider a reading stand an invaluable accessory, especially if they do not enjoy watching television or listening to music. Several companies make these stands, which attach to the handlebars and begin at about $25.

Picking a Road

Look for wide roads with paved shoulders, few stop signs or traffic lights, and a minimum of traffic. Your local cycling club can give you some pointers here—and chances are they conduct some regular training rides that you can join.

Four-lane roads give motorists the option of changing lanes. Interstate highways, where bikes are permitted, are not exciting but they have big shoulders.

Picking a Trail or Dirt Road

Almost any dirt road will do for a fat-tire excursion, but look for those with low traffic—nothing takes your mind off your workout like a faceful of dust and rocks thrown up by passing autos. Many trails are open to bikes, but some are not; they're usually marked as such and should be avoided. Be especially wary of trails frequented by equestrians because horses are not fond of bicycles (some speculate that the buzzing of derailleurs reminds horses of a rattlesnake's warning rattle). Again, your local cycling club can help here and may conduct regular off-road training rides.

Obey the Law

Most cities, counties, and states require cyclists to follow the same rules made for other vehicle operators; some add a few special requirements. In general,

- ride with traffic, not against it, and as far to the right as is practical;

- signal your turns, and be predictable in your movements; don't wander right and left, but keep to a straight line;

- obey all traffic laws as if you were driving your car—that means stopping for red lights and stop signs, yielding to merging traffic, and turning from the proper lanes.

If you're riding off road, follow these guidelines:

- Strive not to damage trails by skidding through corners and descents or spinning out on loose climbs. This accelerates erosion and has led to more than one trail being closed to bikes.

- Announce your presence when you overtake someone (a bell is a nice touch).

- Yield the trail to horses, pedestrians, and other trail users. Don't hammer around blind corners—there may be a hiker coming around the other side.

- Consider taking a day off from time to time to help your local cycling club repair and maintain the area's trail network.

Ride Smart

Think ahead—keep these tips in mind as you head out on your bike:

- Always take at least one water bottle, no matter how short the ride. And drink before you get thirsty—dehydration is a common problem among many cyclists because they don't notice how much they sweat because the breeze they generate evaporates it. Sip frequently, and refill when necessary.

- Take snacks on any ride of 45 minutes or more. Fruit bars, bananas, energy bars, grapes, raisins, orange slices—anything easily digestible will do. Experiment with a variety of snacks.

- Carry extra clothing in your jersey pockets, especially if you live in an area with unpredictable weather. A light rain jacket is a good idea; so are arm and leg warmers, especially in early spring or late fall. Slip some change in there, too, in case you have a mishap and need to phone home, and keep $5 in your seat pack in case you need to buy food, energy drink, or a spare tube to fix a flat.

- When possible, begin your ride into the wind—this may give you a tailwind on the way home, which can be especially welcome after a long, hard ride.

Checking Your Cycling Fitness

Before you begin a workout program, we want you to answer a few questions about your current fitness and health. Many health benefits are associated with regular cycling. Completing this checklist is a sensible first step toward increasing your physical activity. It will tell you whether you are ready for a cycling self-test and with what level of training you may want to experiment. For many of us, physical activity poses no problem or hazard. This cycling readiness questionnaire is designed to identify the small number of people who should seek medical advice about the extent and activity most suitable for them.

Test Your Health/Fitness

Take a few minutes to answer the following questions. Here we offer a self-test that is specific to cycling. It checks both your health history and your fitness habits.

Choose the number that best describes you in each of these 10 areas, then add up your score. The results tell whether your starting line condition is high, average, or low.

Assessing Your Cycling Fitness

Cardiovascular Health

Which of these statements best describes your cardiovascular condition? This is a critical safety check before you enter any vigorous activity. (*Warning: If you have such a disease history, start the cycling programs in this book only after receiving clearance from your doctor—and then only with close supervision by a fitness instructor.*)

No history of heart disease or circulatory problems (3)   _____

Past ailments have been treated successfully (2)   _____

Such problems exist but no treatment required (1)   _____

Under medical care for cardiovascular disease (0)   _____

Injuries

Which of these statements best describes your current injuries? This is a test of your musculoskeletal readiness to start a cycling program. *(Warning: If your injury is temporary, wait until it is cured before starting the program. If it is chronic, adjust the program to fit your limitations.)*

No current injury problems (3) _____

Some pain in activity but not limited by the injury (2) _____

Level of activity is limited by the injury (1) _____

Unable to do much strenuous training (0) _____

Illnesses

Which of these statements best describes your current illnesses? Certain temporary or chronic conditions will delay or disrupt your cycling program. *(See warning under "Injuries.")*

No current illness problems (3) _____

Some problem in activity but not limited by it (2) _____

Level of activity is limited by the illness (1) _____

Unable to do much strenuous training (0) _____

Age

Which of these age groups describes you? In general, the younger you are, the less time you have spent slipping out of shape.

Age 20 or younger (3) _____

Ages 21 to 29 (2) _____

Ages 30 to 39 (1) _____

Ages 40 and older (0) _____

Weight

Which of these figures describes how close you are to your own definition of ideal weight? Excess fat is a major indicator of unfitness, but it's also possible to be significantly underweight.

Assessing Your Cycling Fitness (cont.)

At or very near ideal body weight (3)   _____

Less than 10 pounds above or below the ideal (2)   _____

10 to 19 pounds above or below ideal weight (1)   _____

20 or more pounds above or below the ideal (0)   _____

Resting Pulse Rate

Which of these figures describes your current pulse rate on waking up in the morning but before getting out of bed? A well-trained heart beats slower and more efficiently than one that's unfit.

60 to 69 beats per minute (2)   _____

70 to 79 beats per minute (1)   _____

80 or more beats per minute (0)   _____

Smoking

Which of these statements best describes your smoking history and current habit (if any)? Smoking is the #1 enemy of health and fitness.

Never a smoker (3)   _____

Once a smoker but quit (2)   _____

An occasional, light smoker now (1)   _____

A regular, heavy smoker (0)   _____

Most Recent Cycling Outing

Which of these statements best describes your cycling within the last month? The best measure of how well you will cycle in the near future is what you cycled in the past.

Cycled nonstop for more than 1 hour (3)   _____

Cycled nonstop for 30 minutes to 1 hour (2)   _____

Cycled nonstop for less than 30 minutes (1)   _____

No recent bicycle ride of any distance (0)   _____

Cycling Background

Which of these statements best describes your cycling history? Cycling fitness isn't long-lasting, but the fact that you once cycled is a good sign that you can do it again.

Trained for cycling within the past year (3) _____

Trained for cycling within 1 to 2 years ago (2) _____

Trained for cycling more than 2 years ago (1) _____

Never trained formally for cycling (0) _____

Related Activities

Which of these statements best describes your participation in other exercises that are similar to cycling in their aerobic benefit? The closer they relate to cycling (cross-country skiing, in-line skating, running, for example), the better the carryover effect will be.

Regularly practice similar aerobic activities (3) _____

Regularly practice less vigorous aerobics (2) _____

Regularly practice nonaerobic sports (1) _____

Not regularly active in any physical activity (0) _____

TOTAL SCORE _____

If you scored 20 points or more, you rate high in health and fitness for a beginning cyclist. You can probably handle continuous rides lasting 45 minutes or longer at an easy to moderate pace.

Between 10 and 19 points, your score is average. You may need to take a break or two to complete a 45-minute ride.

A score of less than 10 points is below average. You may need to start cycling slowly, or start your program on a stationary bicycle where you can take breaks off the bicycle.

Test Your Cycling Fitness

Knowledge of your physical fitness level before you begin cycling can help you start at an appropriate level and set reasonable goals.

Your overall health assessment level also provides a baseline against which you can compare subsequent tests as you progress.

Now comes your final exam. This is the most telling of tests, because up to now you've only surveyed your health and fitness with pen and paper. Now you check it where it counts—on the bike. Based on your performance in this test, you will be able to design an exercise program that is right for you.

The cycling efficiency test can provide you with an accurate determination of your fitness level. It offers you a safe way to determine which workout zones to use for effective and challenging cardiovascular exercise. The test can be used by any age group and at any level of fitness, and it only requires your bicycle and a level riding course.

Cycling Efficiency Test

1. Locate a measured 3-mile course at a convenient location (perhaps a residential area of town, a large city park, or a mall parking lot). It can be a straight-out course or a series of loops that make up the 3 miles.

2. Stretch and warm up for 5 to 10 minutes (see below). You should also be dressed comfortably and have your bicycle properly adjusted.

3. Choose a day when the wind is relatively calm and the temperature is not very high. It may be best to perform this test in the early morning or evening, when environmental conditions are usually more favorable.

4. Do not eat for at least 2 hours before your test, and don't participate in vigorous activity the day before.

5. Ride the 3-mile course as fast as you can, maintaining a steady pace. Time your ride to the nearest second. Pace yourself so you can ride the course at a steady pace for the whole distance; if you need to stop or slow way down, keep your watch running during all breaks. Record your time.

6. The time it takes you to complete the 3-mile course will give you an estimate of your relative fitness level. This will help you design your training program.

Fitness category	Minutes for 3-mile ride
Males	
Below average	More than 12 minutes
Moderately fit	8 to 12 minutes
Highly fit	Less than 8 minutes
Females	
Below average	More than 15 minutes
Moderately fit	11 to 15 minutes
Highly fit	Less than 11 minutes

For example, if you are a male cyclist and you ride the 3 miles in 11 minutes and 45 seconds, you are in the moderately-fit category.
Remember, this is your current cycling fitness level and says nothing about your potential.

Retesting

You can retest yourself periodically using this 3-mile cycling efficiency test to establish your gains in performance and fitness. You can retest as often as once a month or on a quarterly basis. To compare cycling efficiency tests, you should ride on the same course, with similar environmental conditions and with comparable bicycles.

Cycling the Right Way

The secret to cycling efficiently is a smooth, relaxed pedaling style that creates a flow that will eat up the miles. But this won't happen if your bicycle does not fit or if you don't pedal correctly. The following information will introduce you to proper position on a bike and how to pedal your bicycle correctly.

There's more to making your bike fit than adjusting the seat height. Proper positioning on a bicycle can provide benefits you probably haven't thought about. You'll feel much more relaxed and refreshed at the end of a day's ride.

Little aches and pains you may now take for granted could be eliminated with careful bicycle setup and pedaling technique. Since you won't be fighting discomfort, you'll ride farther and faster. And you won't be as vulnerable to possible overuse injuries.

Adjusting Your Bike

When you experiment with the following changes, make one adjustment at a time so you can feel what effect it has. And remember, it takes time to get used to a new position. Ride for several days with this new position before you decide whether a change is right or not.

Saddle Height

The saddle height is the most important adjustment you can make on your bicycle. Proper adjustment allows for efficient use of your muscles and ensures greater comfort while cycling. The directions for saddle height fit all three varieties of bicycles. After you have adjusted the saddle height, make sure that at least 2-½ inches of seat post remain in the seat tube for safety. Most seat posts have a maximum height mark on the post; do not exceed this amount.

The height of your saddle is based on your inseam length. Your saddle is correctly positioned when you are sitting squarely on the saddle with your down leg fully extended and the heel of your cycling shoe touching the pedal comfortably. The crankarm should be in line with the seat tube, and someone should be holding the seat from behind to help balance you and the bike. Using your heel to set the height will ensure a slight bend in your knee when you pedal with the ball of your foot. Do not pedal with your heel. Your saddle should be level or slightly tilted with the front of the saddle higher than the rear.

Once the saddle height is correct, front and back positioning can be adjusted on the bicycle. While someone is holding your saddle from the back, put both feet into the pedals with the ball of the foot over the pedal axle, and move the pedals to a level position. Drop a plum line from the center of the knee (behind the knee cap); the string should fall directly in line with the pedal axle. The saddle should be moved forward or backward until the plumb line hits the axle. With your knee lined up over the pedal, you can use the muscles of your upper leg to pedal efficiently.

Please keep in mind that if you make large adjustments to the fore or aft position, you may have to check seat height again. Moving the saddle forward is the same as moving the saddle down; moving the saddle back in effect raises the saddle.

Handlebar Adjustment

On your road or touring bicycle with dropped handlebars, the top of the stem should be level to 1-½ inches below the top of your saddle. On your mountain or hybrid bicycle, the top of the handlebars should be at the top of your saddle or slightly lower.

Like your seat post, there is a maximum height that your stem should be extended out of the steering head tube (head set). Usually there is a maximum height mark stamped on the handlebar stem.

Stem length is the hardest dimension to prescribe because everyone has different back flexibility and upper-body musculature. In general, your stem should be long enough so that the crossbar of the handlebar obscures the front hub when you are seated and your hands are on the break hoods of a road bicycle or on the grips of a mountain or hybrid bicycle. As you gain experience, consider changing to a longer stem to flatten your back and to improve your aerodynamics. Always ride with your elbows flexed slightly; you can better absorb the bumps and vibration of the road, and you will have less fatigue in your arms, neck, and shoulders.

Pulling It All Together

These pointers, of course, are not the last word on fitting yourself on a bicycle. Fitting for the professional cyclist is a complex process that can take up to several months to complete.

If you already own a bicycle, have someone at your local bicycle shop help you, or contact your local bike club for assistance.

Although these adjustments may not seem to affect you immediately, give them time. The more time and miles you put on your bicycle, the more you will appreciate a well-fitted bicycle.

The same adjustments should be made on your stationary bicycle if you plan to buy one for home use. If you use one at a health club, make sure your seat height is set properly.

Riding Correctly

After you have adjusted your bicycle, you need to learn about gearing and pedaling cadence (how fast you pedal, expressed in revolutions per minute, or RPM) to ensure comfort and efficiency, and to put less stress on knee joints.

Pedaling and Gearing

Inexperienced cyclists have a tendency to pedal in gears that are much too high for them, and in a cadence that is far too low. Beginning cyclists should strive to pedal at about 70 RPM. Pedaling cadence can easily be timed by counting the down stroke of one foot for a 15-second period and then multiplying the total by 4.

By maintaining a high revolution rate with a relatively low gear ratio, less muscle strength is required and endurance is increased. In contrast, pedaling in a high gear at a low cadence requires significantly more strength and puts undue stress on the knees and hip joints, which can lead to injuries.

After several weeks, begin to raise your cadence until you can pedal consistently in the 85 to 100 RPM range. Experienced cyclists prefer to ride at these higher cadences. It may take up to 6 months or more before you can pedal comfortably at this cadence.

At first, you may find that raising your cadence seems too fast and literally throws you around on the seat. However, with practice a cadence of 85 or greater can be enjoyable and relaxing.

The Importance of Shifting

To help you maintain a high RPM, you should shift gears when necessary. As the terrain or wind varies, you should switch to a higher or lower gear whenever you feel your cadence is too fast or too slow.

Work with your local bicycle shop to ensure that you have the proper gears on your bicycle to ride comfortably and efficiently in the area where you live. You can purchase replacement chainrings or rear gears.

The terrain you travel should determine the range of gears you'll use. If you live in a hilly area, you'll use lower gears; in a flat area you'll use higher gears. If you live in an area with varied topography, you'll need to be proficient in switching gears.

Learn to shift to a higher gear when you "spin out" (can't keep up with the pedals) and to a lower gear when your RPMs drop. If you consciously do this, it will become automatic; it will also smooth out your pedal stroke and ultimately save you from the pain created by the stress put on your knees by the low RPM pedaling and high torque.

Warming Up and Cooling Down

One of the most appealing aspects of cycling is that it is easy on the body—no pounding, no range of motion extremes, no adverse twisting. Just sit on the bicycle and spin the pedals.

With all the physiological accolades given to cycling, you may wonder why you should bother warming up, stretching, and cooling down. Some cyclists figure they can hop on a bicycle and begin an intense workout without any preparation. Besides, who wants to spend time riding easy and stretching when you could be out riding?

Warming Up

Warming up is a term used to describe a variety of activities—calisthenics, stretching, or easy cycling, for example—performed to prepare your body for prolonged physical activity, such as cycling.

We strongly recommend using a warm-up to enhance your cycling performance. A warm muscle contracts more quickly; oxygen is better delivered to the muscles of the legs, back, and upper body; and metabolic rate is increased.

Considerable research has been conducted on the best way to warm up. Active warm-up involves muscle activity, and passive warm-up involves warming the muscles through external means such as massage or sauna. Passive warm-up, however, is less likely to warm the deep muscles. Also, passive warm-up can be counterproductive. By increasing the surface temperature of the skin and dilating blood vessels, passive warm-up diverts a large amount of blood to the skin rather than to the cycling muscles of your legs.

A good warm-up helps prevent injury and makes your cycling workouts easier. Your body does not like to go suddenly from a state of rest to high-intensity activity. The smoother the adjustment, the easier your body adapts to the cycling workout, especially when exercising in the more difficult zones.

What's the Best Way to Warm Up?

The most effective warm-up consists of riding your bicycle. Begin by riding at a slow, gentle pace, then build gradually to your target heart intensity (the pace at which you'll do the main part of your workout). You may also want to do some brisk walking before you get on the bicycle. You can also begin by riding a stationary bike, or by jogging or walking. Try to involve both the arms and the legs in the warm-up.

How Long Should a Warm-Up Last?

You're probably warmed up if you're just beginning to sweat. If you don't reach a sweat, you should at least feel warm, and the exercise should start to feel easier. This usually occurs in about 5 to 10 minutes. Your heart rate should reach about 90 to 110 beats per minute, depending on your age. You should not feel fatigued after warming up.

The Role of Stretching

Stretching should begin after you have warmed up on the bicycle for a few minutes. If warming up on the bike is inconvenient, do some brisk walking or calisthenics for a few minutes. Stretching while the muscles are not warmed up does little to increase the elasticity of your muscles and joints. Raising the temperature of the muscles is a more effective way to increase muscle elasticity.

The Cool Part of the Workout

The cool-down is not as widely practiced as the warm-up, but it is no less important. Casual athletes, in particular, tend to ignore the importance of cooling down. Your cool-down is a period of low-intensity cycling that follows a moderate or vigorous workout, and it lasts about 5 minutes. A cool-down is like a warm-up in reverse. While a warm-up helps your cardiovascular system and muscles to get into gear, a cool-down helps them return gradually to a resting level.

Why Cool Down?

If you stop cycling abruptly, the blood "pools" in the wide-open blood vessels of the legs. Not enough blood returns to the heart, so the heart attempts to beat faster to increase the flow. You may begin to feel lightheaded as the result of not enough blood reaching the head.

Taking a hot shower or sitting in a hot tub immediately after cycling may compound this problem. As your body dissipates heat by increasing its blood flow to the skin, the amount of blood returning to the heart is further compromised. People have been known to faint while taking a hot shower right after cycling.

During cycling the blood vessels of the legs are wide open to carry oxygen and nutrients to your working muscles. The cool-down helps the blood return to your heart by alternately contracting and relaxing the muscles.

What's the Best Cool-Down?

Pedaling slowly in a lower gear (small chainring in front and larger cog in back) provides a pumping action that helps your body's circulation. After a hard cycling session, pedal in this low gear at about 70 to 80 RPM for 4 to 5 minutes. If you have to get off your bicycle, at least keep walking. Continue cycling until your heart rate has returned to below 120 beats per minute.

Stretch after you have cooled down to a heart rate of 120. This is an ideal time for a few additional stretches because your muscles and joints are warm from the cycling. Slow, static stretches will help reduce your muscle soreness. Be sure to pay particular attention to the muscles of the lower back and the legs.

Stretching for Cycling

Experience shows that individuals who are flexible have fewer injuries to the musculoskeletal system. Experts say muscles that are warmed up and then stretched are more efficient and can produce more strength, thus increasing the efficiency of the athlete in an activity.

Relaxed and gentle movements are the most efficient approach to stretching. Each stretch should be gradual, lasting from 20 to 30 seconds. Try to imagine the muscle stretching, the blood pulsing into the muscle area, and the flexibility increasing. Do not rush in anticipation of the workout.

Despite the obvious importance of flexibility, many cyclists often neglect it. They don't stretch before or after they cycle. That is their loss. Increased flexibility won't improve your cardiorespiratory fitness, but it will let you cycle aerobically with greater ease. Flexibility can also reduce your chances of muscle strain and soreness.

The following are some of the most beneficial stretches for cycling. We suggest that you experiment with several of these stretches for about 5 to 8 minutes before and after your ride. The areas of your body that tend to tire first are the ones you should stretch. If you feel tight during the ride, get off your bike and do a few stretches in the areas of your body that seem to be tired and tight. After the ride, stretch those muscle groups that are sore.

Achilles Tendon

Standing about 2 feet from a vertical surface, place your palms against it shoulder-width apart and just above your head. Lean forward until your elbows touch the surface, keeping your heels on the ground.

Hamstrings

Sit on the ground with both legs extended in front of you. Bend your right knee and slide your heel toward your crotch. Place your heel against the inner side of your left thigh so that a 90-degree angle is formed between the extended leg and the flexed leg. Keeping your left leg straight, bend at the waist, slowly lowering your upper body onto your thigh.

Adductors

Sit on the ground with your knees bent and the soles of your feet together. Grasp your ankles and lean forward, keeping your back straight as you stretch.

Quadriceps

(Don't do this stretch if you have bad knees.) Stand with your right hand against a vertical surface for balance and support. Bend your left leg behind you and grasp the foot with your left hand. Bend your right knee slightly and pull your left heel toward your buttocks. Remember not to overstretch; pull just to the point of tension.

Lie on your back on a table with your left side near the edge. Bend your right leg and slide your foot toward your buttocks; grasp behind your right thigh with your right hand. Lower your left leg off the table and grasp your ankle with your left hand. Slowly pull your left heel toward your buttocks.

Hips

Lie on your back on a table, allowing your left leg to hang over the edge. Bend your right knee, grasp your shin in both hands, and slowly pull your thigh toward your chest.

Buttocks and Hips

Sit on the floor or ground. Bend your right leg and slide the heel toward you. Grasp the ankle with one hand and hook the knee with your elbow. Pull your foot toward the opposite shoulder.

Lower Back

Lying on your back, bend your knees and grasp behind your thighs. Pull your knees toward your chest until your hips come off the ground. Hold for 10 to 20 seconds, then slowly extend one leg, then the other.

Neck

Lie on the ground with both knees bent and your feet on the ground. Lock your hands behind your head and pull your head forward and toward your chest, keeping your shoulder blades on the floor.

Standing with both arms behind your back, grasp your left elbow from behind with your right hand. Pull your elbow to the right across your midline, tilting your head toward your right shoulder (without bending at the waist).

Section 23.2

How Much Should You Ride?

Source: *Bicycling,* January, 1996

By Fred Matheny

Six years ago, Bernie Greenberg, now 41, was a Denver road racer who worked 80 hour weeks at his law firm and trained 2 hours every day. By year's end he was experiencing fatigue, heat intolerance, and vision problems. Eventually he was diagnosed with multiple sclerosis. How could a healthy, hard-charging competitive rider suddenly become so ill? "I think it was a combination of racing and job stress, triggered by injuries from an earlier car accident," says Greenberg—and his physician agrees.

Can too much cycling make you sick? Did Greg LeMond's rare form of an even rarer disease—mitochondria myopathy—result from an immune system pushed too hard by years of elite-level competition and his hunting accident? Less famously—but more to our point—can overtraining coupled with other life stresses suppress the immune system, leading to the colds, flu, and bronchitis that often plague amateur racers and even fast recreational riders?

Cyclists have asked such questions for years.

The first scientific evidence hinting at the danger of riding too much came from a study of 17,000 Harvard alumni by Ralph Paffenberger, Jr., M.D. Paffenberger found that the death rate was a quarter to a third lower among men expending 2,000 calories per week in exercise. But at higher levels of exercise—around 4,000 calories a week—the mortality rate rose.

Aside from this pioneering study, most conclusions about overtraining have been based on anecdotal evidence. Ed Burke, Ph.D., exercise physiologist, member of *Bicycling's* Fitness Advisory Board and head of Project 96, has worked with elite cyclists for 15 years. He says he's become convinced that "chronic, hard, endurance training can depress the immune system. It isn't a healthy situation."

Until now, however, there's been little evidence beyond the one landmark study and some educated guesses. But for the first time, cycling's experts are searching for proof—and solutions.

In Poland, 15 young racers were examined last March and rechecked after 6 months of intense training and racing (averaging more than 300 miles per week, much of it at extreme effort). Not surprisingly, ergometer tests showed marked improvement in their ability to ride stronger and longer. But lab work revealed a significant decrease in several immune system components. As they'd become fitter, their resistance to illness had declined.

In Australia, researchers severely overtrained 5 male runners by subjecting them to 2 intense interval sessions each day for 10 days. After only 6 days, the runners showed significant reductions in the special types of cells that battle illness, as well as progressively declining amounts of body chemicals and substances that help prevent fatigue.

The message is clear. Training too hard will not only harm performance (a well-known relationship that led cyclists to develop the training concepts of tapering and recovery) but might even threaten your health—and, ultimately, your life. The question is: How much riding is too much?

The same studies that reveal the harm of overtraining also demonstrate that moderate cycling doesn't weaken your immune system. In fact, most of the markers of a strong immune system are boosted by moderate training.

But defining moderation is tough because individual reactions to cycling vary greatly. A fast century might strengthen one rider's immune system while plunging other cyclists into illness. That's why professional racers are successful only if they have iron constitutions. The demand for high-intensity riding and lots of miles weeds out racers with relatively weak systems.

Moderate cycling is also relative to the rest of your life. Pro cyclists can complete exhausting stage races because they think of little else but riding, eating, and sleeping. Their other needs are met by the team support people, keeping their overall stress tolerable.

Now consider typical recreational cyclists like Greenberg—or yourself. They probably train a fraction of the miles logged by a pro. But they often have demanding jobs, a family, maybe a stressful auto commute on crowded roads. No mechanic cleans their bikes. Is it possible to overtrain on 150 miles a week when Indurain is logging more than 500? You bet it is. In fact, when total stress is considered recreational riders like us maybe working harder than the stars.

Cycling coach and *Bicycling* FAB member Tom Ehrhard agrees. "Stressors such as job and marital problems, or a poor diet, combine with training to form a total stress equation. Keep this below your individual tolerance point and you'll be healthy and react to training by improving. Past your tolerance point, you're subjected to a fascinating array of sicknesses such as mononucleosis and chronic fatigue syndrome, as well as more common colds and flu."

But how do you know you're overtrained?

Poor performance. If your cycling worsens in spite of hard training, it's almost certainly getting worse because of hard training. Take some time off, maintaining fitness with easy aerobic activities such as hiking or swimming at a heart rate below 70 % of maximum. Ehrhard recommends "putting a big cog on your cassette and noodling up hills." Although the rest needed to recover varies with individual riders, you might try scheduling 2-3 rest days per week for a month when you resume training on the bike.

General fatigue. Day-long exhaustion or lethargy is a sure sign. If you don't have the energy to mow the lawn, you have no business hammering hills with your cycling pals.

Negative emotions. A study done in the '70s by William Morgan, Ph.D., showed that the mood profiles of overtrained athletes are reversed from those of normal people. Instead of being high in vigor and energy, overtrained athletes were high in anxiety, fatigue, and lethargy. This "reverse iceberg effect" is present in all overtrained athletes. In fact, Morgan commented that he'd never seen an overtrained athlete who wasn't clinically depressed.

You don't need a psychologist to tell you when you're fried— family and significant others usually point out your personality change. If you feel irritable and grouchy, short tempered at work and emotionally unstable, you could be overtraining.

Vague physical complaints. "Sore throats or odd sicknesses can be leading indicators of chronic stress," says Ehrhard. So can sore muscles. Unlike impact sports such as running, cycling doesn't normally produce leg soreness. So if your gams are screaming, you've overdone it. Chronic diarrhea or heartburn can mean that your system is so overworked by training that it can't process food properly. Severely fatigued Tour riders often drop out not because they can't keep the pace but because diarrhea takes them off the bike in the middle of a stage.

Disruption of your normal sleep rhythm. Overtrained cyclists often fall asleep easily but wake abruptly in the early morning. Then at 10 a.m. they're ready for a nap. "Our riders chart their sleep, says Dean Golich, U.S. Cycling Federation exercise physiologist. "Poor sleep means it's time to back off on their training."

Elevated morning heart rate. Increases of 10% over several days usually means your body isn't adapting to training (although a few riders might have morning heart-rate fluctuations unrelated to training intensity or volume).

An overpowering desire to buy a new bike. Don't laugh. Severe bike lust might mean you're no longer enjoying riding for the sake of riding. You could be bored and tired, subconsciously craving a different bike to provide the variety and respite from training you crave.

How Too Much Riding Harms You

Weakened immune system.

Think of your immune system as a military unit whose job is to attack intruders—viruses, diseases, and other ailments—and defend your health. You're exposed to something they must fight every day. Some physical activity keeps them in shape and strengthens them so they fight better. But too much marching weakens them so they can't fight effectively. Invaders crash past, causing anything from the common cold to chronic fatigue syndrome.

Free radical attacks

Free radicals are molecules that are unstable because they have one or more unpaired electrons. They try to stabilize themselves by attacking other molecules, damaging them when they steal electrons. When you cycle too much your muscles create lots of free radicals and set them loose in your body. They damage your immune system cells and DNA tissue, leading to sickness and diseases as serious as cancer.

Inflate Your Immunity

You're overtrained? No sweat. Here are 5 steps that will help you stay healthy.

Use antioxidant supplements. Ken Cooper, M.D., who started the aerobics revolution nearly 30 years ago, recently wrote a book called *Antioxidant Revolution*. Cooper contends that intense exercisers can produce free radicals in their bodies that damage their immune systems. For cyclists who regularly exceed 80% of their max heart rate, he recommends daily supplementation with antioxidants, vitamins that offset the negative effects: 1,200 IU of vitamin E, 3,000 mg of C, and 50,000 IU of beta carotene.

Reduce total stress. Parts of your life seemingly unrelated to cycling can make you tired on the bike. "One of my riders was in the doldrums," says coach Tom Ehrhard. "His job was bothering him a lot. I urged him to do something constructive. He not only looked at other jobs but confronted his boss. The boss was receptive and the rider felt like a huge weight had been lifted from him. And his legs came back."

Adjust your goals. If you have a demanding job and want to spend time with your family, don't aim for the Race Across America. Success in club criteriums, road races, and mountain bike events is possible with only 74 hours of training a week. Goals should accurately reflect the time and energy you can invest in meeting them.

Eat enough. Overtraining symptoms are frequently due to chronic glycogen depletion, according to physiologist Ed Burke. And pay attention to a Japanese study that suggests sugar intake during cycling can enhance immune cell function. When cyclists rode at heart rates of 150 beats a minute and consumed a 25% glucose drink, their white blood cells were better able to respond to invading infectious organisms. (As a bonus, their endurance time increased by one-third.)

Become more disciplined. What? Isn't too much dedication what got you in trouble? Yes, but driven cyclists need "tremendous discipline to go easy," says coach Skip Hamilton, "especially when a faster group goes by. You have to resist the urge to jump on. You need to remember your training goals for the day."

This means monitoring your body to keep easy days easy. If you use a heart-rate monitor, set the alarm to beep when you get within 50 beats of your max heart rate. If it screeches, slow down. Or leave the monitor at home and cruise in a gear so low you barely feel pressure on the pedals. Try riding with a friend who is way slower than you. Take a spin on a lightly traveled, flat road in the country. Smell the flowers and talk to the cows.

Moderation in the pursuit of recovery is no vice.

Chapter 24

Running

Chapter Contents

Section 24.1

One Step at a Time: An Introduction to Running

Source: President's Council on Physical Fitness and Sports,
OM 87-0063, 1987.

The Running Revolution

Millions of Americans are running. Young, old, and in-between, male and female, plodders and speedsters, you see them everywhere: loping through parks, pounding city pavements, chugging along suburban streets, and doggedly circling school running tracks.

Running continues to retain its standing as one of the more popular forms of aerobic exercise. Surveys show that more than 26 million adult Americans are running regularly. Most run a mile or two at a time, two or three times a week to improve their overall fitness levels. Many run for competitive purposes, testing their ability against fellow runners in fun runs and road races throughout the year.

The Reasons For Running

Health clearly is the No. 1 reason why so many Americans are running. Studies have shown that regular, vigorous exercise can improve the body's ability to consume oxygen during exertion, lower the resting heart rate, reduce blood pressure, and increase the efficiency of the heart and lungs. It also helps burn excess calories.

Since obesity and high blood pressure are among the leading risk factors for heart attack and stroke, exercise offers protection against two of our major killers.

Possibly more important for motivational purposes are the immediate benefits that beginning runners experience. They almost invariably report that they feel better, tire less easily, and have fewer illnesses.

There are other reasons to run. Some do it because they enjoy it, or because it helps them get rid of tensions. Others do it for the competition, or to prove something to themselves. Many do it to shed pounds and tone flabby muscles.

Experienced runners say they develop a "positive addiction" to running and don't feel right if they don't do it. Ask almost any runner why he or she began and you will get an answer something like this: "To get in shape and lose weight. " Ask them why they continue and you will be struck by a subtle difference in the reply: "Because I enjoy it. " "I feel I'm cheating myself when I don't do it." "I like knowing that I'm capable of running five or six miles."

Running also exerts a favorable influence on personal habits. For example, smokers who begin running often cut down or quit. There appear to be two reasons for this. One, it's difficult to run if you smoke, and two, improved physical condition encourages a desire to improve other aspects of your life.

Several forms of endurance exercise—cycling, swimming, and cross-country skiing among them—are as effective as running, but running's immense popularity is due to its unique advantages. Some of these are:

Almost everyone can do it.

You don't have to take expensive lessons to be a runner. If you can walk, you probably can work up to running. You can learn what you need to know from magazines, books, and acquaintances who are runners.

You can do it almost anywhere.

Running doesn't require expensive facilities. You can run in parks, on streets or country roads, in gymnasiums, or on the tracks and running trails found in almost every community. (If you run on roads or streets, stay on the shoulder or close to the curb and run facing traffic. A few localities have banned runners from road ways, so you should check to see if yours is one of them.)

You can do it almost anytime.

You don't have to get a team together to run, so you can set your own schedule. Weather doesn't present the same problems and uncertainties that it does in many sports. Running is not a seasonal activity, except in the most extreme climates, and you can do it in daylight or darkness. (Wear light-colored or reflective clothing and exercise extreme care if you run at night. Several runners are struck and killed each year by autos.)

It's inexpensive.

You don't have to pay to do it, and the only special equipment required is a good pair of running shoes.

Running Style

In most sports we are taught to run for speed and power. In running for fitness the objectives are different and so is the form. Here are some suggestions to help you develop a comfortable, economical running style:

- Run in an upright position, avoiding excessive forward lean. Keep back as straight as you comfortably can and keep head up. Don't look at your feet.

- Carry arms slightly away from the body, with elbows bent so that forearms are roughly parallel to the ground. Occasionally shake and relax arms to prevent tightness in shoulders.

- Land on the heel of the foot and rock forward to drive off the ball of the foot. If this proves difficult, try a more flat-footed style. Running only on the balls of your feet will tire you quickly and make the legs sore.

- Keep stride relatively short. Don't force your pace by reaching for extra distance.

- Breathe deeply with mouth open.

What To Wear

The most important item of apparel for the runner is a pair of sturdy, properly-fitting running shoes. Training shoes with heavy, cushioned soles and arch supports are preferable to flimsy sneakers and racing flats. (Several running magazines annually rate the major brands and popular models.)

Weather will dictate the rest of your attire. As a general rule, you will want to wear lighter clothing than temperatures might seem to indicate. Running generates lots of body heat.

Light-colored clothing that reflects the sun's rays is cooler in the summer, and dark clothes are warmer in the winter. When the weather is very cold, it's better to wear several layers of light clothing than one or two heavy layers. The extra layers help trap heat, and it's easy to shed one of them if you become too warm.

You should wear something on your head when it's cold, or when it's hot and sunny. Wool watch caps or ski caps are recommended for winter wear, and some form of tennis or sailor's hat that provides shade and can be soaked in water is good for summer.

Don't wear rubberized or plastic clothing. Such garments interfere with the evaporation of perspiration and cause body temperature to rise to dangerous levels.

If you dress properly, you can run in almost any weather, but it's advisable not to run when it's extremely hot and humid. On such days, plan to run early in the morning or in the evening.

Setting a "Green Light"

Before you begin running you should have a complete medical examination. Chances are that your physician will give you a go-ahead. Even persons with serious organic disorders, including many heart attack victims, are able to run under carefully prescribed conditions.

If you have a history of cardiovascular problems, or if you have reason to suspect the existence of such problems, it's a good idea to have an exercise, or stress, electrocardiogram (ECG). It will help your physician detect any complications that might be provoked by prolonged, strenuous exertion.

"Warming Up" and "Cooling Down"

Now you're ready to begin running—or almost. Elsewhere in this section you will find a set of six stretching exercises. These should **always** be done after you warm up your body by doing some low-level limbering exercises like walking in place, arm circles, and knee lifts for a few minutes. Stretching "cold" muscles can lead to injury. The exercises in this booklet will stretch the muscles you use in running and prepare the joints for movement through a full range of motion.

The six stretching exercises should be repeated during a "cooling down" period following each run When you have finished running, walk until breathing returns to pre-exercise levels and then do the exercises. This will help prevent muscle soreness and also aid the return of the blood from the extremities to the heart.

Running

Now that you really are ready to run, you may find that you have to begin by walking. If so, don't be discouraged. Few beginners are capable of running continuously for any distance. It probably took you several years to get in the shape you're in, and it will take awhile to repair the neglect. Patience is the key to success.

The "walk test" will help you determine where to begin. If you can comfortably walk three miles in 45 minutes, it's okay to start running. Or, more precisely, alternately running and walking. If you can't pass the test, walk three miles a day until you can.

In the beginning you should alternately run and walk continuously for 20 minutes. Speed is not important, but the amount of time is. It takes about 20 minutes for your body to begin realizing the "training effects" of sustained, vigorous exercise.

No one can tell you exactly how far you should run/walk at the beginning. Exercise capacity varies widely, even in individuals of similar age and build. Here's a rule of thumb to follow:

> After your warm-up, walk briskly until you are moving easily. Run at a comfortable pace until you begin to become winded or tired or both. Walk until you're ready to run again. Repeat the cycle until your 20 minutes are up.

The more often you run, the faster you will improve. At least five workouts a week are recommended for persons trying to raise their level of fitness. Three workouts a week generally are considered to be the minimum number needed to maintain a desirable state of fitness.

The "talk test" can help you find the right pace. You should be able to talk while running, or while alternately running and walking. If you're too breathless to talk, you're going too fast.

When you first begin running, progress will seem slow, but gradually in the weeks ahead you will become aware that your strength and staying power are increasing. After eight or 10 weeks, if you work out faithfully, you should be able to run the full 20 minutes at a reasonable pace, although this process may take somewhat longer for older persons.

After you have completed the reconditioning phase, you should extend your run to 30 minutes. Remember, the amount of time you invest is more important than your time for a specific distance.

Stretching Exercises

To minimize the chances of injury or soreness, the following exercises should be done before and after running. If you find the exercises difficult to perform, you may want to do them twice when warming up to increase flexibility. Stretch slowly and do not bounce to attain prescribed positions. If you feel pain ease up on the stretch.

Achilles Tendon and Calf Stretcher

Stand facing wall approximately three feet away. Lean forward and place palms of hands flat against wall. Keep back straight, heels firmly on floor, and slowly bend elbows to hands, and tuck hips toward wall. Hold position for 30 seconds.
Repeat exercise with knees slightly flexed.

Back Stretcher

Lie on back with knees bent and arms at sides with palms down Slowly pull right knee toward chest, keeping left foot on floor. Hold position for 30 seconds.
Repeat exercise with opposite leg.

Thigh Stretcher

Stand arm's length from wall with left side toward wall. Place left hand on wall for support. Grasp right ankle with right hand and pull foot back and up until heel touches buttocks. Lean forward from waist as you lift. Hold for 30 seconds.
Repeat exercise with opposite hand and foot.

Modified Hurdler's Stretch

Sit on floor with one leg extended straight ahead Bend other leg at knee placing heel against inside of extended leg. Slowly bend forward sliding hands along extended leg. Bring chest toward knee and keep back straight. Hold for 30 seconds.
Repeat exercise with opposite leg.

Straddle Stretch

Sit on floor and spread legs at a comfortable width apart. Keeping back straight, slowly bend forward sliding your hands along the floor until you feel a stretch on the inside of your legs. Beginners can bend knees slightly. Hold for 30 seconds. Return to starting position. Slowly stretch forward over right leg, bringing your chest toward your knee until you feel a stretch in the back of your leg. Hold for 30 seconds.

Return to starting position. Repeat second step of exercise to left side.

Leg Stretcher

Sit in same position as in preceding exercise. Rest left hand on left thigh and grasp inside of right foot with right hand. Keep back

Section 24.2

AR&FA's Guide to Running and Racing

Source: American Running and Fitness Association, 1994.
Used by permission.

Do you have the urge to start running? Are you a runner who gets injured frequently? Do you feel you are not running your best? Training smart is the key to beginning, enjoying and maintaining a running program. Novices as well as seasoned runners can enhance their running and reduce their risk of injury by adhering to some basic training principles.

Training Methods

Long Runs

No more than once a week, but at least once a month, incorporate a long run into your schedule. The long run often equals about 20% to 30% of your total weekly mileage. Long runs help build endurance (the ability to withstand fatigue over a certain amount of time) and will make shorter runs feel easier. The pace for a long run should be slow and comfortable. Concentrate on finishing the distance. If you have raced before, the long run should be about 90 seconds to two minutes slower than your 10K race pace. Long run distances can be increased by 10% a session. Don't feel compelled to do a long run just because it's on your schedule. If the run feels unusually hard after just a few miles, then cut the run short and try it on another day. Also be sure to drink plenty of fluids before, during and after the run.

Hill Runs

Hill running (or stair climbing if there are no hills in your area) helps runners build strength. Use a hill that rises one foot in 15 and not steeper than one In 10. Anything steeper may cause you to lose good form. Your hill should be from 100 to 300 yards long. Run up the hill at an intensity that feels like 5K to 10K pace. This will be fast enough to be effective, yet will allow you to run with good style and rhythm. Jog down the hill for recovery.

Speedwork

You can use speedwork if you decide to race, or if you just want to be a faster runner. The three most popular types of speedwork are intervals, fartlek and tempo runs.

Intervals refer to a structured type of speedwork that you do on a measured track. You go the measured distance at a pre-set time goal, and you never completely recover after each burst of speed. You're only restricted by your own creativity in constructing interval workouts. See the chart (below) for general guidelines.

Fartlek or speed play, is where you begin your run at a comfortable pace, Once you are warmed up, increase your speed and run for a few minutes until you begin to feel fatigued, then slow down and run at a comfortable pace until you get your wind back. Then speed up again. Repeat these speed burst/recovery runs for most of the distance you plan to run for the day. In time you will notice your speed bursts lasting longer and going faster. Use fartlek during any phase of your training.

Are You Overtraining?

Check for these changes...

Increases in Resting Heart Rate.	Take your pulse each morning before you get out of bed. If your pulse is up five to ten beats per minute from your normal rate, you may be overtraining.
Increased Thirst.	If you seem to be thirsty all of the time, you may be overtraining.
Weight Loss or Weight Gain.	If you notice large inexplicable fluctuations in your weight, you may be overtraining.
Changes In Sleep Patterns.	If you notice you're not sleeping as well as normal, or that you're not sleeping as long as normal, you may be overtraining.

Tempo runs build your ability to maintain long, hard running as you must do in a race. After warming up, run for 20 to 30 minutes at a "comfortably hard" pace, about 15 seconds per mile slower than your 10K race pace. To get the maximum benefits out of tempo runs, do them at as even a pace as possible. Monitor your improvement by noting how much easier they feel, rather than by doing them faster.

Don't Forget

Warm up

Warm up by walking briskly or jogging slowly until you begin to sweat or feel warmer. This will warm your muscles before vigorous activity, thus reducing your risk of injury. It's more difficult to strain or pull a muscle that has been warmed up.

Cool Down

After running, cool down by walking briskly a jogging slowly. Cooling down allows you to slowly bring your heart rate back to normal.

Interval Training Guidelines

Determine your goal time for a race. Next, figure out how fast you have to run per minute. For example if you would like to run a 7-minute mile, you will need to run 400 meters in 1'45". Finally, determine how fast each interval needs to be.

Length of Interval	Speed of Interval
1 mile	at 5K to 1 OK race pace
800	meters at 5K race pace to 5 seconds faster
400	meters 5 to 7 seconds faster than 5K to 10K pace

Interval	Repetitions	Duration	Work/Rest Ratio*	Heart Rate % Max
Long	4–6	3–10 min	1:1	90-95
Medium	8-12	1-3 min	1:2	95-100
Short	16-25	30-60 sec	1:3	100
Sprint	25 +	10-30 sec	1:3	100

*1:3 means rest is 3 times as long as work (in time)

Stretch

After cooling down, do some gentle stretches of the Achilles tendon, calves, hamstrings and lower back. These areas contract when you run and stay in that position until you stretch them. If you do not stretch, you run the risk of pulling the muscle later. Stretching should always be done when your muscles are warm. Stretching a cold muscle can invite injury.

Shoes

Purchase a good pair of running shoes. If you need help with shoe selection, the American Running and Fitness Association's Running Shoe Database can help. Call 1-800-776-ARFA for more information.

Check-Up

If you're sedentary, overweight, a smoker or have high blood pressure or blood lipids, check with your doctor before starting a running program.

Hard/Easy Concept

Hard Runs

A hard run one day should be followed by an easy run the next. Exercise stresses muscles and they need time to repair themselves. If given enough rest, muscles come back stronger than before. This is how runners grow stronger and faster. If, however, muscles aren't given time to rest and repair themselves they run the risk of being injured.

A "hard" run is defined as one that includes more distance or speed than usual. A hard run means something different to every runner. For the novice who has never run for 10 minutes without stopping, a 10-minute run is hard. For the seasoned runner who has never run a seven-minute mile, then running a seven-minute mile is hard. If a run feels hard, go easy the next day.

Easy Runs

An "easy" day can mean that you take an entire day or two off, or that you run at a distance and pace that feels comfortable, enjoyable and relaxing. During easy days, you should be able to carry on a conversation while running. Some easy days could also be days when you are training hard, but not with the same muscles you use in running. Cross training on a bicycle is a good complement to running because bicycling strengthens muscles that are not used much in running. In this way, you can train hard more often and still use the hard/easy concept.

Total Concept

The hard/easy concept should be incorporated into all phases of training. Easy days follow hard days: easy weeks follow hard weeks: easy months follow hard months: and easy years follow hard years.

Duration

To strengthen your heart and lungs, exercise for at least 25 to 35 minutes, three to four days a week, or every other day. Additional mileage depends on your goals. Runners typically run more than the minimum to train for a race, reduce stress, aid in weight loss or for pure enjoyment.

10% Rule

Do not increase mileage by more than 10% per week, or 20% every two weeks. Exercise places stress on the body. The body grows stronger if it is stressed in small increments, but breaks down if stressed too much. Studies show that increasing mileage by 10% a week helps most people grow stronger and avoid injury. Follow the 10% rule whether you increase your weekly running from five minutes to 25 minutes, or from 40 miles to 60 miles. if you stop running for more than two to three weeks, build mileage back slowly.

Training Specificity

Training is specific to the sport. Swimmers improve by swimming. Runners improve by running. The type of running is also specific. To run fast, incorporate fast runs into your training. To run long distances. incorporate long runs. It is best, though, to incorporate all types of running in your program and allow your goals to dictate what type of running gets the most emphasis. For example, if your goal is to run the fastest mile you can, you would not train by just running one mile every day at a fast pace. Longer runs would give you stamina to sustain a fast pace and keep you from fatiguing. Shorter runs help you build speed. On the other hand, marathoners benefit from doing shorter, faster runs as well as longer runs.

Section 24.3

Women on the Run

**Improving bone strength for runners who increase
the intensity of their workouts.**

Source: *American Fitness,* November/December, 1995.

By Anna Kreiner

Thousands of women regularly hit the track in pursuit of good health. But make sure you're not breaking your bones to help your heart. Too much pounding on even a healthy frame can be a prescription for disaster.

Moderate exercise is essential for strong bones. But overtraining increases a runner's chances of injury. And female athletes who stop menstruating due to overtraining may be at even greater risk for irreversible bone loss.

A woman shouldn't sacrifice her bone health. Sticking to a reasonable training plan, getting enough calcium and maintaining proper hormonal levels are the keys to achieving high-quality athletic performance.

Anyone in an intense exercise program who puts constant strain on their limbs is likely to suffer from stress fractures (small hairline breaks in the bones of the ankles, feet and lower legs). "even normal, healthy young men are susceptible to injury during training," says Theodore Hahn, Ph.D., professor of medicine at UCLA and director of the Geriatric Research, Education and Clinical Center at Veteran's Administration Medical Center, in Westwood, California.

Indeed, the more you run, the greater your chances of getting hurt. According to a recent study in *Sports Medicine*, women who log 50 kilometers per week are twice as likely to be injured as those whose weekly distance is under 15 kilometers.

Female runners may find themselves in big trouble if they stop menstruating during training. Amenorrheic women are more likely to develop osteoporosis, a skeletal disorder characterized by low bone density. There is no cure for this syndrome, which can lead to fractures, long-term disability or even death.

Many amenorrheic athletes fail to gain the benefits of exercise, according to Barbara Drinkwater, M.D., a research physiologist at

Pacific Medical Center. Drinkwater has conducted several studies on female athletes and bone strength. Female athletes' bone density is often 10 to 12% lower than normal and may decrease at a rate of 3 to 4% each year. "When you're talking about young women, even losing 1% is losing a lot of bone," says Drinkwater. "And bone loss following prolonged amenorrhea may be permanent."

With the growing number of women runners, amenorrhea-induced osteoporosis could soon become a widespread problem. Approximately 2 to 5% of women have irregular menstrual cycles. Among female athletes, the figure may be closer to 50%.

The exact relationship between an athlete's training regimen and the onset of amenorrhea remains unclear, but researchers have found some consistent patterns. Amenorrheic athletes tend to consume less food and weigh less than menstruating women. Women who suddenly increase the intensity of their workouts or lose weight rapidly are also more likely to experience irregular periods. Genetic factors and pre-training menstrual patterns also influence a runner's cycle.

What can you do to protect your bones and athletic performance? Prevention is the best strategy. Bone mass increases until age 25, and eating enough calcium throughout childhood and adolescence can go a long way toward building a healthy skeleton. It's also important to keep up calcium intake throughout adult years.

Almost all women can benefit from the bone-strengthening effects of moderate weight-bearing exercise. But devoted runners who enjoy more rigorous training should take extra precautions to prevent osteoporosis.

Some risk factors for osteoporosis apply to all women. Small-boned women, women of Asian or Caucasian descent, cigarette smokers and women with low calcium intake are particularly likely to develop the disease.

Calcium

Calcium is the chief element in bone, and lifetime calcium intake has an important influence on long-term bone health. Doctors recommend consuming at least 1,000 mg, preferably 1,500 mg of calcium per day. (A glass of skim milk contains approximately 300 mg.) Many women, however, get less than one-half the recommended allowance every day—putting themselves at risk for serious bone problems down the line.

Lactose intolerance, a fear of high-fat dairy products or a dislike of calcium-rich foods keep many women from eating enough calcium. But you can get all the calcium you need without clogging your arteries or putting on extra pounds. Concentrate on low-fat or skim dairy products, leafy green vegetables, calcium-enriched orange juice, canned sardines and salmon (eaten with the bones). If you can't get enough calcium through diet alone, ask your doctor about oral supplements. Doctors usually prescribe calcium carbonate or calcium citrate.

Hormones

You won't benefit from a high calcium intake if your estrogen level is too low. Most physicians recommend female athletes who stop menstruating engage in a less-intense exercise program until they resume their regular cycles. But many committed athletes are unwilling to alter their training schedules, according to Robert Marcus, professor of medicine at Stanford University. These women should consider estrogen replacement therapy, which uses estrogen and progesterone to induce menstruation. The hormones can also be taken as an oral contraceptive.

Some elite athletes refuse hormone replacement therapy out of fear of losing their competitive edge. "There is no evidence of impairment from the use of estrogen," says Marcus. "Yet, the subtleties of changes in performance and mythologies among athletes about the effects of estrogen therapy keep many female runners from taking the hormones."

Runners are advised to begin estrogen replacement therapy within six months to a year after the onset of amenorrhea. Prolonged amenorrhea may lead to permanent bone loss. "Women can undertake heavy training regimens with no ill effects if they are willing to use estrogen replacement therapy," says Marcus. "But there is still concern replacing estrogen is not the same as regaining normal menses."

Exercise

Aerobic exercise, such as brisk walking, performed three to four times a week for 30 to 60 minutes, should be adequate to promote cardiovascular fitness and bone health. But what about women who enjoy more extensive training? Marcus advises women not to exercise so intensely that they stop menstruating.

Hahn cautions all exercisers against increasing the intensity of their workout suddenly or losing weight too quickly. Even overweight women who undergo rapid weight loss are more likely to become amenorrheic than those who take off the pounds over a prolonged period of time. "The secret is not to suddenly go all out," says Hahn. "Build up gradually." Proper exercise technique, posture and the use of correct footwear can also help prevent injuries.

Strong bones are important for overall health, flexibility and strength. So far there is no remedy for the debilitating condition of osteoporosis. As the old saying goes, an ounce of prevention is worth a pound of cure. Adequate calcium intake, proper hormonal balance, and a reasonable training regimen are the best ingredients for keeping you on track to good performance and healthy bones.

Boning Up on Good Health

Human bone contains two types of tissue—cortical and trabecular. The dense cortical tissue makes up three quarters of the skeleton and forms the outer layer of bones. The spongy and highly vascularized trabecular tissue is found in vertebrae, flat bones (including the hips), and the ends of long bones.

Human beings build new bone until age 25 or 30. After that, new bone mass is no longer added to the skeleton. However, bones undergo a constant process of remodeling. Cells called osteoclasts resorb the old bone, and osteoblasts on the bone surface produce new tissue. This new bone becomes hardened and strengthened during the process of mineralization. Each remodeling cycle lasts approximately 200 days, and any bone lost during that period cannot be replaced once the cycle is completed.

After age 40, bone loss occurs at the rate of approximately 1 to 2% per year. Hormonal factors play a key role in bone physiology. Estrogen appears to act directly on osteoblasts to activate bone formation and indirectly on osteoblasts to inhibit their resorptive activities, according to Theodore Hahn, Ph.D. at UCLA. After menopause, women undergo amuch more rapid rate of loss for five to eight years. Their low estrogen levels fail to inhibit bone resorption.

The exact mechanisms of osteoporosis remain unknown. But the condition seems to result from an imbalance in the resorption and formation phases, which leads to decreased bone mass and density. Trabecular tissue is most impaired, accounting for the high prevalence of vertebral and hip fractures among osteoporotic women. Since there is no cure for osteoporosis, treatment measures focus primarily on preventing injury and further bone loss.

Anna Kreiner is a freelance writer who's been published in Newsweek *and* Kids Today. *She also designs nutrition education materials for the Women, Infants and Children program in Los Angeles, California.*

Chapter 25

Swimming

Chapter Contents

Section 25.1

Fluid Movement

Source: *Men's Health*, November, 1995.

Face it, it's going to happen again this year, just as it has every other: The wind and the snow and the ice will whip up, and every third idiot neighbor will decide he doesn't feel much like shoveling his sidewalk this time around. You'll be too scared to venture out, much less don running shoes and practice intervals, lace up your in-line skates and take to the streets or hop on your bike and steal away.

The problem is obvious. You need a new form of exercise. One that keeps you indoors, away from the cold. One that avoids the endless boredom of the weight room or the basement, one that's fun and interesting and one that, most important, you already know how to do. Something like, well, swimming.

Swimming. Go ahead, jump in. But we suggest you pause and read this article first. Because while you may swim well enough to keep from drowning, you probably can't swim well enough to get any real fitness benefit. "Studies show only 2 percent of those who say they can swim can actually go as far as a quarter mile nonstop," says Terry Laughlin, director of Total Immersion swim camps. "That's 18 laps and it's probably a reasonable minimum for fitness swimming."

Of course, there's another reason it's crucial to sharpen your technique: It's the only way to look good. "You want to burn calories, but you don't want to look ridiculous doing it," says Emmett Hines, head coach of the H_2Ouston Swims Masters Swim Club and the 1993 US. Masters Swim Coach of the Year. "You want to be the guy who's taking 10 or 11 strokes per length and swimming along twice as fast as the other guy, while making it look effortless."

Forget Your Arms and Legs

Both Laughlin and Hines are disciples of Bill Boomer, a revolutionary swim theorist and movement scientist who took over the swimming program at the University of Rochester 30 years ago. "In swimming, hoary traditions get handed down from coach to coach," Laughlin says. "And Boomer came in and saw things entirely differently." Hines and Laughlin now work to bring the guru's teachings to the masses.

The first step to becoming a better swimmer is to lose your preconceptions about what propels you through the water. "The typical novice is maybe 10 to 20 percent as efficient as a world-class swimmer," Laughlin explains. But you can close the gap-to maybe a 20 percent spread-simply by streamlining your movements.

"If you're running, with every stride you get to push off solid ground," Laughlin says. "A huge amount of the energy you're expending gets returned to your foot. In the water, you're pushing against a moving medium, so an awful lot of that energy gets dissipated. Swimming is like trying to run across a field of Jell-O into a gale-force wind. You've got to balance your body and streamline."

Both Laughlin and Hines recommend a few crucial first steps to swimming efficiently:

Try being top heavy. Our bodies are designed to be balanced on land, which is why we're dense and heavy from our hips down and lighter on top. To balance yourself in the water, you need to transfer some of your body weight to your upper body. To do this, imagine you've got a line running down the center of your body and another crossing it from shoulder to shoulder. When you're swimming, you want to concentrate on pressing the "T," the point where the two lines meet, into the water. It's like adding weight to one end of a seesaw— your hips and legs should rise automatically toward the surface.

"If I put a swimmer on his stomach in the water and have him kick slowly," Hines says, "I should see his shoulder blades just touching the surface of the water, the back of his head just out of the water, and the cheeks of his butt kissing the surface. You'll get this by distributing more weight toward your upper body with each stroke "

Lengthen your boat. It's an ironclad rule of clipper-ship design— the longer the boat is at the waterline, the less drag it has and the faster it goes. Laughlin estimates that, all other factors equal, a 9-foot vessel can move through the water a full 25 percent faster than a 6-foot vessel. But, of course, we can't do anything about how tall we are, right? Not exactly.

The trick is to maximize the time you extend your arm. As soon as your hand enters the water, stretch it forward as far as possible. Then pause that hand at full extension for a moment before you begin your stroke.

Do the twist. "The biggest mistake people make in all strokes is that they try to do their work with their arms and legs and ignore the torso," Hines says. "You should actually look to use the arms and legs as a way to transmit the energy that's been created in your engine, the torso." Think of your hands as the threads on a screw, holding onto a spot in the water as you generate the power to drive through it by rolling your body back and forth.

As your right hand enters the water, roll your body-including your hips-at least 45 degrees, and preferably as much as 60 degrees, toward your right side (so that you'd be looking left). Roll back toward your left side as you execute the left stroke. Besides generating power, this rotation streamlines the body as it slips through the water, keeping one shoulder out of the water most of the time. "To reduce drag, you want to spend the most time swimming on your side," Laughlin says. "And as little as possible on your stomach."

Unload your arms. Once you're properly using body rotation for propulsion, the roll of your body should drive your arms forward into the water. "If you swim flat and try to reach out in front to try to take a stroke, you have to do it all with your arms and shoulders," says Hines. "This gives you a real poor mechanical advantage." If, however, you let body rotation drive your arms through the first part of the stroke, you can then generate enough force to push down hard in the follow through.

Swim at attention. Pretend that your neck has lost its flexibility, and that your head is firmly attached to the rest of your body. When you rotate to your side, look to the side-and take your breath then. "You tend to lift your head to breathe when you're on your stomach," Laughlin says. "But doing this is what most commonly breaks down form—your hips and legs just sink."

Breathe bilaterally. Most of us never learned to breathe on both sides of the stroke, but doing so will balance the stroke and, by keeping your breath longer, make you more buoyant. Practice breathing on every third stroke.

Perfecting the Stroke

Now that you've gotten the rest of your body working right, it's time to focus on the motion of your arms. The object of any effective stroke is to get as close as you can to the sensation of swimming down an exceedingly narrow trough—the idea being to streamline your body as tightly as possible. With that in mind, here is a five-step program for developing proper stroke technique, courtesy of legendary triathlete Dave Scott.

1. **Entry.** "Where your hand enters the water is critical," Scott says. The optimum place to put it is about 8 to 12 inches short of a full arm extension. "You don't want your arm to be completely extended until after it's in the wake. If you do that, your elbow and hand hit the water at the same time, you push down, and you trap a lot of water." Slip the hand in at about a 30-degree angle to the water, thumb and index finger first, with your palm facing away from your head—other wise, your hand traps air bubbles and slows you down. And don't cross the imaginary midline extending out from the center of your head. "If you overreach, it causes your hips and feet to wag back and forth and increases resistance," Scott says.

2. **Down sweep.** After entry, fully extend your arm. Your shoulder should come downward into the water as you do this, and help you rotate your hips and shoulders.

3. **Inward sweep.** Now, turn your hand so your middle and ring fingers start coming back toward your body. "If you had an eyeball in the middle of your right palm, that eyeball would be looking back at your left toes," Scott says. Keep your elbow up and pull your hand back toward the midline of your body at your waist.

4. **Upsweep.** "For most people, the biggest weakness is not finishing the stroke," Scott says. "After your hand passes your lower ribs, push back with the heel of your hand, not your fingertips, and rotate your wrist so your pinky leaves the water first."

5. **Recovery.** The recovery is when you get to relax your arm and prepare it for the next stroke. If you can't wiggle your fingers as you swing your arm forward, you're too tense.

And don't windmill. Raising your arm straight over your head will weigh you down and rock your body, creating drag. Instead, pretend that you're a marionette and a puppeteer has a string attached to your elbow, pulling it out of the water. Your forearm and upper arm dangle from it and swing forward into the water.

Do the Drill

"The big misunderstanding for a lot of people is that swimming is sort of a wet cousin of running or biking," Laughlin says. "If you run or bike and want to get better, you basically do more miles. In swimming that doesn't work. The more laps you do without having learned the basic skills, the more you're practicing your mistakes, and the only thing you get better at is making them."

Laughlin's prescription for improvement is to spend most of your time in the pool perfecting the new techniques by doing drills—25- to 100-yard lengths that focus on one skill at a time.

Following is a sampling of the drills Laughlin uses:

- Swim single laps just kicking, with your arms together out in front of you in a streamlined position, until you feel comfortable with getting your body in balance. (Remember to concentrate on pressing that "T" into the water.) Breathe by moving your chin forward, and work to find your balance again as quickly as possible after each breath.

- Swim 25s, stroking with only one arm and keeping the other out in front of you. As you swim with your right arm, turn your belly button completely to the left side on each stroke. Then repeat with the other arm. This will also make it easier to learn to breathe on both sides.

- Practice the catch-up drill. Keep your right arm outstretched all the way through the left arm's movements, until your left hand enters the water and covers the right. Then begin moving your right arm and keep your left arm outstretched throughout.

- Play pool golf. Swim 50s, timing yourself and counting your strokes (the number of times each arm pulls). The number of strokes plus the number of seconds is your score, so if you swim two laps in a minute, using a total of 40 strokes, you'll score 100. As your score declines, your skill level is increasing; the idea is to go as fast as possible using the fewest strokes necessary.

Section 25.2

Swimming for Life

Source: *Fitness Swimmer*, December, 1992.

By Terry Laughlin

Last spring I was reunited with a group of swimmers, now in their mid-twenties, whom I coached as teenagers. I was delighted when several of them mentioned that I look younger at 41 than I did 10 years ago.

Even more gratifying is the fact that I can honestly say I feel far better now than I did at 30. I know that I owe it all to having resumed swim training four years ago, after a 17-year layoff.

Besides the fact that I love looking and feeling younger, another reason I'll swim more than 400 miles this year is that I want to continue to improve competitively. After a fairly undistinguished college swimming career, I'm thrilled with my "elite" status as a Master. My times have gotten better each year, and I've placed as high as second in a United States Masters National Championship. It's a matter of faith with me that I can continue to refine my stroke, improve my workouts, take off a few more pounds. and build strength for several more years.

Ultimately, I plan to surpass my old college times (dating to 1970) and win a National Masters Championship. I'm not alone in my belief that swimmers can continue to perform well—and even improve—with age. At every clinic and camp I conduct, I meet swimmers in their forties and beyond who are still excited about getting faster, and eager to learn everything they can about how to do so.

Perhaps the best thing about working with these people is that their enthusiasm is tempered by maturity. They are aware—as I am—of the dangers of too much of a good thing. Sure, fast swimming is exciting. But to most fitness swimmers over 40, remaining healthy and having fun matter much more.

Fortunately, it's possible to train in ways that balance peak performance periods with long-term, continuous fitness and, of course, fun.

John Flanagan has struck this balance successfully for 25 years. The 46-year-old swimming coach from Arlington, Virginia, trains hard from September through April each year. During this period he swims more than 30,000 yards per week and competes in one or two Masters meets per month. From May through August, however, Flanagan stays out of the water.

Instead, he bicycles more than an hour to and from his coaching job every day (weather permitting), and paddles his kayak several days per week. This pattern of including both work and rest phases in a training cycle is called periodization. It is fundamental to long-term success in any physical activity.

Flanagan knows this well. "Fifteen years ago I set a goal of being in this sport when I'm 80," he says. "I realized that the only way I could do that would be to take time off—not willy-nilly, but by breaking each year into programmed cycles of work and relaxation."

This approach has paid off spectacularly. Flanagan has seen virtually no decline in his performances over the past 25 years.

In fact, last year he set a national age-group record of 10:46 in the 1000-yard free—more than a minute faster than he swam in college. He has never missed training because of injury, and he returns to the pool each September with a fully restored appetite for swimming.

"When I'm swimming, I'm competitive," he says. "I work out hard and I swim to win. But I realize I can't maintain that intensity constantly for another 40 years. So I do my summer activities strictly for fun, fitness and relaxation."

Flanagan's approach illustrates several strategies that can help any swimmer achieve success in competition but still maintain enthusiasm for the sport for 20 to 50 years:

1. Follow a pattern of periodization. That is, alternate cycles of intense, goal-oriented training with periods when you swim more for pleasure than for performance, or drop swimming altogether for other fitness pursuits, as Flanagan does.

Your training cycles can last for weeks, months, or even years. To get the maximum pay-off from each cycle, first set a baseline average number of weekly hours or yards of swimming you must perform to maintain general fitness. For most people, this can be accomplished in 6,000 to 10,000 yards per week, or 300,000 to 500,000 yards per year.

Next, determine your top training level, how long it takes you to reach it, and how long you can sustain it. You will learn these things gradually, by paying constant close attention to your body's feedback. A typical buildup might be a period of three to five months during which total weekly yardage increases by 50 to 100 percent. Only a handful of top Masters swimmers log the 30,000 yards weekly that

Flanagan does in preparing for Nationals. A training load of 10,000 to 15,000 yards per week during intensive training is more common.

Finally, plan cyclical rest periods following your times of intense training. During this time, you might reduce your average weekly yardage by anywhere from 30 to 100 percent. Substitute other activities if you wish (see next point), or rest completely for brief periods. Watch your weight and caloric intake during downtime.

2. Cross-train for total fitness, especially during the less intensive phases of your training. "Masters athletes can't sustain a high level of training for very long without risking injury or staleness," says Stan James, M.D., an orthopedic surgeon in Eugene, Oregon, and advisor to some of the world's top over-40 runners. He endorses Flanagan's seasonal multi-sport approach. "I tell my runners to maintain fitness with a variety of activities for most of the year, then follow a more structured, specialized program for a few months before a big competition."

As a swimmer, you can substitute running, cycling, in-line skating, rowing, kayaking, or any other aerobic sport that you enjoy between swim seasons. In addition, feel free to continue resistance training (either with weights or the weight of your body) year-round.

3. Watch out for fatigue, pain and injury. Building yardage and intensity during performance-oriented training increases your risk of overuse injuries like tendinitis. Jim Miller, M.D., a Masters coach in Richmond, Virginia, warns that ignoring pain signals for as little as one to two months can allow an overuse injury to progress to the point where one to two years of rehabilitation may be needed for a return to previous performance levels.

Listen to your body and learn to discern the difference between acceptable training-related soreness and the kind of pain and fatigue that signal the need for a break.

4. Don't stake your pride on continually improving your best times, or on beating the younger competition. This approach will eventually lead to frustration. Instead, compete with your peers, setting reasonable, realistic, long-term goals that you can adjust as you age. The success you will experience by training in this way will keep you motivated. By staying active, you will enjoy your fullest physical and mental potential for the long run.

5. Remember that it's never too late to embark on a "lifetime of swimming." Tony Lopez, 92, of Poughkeepsie, New York, didn't learn to swim until he was over 80. Crippled by arthritis, he began water exercise on his doctor's advice. The most tentative therapeutic movements evolved into swimming strokes as he gained strength and mobility.

When the local Masters coach saw Lopez swimming lengths of the pool, he invited him to join the team. Now Lopez is a national champion and record holder in the 90 to 95 age group. Last summer, 10 weeks after cancer surgery that removed his stomach, he won several titles in the Masters World Championships in Indianapolis.

Another of my heroes is Tom Lane, 98, of San Diego, who learned to swim in the 1890s, but never competed until the 1980s. Though legally blind, he swam six events (including the 400-meter freestyle) in one meet.

Terry Laughlin is the director of Total Immersion Adult Swim Camps & Clinics, and the Fitness Swimming Specialist for Speedo America.

Section 25.3

The Right Way to Teach Kids to Swim

Source: *Fitness Swimmer,* December, 1992.

By Rob McKay

A commercial aired during the Barcelona Olympic Games grabbed my attention. It was a footwear ad showing young hopefuls at basketball team-tryouts. It ended by asking "You got the love?"

To apply that question to learn-to-swim programs for kids, I'd ask "You got the joy?" By that I mean the joy of moving in the water that can make swimming an experience to last a lifetime. As an instructor of youngsters aged eight months to 12 years, I put that joy at the top of the list of elements of a successful swimming program.

Why Every Kid Should Learn to Swim

Introducing children to water at an early age makes sense. After all, water is part of our very essence. It surrounds us in the womb, and nourishes and cleanses us throughout our lives. On a more practical note, teaching a child swimming skills promotes safety, recreation, fitness, competition rehabilitation relaxation, self-esteem and more.

Our Lifestyle Swim School, located at the Boca Raton Resort and Club, is bordered by the Atlantic Ocean on one side and by the Intracoastal Waterway on the other. The whole of South Florida is laced with canals and dotted with millions of backyard and commercial pools. Children's safety in and around the water is a big concern. Parents want their kids to learn to swim so they won't drown.

Unfortunately, some so-called "drown-proofing" programs can be an intimidating introduction to the water. Some parents believe that this is the only way to protect their kids. However, children can acquire aquatic safety skills in a positive, loving way. In good swim programs, safety in the water naturally follows from feeling at home, relaxed and confident in the aquatic environment.

For swimming to appeal to children, the teaching, philosophy, goals and methods must be centered upon the child's well-being. Only if instruction is age-appropriate and designed in a positive, nurturing way, can there be a marriage between the water and a child's learning experience within it. (Note: No child, no matter how skilled, is "drown-proof." Always watch children carefully in and around the water.)

The Power of Positive Swimming Lessons

Infants and toddlers can learn to move in the water even before they start walking. Stimulating coordination and fitness in the water at a young age makes swimming an activity that lasts from infancy to old age. Few other sports can make that claim.

For many children, swimming lessons are among their first organized activities outside the home. Even for those youngsters who've had instruction in other areas, swimming offers exposure to a different environment. Teaching swimming is therefore an opportunity not only to introduce children to water, but also to teach them to trust adults and the world around them. Positive swimming lessons—those that treat children with dignity, patience, kindness and respect—help children expand and grow as swimmers and as total human beings.

Lessons that put the instructor's time frame and goals before the child's can have disastrous consequences. Vomiting, stuttering, nightmares and other negative reactions may occur, or a child may develop a fear of the water, of instructors, or even of all adults. The need for patience and setting appropriate goals cannot be overemphasized.

The Benefits of a Water-Loving Child

Once children learn to swim, swimming can be a recreational activity for the entire family. What other activity can be enjoyed by everyone from age eight months to 80 years and beyond? One mother in our program told me that the lessons not only brought her, her husband and their two-year-old son closer, but that the 20-mile drive to and from class also provided a welcome time for sharing.

Water, a most forgiving and cushioning medium, can also help children with special physical needs. We've worked with infants who were born prematurely and children with broken bones. Water can contribute to the growth and healing of these children. In addition, water can provide a comforting learning and play environment for physically disabled kids, who may be able to move more freely in the water than on land.

Older children whm have mastered swim skills are candidates for competitive swimming. Good competitive swimming programs teach children how to handle success and failure, and how to set and work toward clearly defined goals.

Swimming also can prepare a child for other aquatic sports such as sailing, snorkeling, diving, fishing and others. But even children who choose never to pursue other water sports gain self-confidence from learning to swim. You can see it in their eyes. One father in our program was amazed at the changes in his five-year-old daughter. After her swimming lessons she would come home happy, and clean her room and do chores without being asked.

Parents' Role in Teaching Kids to Swim

A swim program should involve one or both parents (or whoever is the child's main caretaker). When kids have their parents in the water with them, they feel more secure in an unfamiliar environment. This proximity creates a strong parent/child bond—swimming lessons ensure "quality time" that busy parents can spend with their children. The time together can be a period of growth and discovery for both parties.

Most parents in our program love the interaction with their infants and children. The water's buoyancy makes children light and easy to handle—they can be held comfortably face-to-face and eye-to-eye for extended periods.

Besides encouraging parents to join their children in the water during lessons, we urge parents to practice water skills at home with their children. This helps reinforce the skills learned in class, and allows the lessons to be more efficient.

How to Recognize a Good Learn-to-Swim Program

A successful learn-to-swim program should foster a positive learning environment. Good programs recognize that learning to swim is a long process that takes patience, practice and more patience. Never rush a child in swimming lessons for any reason, be it to save money, time, or the teacher's or parent's sanity. Some children will take to water like fish, others like trembling puppies. If the teacher and parent impose no time constraints or limitations, then the child won't feel anxious or coerced. Your child will tell you if he or she does not want to return to class. That's your signal to slow the pace, or to ask the teacher to take a more relaxed, low-key approach.

While private lessons can be effective, a group class is best for most children, particularly those aged four and under, and for frightened children up to age 12. Group classes are stimulating and fun. An "all for one and one for all" spirit predominates, and the process of individual learning becomes part of the progress of the whole group.

Our program does not exceed a teacher/student ratio of one to six. We encourage students to demonstrate their individual progress in order to get them more involved. In a class of 12 children, at least one student is always ready and willing to demonstrate. We consider this "peer learning" essential to the success of our program.

A child should never be forced to participate in a particular activity. If a child is crying or frightened, neither the teacher nor the parent should force him or her to stay in the pool. Let the child play alone—keeping an eye on him or her, of course—until he or she is ready to join in. The teacher and parent can work together to draw the child into the class a little more each day.

A program can promote self-esteem by making each child feel special. Teachers should know each child's name and use it both in and out of the water. It's rare that a youngster who feels confident and secure doesn't eventually learn to swim. Using force can actually slow a child's learning rate. No one can make a child learn to swim.

Water adjustment is the biggest hurdle for most young swimmers. About one out of every 10 swimmers we teach does not like water in his or her face. It takes some children up to 32 lessons before they can tolerate having water splashed on their faces, let alone submerging their faces in the water.

Good programs use distraction, demonstration and reward to guide frightened children through water adjustment. Squirt guns, puppets, squeeze toys, nerf balls, beach pails and other toys are used in a spirit of fun and gentleness to accustom students to having water on their faces. We use humor and songs ("If you're happy and you know it wash your face") to diffuse the children's fear. Often the best way to overcome fear is to watch a classmate or an older sibling put their face in the water. Some children feel better if they can wipe their faces with a towel after they get wet. Goggles may be helpful for children aged two and a half years and older.

Keeping Kids Comfortable in the Water

For children under 12, lessons should last about 25 to 30 minutes. Kids over four can build up to a 45-minute lesson if they wish.

The more often classes meet, the better—as long as the child doesn't feel rushed. Consistency is especially helpful for beginners. Students who attend class four days a week progress twice as fast as those who attend twice a week, and those who come twice a week learn twice as fast as those coming only once a week. However, all beginners will see major progress by the 16th lesson. Except for some very frightened students, all kids from eight months to 12 years will be propelling themselves some distance through the water by the end of a 16-lesson series.

Of course, not all kids (or parents) can attend class four days a week. However, a frightened child will benefit from coming to class as many days in a row as possible, and babies will learn to hold their breath more quickly if they can attend class more often.

The ideal water temperature for children to learn is 90 to 92 degrees, which will feel warm for adults. Most children can tolerate water as cool as 82 degrees if the air is still. Although a T-shirt or wet suit can help keep a kid comfortable in cool water, lessons should be cut short if children are cold.

Keeping the Accent on Fun

If learning to swim isn't fun, why bother? Fun eases kids' initial fears of the water and makes them want to keep returning to it. When your child grabs his swimsuit and stands at the door saying "pool," you know he's having fun.

Teachers and parents can keep swimming fun by making learning a game. Games impart skills without kids even realizing that they are learning. Even the most frightened child will want to jump through a hula-hoop, do the "alligator walk" on the pool steps, play water basketball, or negotiate an aquatic obstacle course.

There's nothing quite like seeing a child experience the joy of moving in the water. Fortunately, it's a joy that just about every child can have. In a supportive, child-centered atmosphere where the accent is on fun, children can master the swimming and water safety skills that will give them joy for a lifetime.

Rob McKay is the founder of Lifestyle Swim School and Lifestyle Video Productions in Boca Raton, Florida. He is an ASCA-certified Level IV swim coach, a certified Water Safety Instructor, and a charter member of The National Swim School Association.

Section 25.4

Toys of the Trade

Source: *Fitness Swimmer*, March 1993.

By Doug Stern

Kickboards, pull buoys, hand paddles and fins. You see these training aids at pools all the time, but do you know how they work and what they can do for your swimming? When used correctly, these "toys" reinforce and enhance proper stroke technique, isolate and challenge swim-specific muscles and add variety to workouts.

Whether you swim seriously or just love to play in the water, training aids can make your workout a great learning experience and a lot of fun. Knowing what to use and when to use it can make the difference between sore muscles and progressive conditioning, and it can do wonders for your technique.

I play at swimming, and I think of training tools as my toys. My kickboard is a speedboat with me as the motor. Pull-buoys allow me to rest my legs and float like a cork as I skewer through the water. Wearing hand paddles, I plane on the surface while powering down the pool.

Dozens of new toys are introduced each year, but most are variations on established themes. Paddles now come in multiple shapes, sizes and surface areas, for instance, and fins have recently been cut down to increase leg turnover. Coaches and experienced swimmers often modify their equipment to gain a competitive edge, and their modifications often become tomorrow's standard.

Let's look at some of these toys and how they work.

Kickboards

This old standby is most commonly used to isolate and overload the feet and legs. You've probably done the basic kickboard drill: Straighten your arms in front of you, rest them on top of the kickboard and grab the far end. Push off the wall and kick, using any motion you wish. A variation on this drill, which I call the "scooter," strengthens your upper body. To do the scooter drill, you extend one arm down the center of the board, grip the far end with that hand, and use the free arm to pull yourself through the water. This drill gives the muscles of the stroking arm a terrific workout, reinforces proper hand entry and works your legs

Have you always secretly wanted to be a surfer? Try standing on your kickboard with a drill I call "surf sculling." In the shallow end of the pool, place the board under your feet with your knees bent so the board hovers over the bottom. Using a tiny breaststroke, pull yourself through the water. Surf sculling is a great way to end a group workout with some fun and competition. Line up your buddies in the shallow end, on kickboards, and race across the pool at the word "Go!" Anyone who loses a kickboard must stop and reposition it before continuing.

Pull-Buoys

A pull-buoy is to the arms what a kickboard is to the legs. It allows you to isolate and condition your upper body. Made from two cylindrical floats held together by an adjustable rope or nylon strap, pull-buoys come in a variety of sizes, with the largest providing the most flotation. Big, muscular swimmers usually opt for large pull-buoys, while smaller swimmers (including most women, who have more body fat than men,and therefore float better) use small ones.

To use a pull-buoy, place it between your thighs as high as possible and hold it in place by squeezing your legs together. The buoy will hold your lower body on the surface while you stroke with your arms and rest your legs. Your first efforts may feel awkward because the buoy makes your body ride higher in the water than you're used to. Once you find the right size (a buoy that holds your body at or near the surface) and practice, you should feel comfortable.

Women (and men with a lot of body fat) who feel that a pull-buoy pitches them too far forward should try a smaller size. Men's muscular bodies don't float as well as women's, so they tend to like the "lift" a buoy provides. In fact, some men become dependent on a pull-buoy because they love to cruise through the water without kicking. Don't fall into this pattern if your kick is weak due to poor ankle flexibility. Instead, use a kickboard or other kick toy to improve your kick.

Besides strengthening the upper body, pull-buoys enhance your sense of body rotation in the water. When I introduced pull-buoys to one of my classes, participants felt as though they were rolling over when they swam the freestyle. Using a pull-buoy forced them to keep their legs close together; their feet couldn't stop their bodies from rolling as each arm reached forward. You will get used to this feeling, and your arms will counter the tendency to roll as they get stronger.

To keep the pull-buoy from slipping toward your knees on a long pulling set, loop a shoe lace through the bottom of your swimsuit and around the buoy. When I do this I can flip all my turns and never lose the pull-buoy.

Fins

Put on a pair of fins and you'll feel like a world-class swimmer. Like a kickboard, fins are used to overload and strengthen your legs. They also force you to point your toes and increase ankle flexibility. As a teacher and coach I use fins for both sprint-assisted training and neuromuscular learning (explained below).

There are three basic types of fins on the market today. Regular-size fins are used by scuba divers, surfers and general-purpose swimmers; small or "cut-down" fins are used in high-speed swim training;

and large "monofins" are used in underwater fin racing. Your choice of fins depends on your goals.

I use regular-size fins when I teach adult beginners to swim because my goal is to give them confidence and provide instant movement. A beginner's main concern is getting from point A to point B without drowning, and regular-size fins provide an easy form of propulsion. A beginner can put them on and move to swimming drills after just a few minutes of kicking and streamlining practice. With fins, beginning swimmers are able to reduce their learning time significantly.

I use small fins to work on ankle flexibility because they force me to point my toes. Regular-size fins and the new stiff small fins stretch my ankles too much, which can lead to stiffness and inflammation of the tendons. You can wear small fins to do kicking sets. Extend your arms in front of you and rest them on the water (no board), keeping the water at eye level.

I also use small fins for sprint-assisted interval workouts. My favorites are small high-speed training fins. Their light weight and thin construction allow for a quick kick, which coordinates well with my arm turnover. In addition, fins encourage neuromuscluar learning, which is a key ingredient of fast swimming. Conditioning your body is only one aspect of developing speed. Another is neuromuscular conditioning— teaching your muscles to respond. The only way to do this in swimming is to practice swimming fast, which is what wearing fins allows you to do. When I take my fins off I always swim my fastest times.

Hand Paddles

You can use hand paddles to overload your upper body, lengthen your stroke and reinforce proper pull pattern. If you own hand paddles, don't read any further until you inspect them. If yours have a finger and wrist strap, remove the wrist strap now. Since the straps prevent the paddles from falling off or shifting positions when you swim with faulty technique, you will not be able to identify poor technique if your paddles have them.

Wear your paddles the next time you do a pulling set. Notice how they move through the water, and be aware of when and if they fall off. Did it occur on hand entry or was it when you tried to lift your hand out of the water? You will only be able to discern this with strapless paddles.

Hand paddles, generally made of molded plastic, come in many shapes and sizes. Some are solid, some are perforated and some even have fins on the underside. Rectangular paddles are excellent for working on your stroke "catch." As you slip your hand into the water, you can feel the lift as you press into the stroke. Some world-class swimmers use serving-platter-sized paddles to work on their catch.

Ease into using rectangular paddles. They put tremendous stress on the muscles of the fingers, wrists and forearms, and can cause swimmer's shoulder if used too much, too soon. I like sprinting short distances with these paddles. They're great for strength and feel.

Tapered paddles are shaped like hands in that they're narrow at the fingertips and wider over the palm and wrist. This shape puts less stress on the hand, wrist, forearm and shoulder than rectangular paddles, but the tradeoff is less "feel" for the water. I can do long pull sets with these paddles with no shoulder discomfort, but since there is some overload of the large muscles of the chest and back, ease into using tapered paddles as well.

Webbed gloves and so-called "swim mitts," made from neoprene or lycra, can be used to increase the hand's surface area, just as paddles do. They do a good job of overloading the muscles during swimming and other types of aquatic exercise. However, I don't recommend gloves for improving your swimming technique because once they're on, they'll stay on, so you don't realize when your hand has entered the water incorrectly. Also, the webbing between the fingers changes the way water flows over your hand, creating turbulence as your hand enters the water.

A Few More Tricks

Here are some simple ways you can build strength without altering your stroke technique:

- Wear two bathing suits.

- Place small sponges in the sides of your suit.

- Wear a light T-shirt with cut-off sleeves.

- Swim wearing a pull-buoy fastened to your ankles with a large rubber band.

Toys make workouts fun. Remember, though, that they're only a part of the total plan. Their purpose is to make you a stronger equipment-free swimmer. Toys stress your muscles and must be used judiciously—staying injury-free should be your goal. Use toys a little at a time and build yardage slowly. Don't become a toy "junkie," doing all your long sets with them.

With these caveats in mind, play on!

Doug Stern has been teaching swimmers, triathletes and water runners for more than two decades.

Section 25.5

Swimming Through Your Pregnancy

Source: *Fitness Swimmer,* December 1993.

By Mary Bolster

Tink Murdoch started swimming laps just before the birth of her 11th child in 1965 and continued swimming through her last three pregnancies. Looking back on those days, Murdoch, now a 65-year-old triathlete from Princeton, New Jersey, says her doctors: didn't object to her swimming while pregnant but they didn't know much about its effects on the fetus, either.

Today, doctors know much more, thanks to interested sports physicians and obstetricians and to women, like Murdoch, who just know they feel better exercising through their pregnancies. Together, they continue to challenge conventional wisdom and push the parameters of currently accepted levels of exercise during pregnancy.

Changing Tides

Twenty five years ago women were encouraged to stop exercising once they became pregnant. Eight years ago the American College of Obstetricians and Gynecologists (ACOG), in Washington, D.C., issued guidelines that, for the first time, officially addressed the issue of exercise during pregnancy. Last year ACOG updated those guidelines and fully endorsed exercise, even for pregnant women who were previously sedentary.

Exercise Energizes

In its guidelines, ACOG suggests that staying active can reduce discomforts associated with pregnancy such as back pain, constipation and fatigue. In addition, ACOG says, regular exercise throughout: pregnancy helps women adjust to added weight, improves their sense of well-being and self-image and gives them more energy.

Paula Radulski, a 37-year-old swimmer from Londonderry, New Hampshire, has never read the ACOG guidelines but her experience of exercising while pregnant confirms much of what is included in them. "As I got heavier—I gained 31 pounds—swimming was wonderful. Once I got in the water, I felt like I was on the moon. I had more energy. I felt more euphoric."

Another swimmer, 35-year-old Ann Marie Resnick from New York City, offers a similar testimonial: "I was never, never tired, even up to the end, because I was in such good shape. I had the easiest pregnancy and I think it's because I swam."

Take a Load Off

These women and other water enthusiasts are finding increasing support for their decision to continue exercising through their pregnancy. Elsewhere in its guidelines, for example, ACOG urges pregnant women to avoid exercise that is high impact or involves jerky, bouncy movements, particularly in the last trimester. This is because during pregnancy, women release three hormones—relaxin, progesterone and estrogen—which loosen the tissue that connects muscles and joints in preparation for delivery. High-impact exercise can cause ligament damage or soreness.

Dr. Pat Kulpa, an obstetrician and sports physician in private practice in Tacoma, Washington, has studied the effects of exercise on more than 140 pregnant women. She has convinced many of her patients who run to switch to swimming in the third trimester because it gives them a good workout without as much wear and tear on their bodies. She even recommends it to non-swimmers. "It's an excellent time to learn to swim because you're so buoyant," she says.

Valerie Raffle's doctors had a similar attitude so the 33-year-old New Yorker switched to deep-water running in the fifth month of her pregnancy. "My doctors were against running on the road but said, 'swim all you want,'" she says. She found the pool soothing and completely comfortable. "[Deep-water running] didn't bother me at all.

There was no bouncing around. I couldn't shake. The float around me just had to get bigger," Raffle recalls.

Pam Ward, 37, preferred aerobics to running but now that she's pregnant she feels uncomfortable jumping up and down in class. "I prefer swimming. It eases the load. I have big babies and I'm not a big person so I get back pain. Swimming relieves everything," she says.

Avoid the Heat

Doctors such as Raffles', who follow ACOG guidelines, encourage their patients to exercise while pregnant, but not to the point of overheating. Although ACOG admits there is no conclusive proof that a mother's overheating negatively affects the fetus, it is concerned that prolonged hyperthermia—very high body temperature—during the first trimester may cause birth defects. Exercising in water may be an effective way to avoid overheating.

Research by Dr. Robert McMurray at the University of North Carolina in Raleigh appears to support water's anti-overheating property. He measured the core body temperature of seven pregnant women after they'd exercised at moderate intensity for 20 minutes on a stationary bike on dry land; he then repeated the process with them except he had them cycle in water. (Normal core body temperature for pregnant women is roughly 37.2 degrees Celcius.) He found that, while the women's core body temperature rose in both cases, the increase was less in water: 0.5 degrees Celcius on land and 0.1 degrees Celcius in the water.

Based on such findings, the Melpomene Institute in St. Paul, Minnesota, encourages pregnant women to exercise in a pool or air-conditioned health club to avoid overheating. A non-profit organization founded in 1982, the Institute researches and reports on the links between physical activity and women's health. It has produced *Exercise and Pregnancy*, a comprehensive packet on the subject.

The Institute may have to qualify its recommendations about overheating, however, in light of new findings from a recent study at the MetroHealth Medical Center in Cleveland. When the study's researchers, Drs. James Clapp and Kathy Little, compared the core body temperature of 22 pregnant women when they swam laps to when they rode exercise bikes, the results were slightly different.

According to Dr. Little, the women's core temperature increased more after swimming for 20 minutes (up 0.5 degrees Celcius) than after biking on land for 20 minutes (up .25 degrees Celcius). When asked about the discrepancy between these findings and those of McMurray's, Little admits varying water temperatures could have been a factor. However, she feels additional studies need to be conducted with larger test groups to look at how different types of exercise may affect blood flow and core temperature. In fact, she and Dr. Clapp are just starting to research pregnant women who have taken up deep-water running.

Target Practice

Research is still needed to determine a safe target heart rate for pregnant women during exercise. At the moment, there is no consensus among doctors. ACOG guidelines, which many sports physicians consider conservative, advise pregnant women not to exceed a target heart rate of 140 beats per minute.

Dr. Gloria Cohen, an obstetrician in private practice who specializes in sports medicine in Vancouver, British Columbia, thinks a better guide for determining a pregnant woman's target heart rate is her pre-pregnancy fitness level. "ACOG is on the conservative side which is important, but you should assess each patient individually," she says.

"Elite athletes are a different group. You can't generalize about them," notes Dr. Dan Ferrante, an obstetrician at Morristown Hospital in New Jersey. He and many other obstetricians and researchers recommend ACOG guidelines mainly for pregnant women who are sedentary and/or recreational athletes.

Stop and Listen

"You've got to individualize. That's one of the drawbacks of the guidelines," says Dr. Kulpa, who recommends the Borg's Rate of Perceived Exertion scale (see below) as an effective exercise determinant for pregnant women because it helps put them in tune with their bodies. When pregnant women listen to their bodies, they're better off, according to Kulpa. "My patients slowed themselves down. They did it without me telling them. Their bodies were telling them to slow down," she says.

That's what happened to Arlene White, a 37-year-old Masters swimmer from Fairfax, Virginia. "I was starting to swim slower, especially after my weight gain. My times were slower even with the same energy but I still felt good," White explains.

Kate Barbour, a 29-year-old who swims with Murdoch in Princeton, had a similar experience during her pregnancy. "I didn't strain myself. I just hung back. I swam with a slower group. As long as I didn't push myself, I could go forever," she remembers.

Huddie Walsh Murray is another swimmer who adjusted her workout pace during pregnancy. "I certainly got out of breath more easily but I still did some pretty hard sets," admits this 36-year-old Texan and mother of six. She was careful, she says, not to get her heart rate up too high for too long. "Butterfly was the easiest stroke for me but I didn't do it too hard," says Murray, who, in the 1970s, was ranked among the top 25 in the world in 200 butterfly.

Swimming Suits You

The benefits of water exercise and swimming are obvious to these women and, although swimming's effect on core body temperature is still being debated, its positive effect on ligaments and joints is crystal clear to many physicians.

"Swimming is an ideal sport," says Dr. Ralph Hale, executive director of ACOG and a member of the sports medicine team for the U.S. National Women's swimming team. "There are no contra-indications as far as I'm concerned. Water aerobics is [also] an excellent exercise. There's no stress on the hips or joints."

Ann Moore, MS, a nurse midwife in New York City with a degree in exercise physiology, echoes these sentiments: "Swimming is wonderful during pregnancy because of non-stress on joints. The horizontal position is also good. Swimming also helps to get rid of edema [swelling] during pregnancy."

"It's certainly a lot better than bronco-busting or downhill skiing," quips Dr. Lawrence Longo, a professor of obstetrics and gynecology at Loma Linda University School of Medicine in Loma Linda, California. "If one were looking for an ideal exercise during pregnancy, swimming would be it."

It was for Barbara Nathan, a 33-year-old technical writer from Bethel, Connecticut, who swam through her two pregnancies. "Swimming was great. It was therapeutic. The nice part was getting off my feet. I would get in the water and do some stretching," she says.

Moms Movin'

Eager to reap the benefits of water exercise, Tammie Thompson Perkins, a 35-year-old freelance writer from Truckee, California, joined an aquatics fitness class in nearby Tahoe City. Called *Movin' Mothers*, the program is designed specifically for pre- and post-natal women. "I thought the program was great, especially from a mental standpoint. It gave me the chance to talk to other women my age who were having kids," she says. Perkins also felt the program's founder, Sarah Lowis, was a particularly effective instructor. "Sarah knew her anatomy. She told us when to take it easy and when to push," she explains.

In an ideal world, all women would be exercising during pregnancy, but in reality, as Dr. Longo points out, "we still live in a society where 20 percent of pregnant women smoke and drink. I think a moderate exercise program should be part of a whole gestalt of how one approaches pregnancy."

Dr. Ferrante concurs, emphasizing that exercise benefits pregnant and non-pregnant women in the same way—lowers cholesterol levels, reduces the risk of heart disease and osteoporosis and increases energy levels. Also, studies published in *The American Journal of Obstetrics and Gynecology* and *Experientia* among others suggest that women who exercise during pregnancy cope much better with labor pains.

Dr. Kulpa says there is also evidence that exercise during pregnancy reduces the risk of gestational-induced diabetes. "Because exercise burns off glucose it helps to regulate sugar levels. Regular exercise isn't going to help all pregnant women reduce the risk, but it will help those who are borderline," she states.

Exceptions

Despite all the talk about the positive effects of exercise during pregnancy, a significant warning remains: Women with high-risk pregnancies should not exercise, regardless of their pre-pregnancy physical history and fitness. These guidelines and recommendations are tailored for women at low or no risk for complications during pregnancy.

The following tips, the medical community agrees, are useful for pregnant women who are considering swimming or some other form of exercise:

- Consult your doctor before starting an exercise program.

- Do not begin a rigorous training program during your pregnancy.

- Do not exercise to lose weight.

- Eat sensibly and regularly.

- Avoid overexertion.

- Listen to your body and learn to identify warning signals to stop or modify your exercise regimen.

- Do not dive or jump into the water and avoid water-skiing.

- If you feel contractions or joint pains, either stop swimming or choose a different stroke or style (e.g. sidestroke, breast stroke, kicking).

- Swim according to your abilities.

As Judy Mahle Lutter, co-founder of the Melpomene Institute, says, "Some [pregnant] women have been scolded by strangers for exercising, but intelligent women are still looking for scientific confirmation to bolster their instinct that this [exercise] is right."

Movin' Mothers' Lowis is providing some of that scientific confirmation. She's conducting research at the University of Nevada in Reno to determine the effects of water exercise. "We're finding that women can get in the water with very little risk [to the pregnancy]. The cushioning effect of water is protective to her joints...I'm not trying to be biased but the data are suggesting that water is better for the body," she says.

Apparently, pregnant women who swim or do water exercise don't need data to convince them of that.

Borg's Rate of Perceived Exertion (RPE)

Many exercisers measure their heart rate at the end of their workout to determine how hard they've pushed themselves. For some of you, this may be confusing, impractical or even inaccurate. Gunnar Borg, a Swedish psychophysicist, has devised a Rate of Perceived Exertion (RPE) scale which purports to be much simpler and just as accurate. In his research on physical exertion, he found that participants were able to determine their heart rate readings based on how hard they felt they were working during a given exercise. He then matched the feelings with numbers and found that when exercisers said they were working somewhat hard (a rating of between 12 and 13), they were working at 60 percent of their maximal heart rate reserve. Borg's research showed that the RPE scale correlated closely with heart rate, ventilation, oxygen consumption and blood lactate concentration. An RPE scale is particularly useful for swimmers and water exercisers since the heart rate is not a reliable measurement of exertion for aquatic exercise.

6	
7	Very, very light
8	
9	Very light
10	
11	Fairly light
12	
13	Somewhat hard
14	
15	Hard
16	
17	Very hard
18	
19	Very, very hard
20	

The numbers in the left-hand column correspond to a six-second land-based exercise heart rate.

Mary Bolster is Fitness Swimmer's *associate editor.*

Section 25.6

Taking It to the Water

Source: *Fitness Swimmer,* December 1993.

By Colleen Mogil

Aquatic Workouts are Making a Splash!

As a trained fitness instructor, I would never have considered including water aerobics as part of my high-intensity workout regimen. I thought water aerobics was for injury rehabilitation purposes and for pregnant women or the elderly who couldn't handle the sweating, grunting and oxygen-debt I'd come to associate with a "real" workout.

Naturally, I wasn't worried when I agreed to take over a colleague's aqua aerobics class while she went on vacation. At the time, I was teaching high-impact land aerobics to conditioned athletes in a posh fitness club. I figured I'd sit in on one of her classes and learn the routine.

As I expected, the movements mirrored many land aerobic exercises. What surprised me was how deliberate and challenging even the simplest moves became in the water. The workout proved tougher than I expected. At the same time, the water had a curious soothing effect on me. I felt unusually relaxed; a pleasant sensation I didn't normally associate with vigorous exercise.

In the U.S. alone, an estimated five million men and women seem to feel the same way. No longer considered to be a sport for just the elderly or injured athletes, aqua aerobics, people are finding, provides a complete training program by itself.

Colleen Brenan, a member of the Fort Lauderdale, Florida-based American Swim Coaches Association and a water aerobics instructor at several Philadelphia fitness clubs, says that aqua-aerobics has grown so popular that her classes have a three-session waiting list. According to Brenan, many of her students originally tried a class as part of injury rehabilitation. Once recovered, they just never gave it up.

"A few years ago, we couldn't get many people to take classes," says Kim King, M.S., aerobics director at The Sports Club/LA in Southern California. "Aqua aerobics was considered to be a 'wimpier' version of swimming or land aerobics. Even after we got some of the land-aerobic diehards into the pool, they often complained that they weren't getting a good workout." King says this is because the water has a cooling and soothing effect which camouflages the "burn" effect most land-aerobic diehards are used to feeling.

King, who holds a master's degree in kinesiology, says water's low-stress impact on the skeletal system is one of the main reasons her clients are switching to aqua aerobics, and to water sports in general. Since there is less impact, injury is very rare.

Aqua aerobics has a lot going for it. It's effective for cardiovascular conditioning because the water pressure increases the amount of oxygen the body absorbs. Your heart also works 17 beats less per minute in water than it does for comparable effort on land.

By exercising in the pool, you also help improve your circulation due to the water's massaging action. You'll also find you're more flexible during water exercise, allowing for greater range of motion. And, since water is 12 times more resistant than air, you'll build strength more easily. Finally, water exercise can help reduce your body fat. Studies have shown that people can burn more fat in water than on land, again due to water's resistance. Aqua aerobics can be as strenuous and intense as participants want to make it, according to Jan Berkbigler-Burke, owner of the Fit Bodies By Jan spa in Los Angeles and an instructor at The Sports Club LA. And, there are many resistance devices you can use to make your workout more challenging. For instance, webbed gloves help increase the intensity of upper-body moves by causing greater resistance. Curls and presses become more difficult when wearing gloves.

Foam dumbbells are also effective for upper-body toning. The arm exercises are done under the water with the dumbbells submerged. The water slows the motion, and the toning effects are similar to those found by doing light free weights. Buoys are another common device. They are placed under each arm for flotation during lower-body toning exercises. The newest pool flotation accessory is the "horse," a curved cylindrical tube that you can straddle or sit on as you work specific muscle groups.

Even step aerobics has gone aqua. Several companies, including swimsuit giant *Speedo Authentic Fitness*, have introduced step benches that rest on the bottom of the pool. Many class participants

347

claim he step provides a great lower-body workout, and that the effects are nothing short of amazing. "When my friends see how toned my legs have become, they always assume I've taken up weight training. Actually, all I do is a water step class twice a week," says one fan.

A typical Berkbigler-Burke class begins with a 10-minute walking-and-jogging warmup. This is followed by a 20-35 minute cardiovascular segment featuring vigorous moves (e.g. jumping jacks, knee lifts, skips, jogging, strides) designed to get the heart rate up. Lastly, there's a five- to 10-minute cardio-cooldown and stretch. Toning of specific muscle groups comes at the end of the class, and it is during this segment that the resistance equipment is used. To liven things up, instructors rely on good choreography, hot music and resistance tools. Berkbigler-Burke recommends that participants wear some type of cushioned, high-traction footwear so that the foot lands with more stability. There are several brands of footwear made specifically for water aerobics. You may also get by with aqua socks or sailing/rafting shoes.

Over and over again I heard participants say how much they enjoyed the social aspects of a water-exercise class. Since their breathing isn't labored, they find it easier to talk to one another.

"Yes, aqua aerobics keeps me in great shape," says one The Sports Club LA participant, "but it's the social aspect that keeps me coming back. These classes are not a chore. They're actually fun."

Water Workout

Jump on the water exercise bandwagon! To get you started, *Fitness Swimmer* asked deep-water exercise trainer Diahanne Bedortha to devise an aquatic circuit training program that offered a balanced, full-body workout for athletes of different fitness levels. The result is a fun, effective and simple way to achieve muscular and aerobic conditioning and strengthening. What's more, it can add a refreshing splash of variety to your existing exercise regimen, help with weight reduction, and is easily modified to higher- or lower-intensity levels.

An adaptation of the *AquaJogger Water Workout Gear Handbook*, Bedortha's circuit workout, designed for deep water, requires the use of flotation devices and resistance equipment. It consists of five stations, each with four exercises. All five stations should take you about 25 minutes. When finished, repeat all five stations once more for a total of a 50-minute workout.

Depending on your fitness level, you can increase the intensity of the work-out by increasing the speed of repetitions within each four-minute station, according to Bedortha. She recommends doing 10 repetitions of each move for an easy workout; 15 to 20 repetitions for a moderate workout; and 30 repetitions for a hard workout. Less fit individuals may want to adjust their work-to-rest ratios, slow the pace of the workout and employ larger movements, she adds.

You can perform the circuit on your own or as part of a group. In the former, you simply warm up and proceed through the circuit format. In group circuits, the group is divided evenly for each station and, after the warmup, each group rotates from station to station. Don't compete with someone on the same circuit who is fitter than you. You'll find yourself doing the exercises incorrectly just to keep up, getting discouraged or-worst of all-injuring yourself.

You do not have to follow the circuit in a specific order or format. Just make sure to include an adequate warmup and warmdown. Also, remember to follow the perceived exertion scale that is appropriate for you (see below) and to check with your doctor before starting this or any exercise program.

The Circuit

Warmup (five minutes)

You'll want to warm up in the deep end. Wearing your flotation belt, begin by simulating cross-country skiing for one minute, then work on abductors (moving arms and legs away from body) and adductors (moving arms and legs toward body) for 30 seconds. Follow with cross-country skiing for 30 seconds; heels behind (see **Station IV, exercise 4**) for 30 seconds; cross-country skiing for one minute. Finish up with straight-leg toe touch (see **Station I, exercise 4**) for 30 seconds

Station I: Aerobic/Endurance

Benefits: increases cardiovascular endurance, improves body composition, burns fat

Intensity: moderate

Duration: one minute each

1. Rock Climb

This is similar to running except the movement is like climbing a ladder diagonally. Reach forward with one arm, place it in the water and pull it through past your hip. Bring your opposite knee forward toward your chest while simultaneously pushing the other leg straight back until it's fully extended.

- Cup your hand to increase resistance.

- Avoid leaning forward.

- Do not lie on your stomach as you would when swimming. Instead, lower your hips so that you are working at an angle.

- Tighten your abdominals when you pull your knees to your chest.

2. Tires

This is similar to the football drill of running through two parallel lines of tires. Start with your body in an open and vertical position. Turn out your legs and flex your feet as you alternate pushing down with each leg.

- Try breaststroke arms, or scoop the water in toward your chest.

3. Bent-knee Cross-Country Ski

Your body is vertical in the water with legs bent to accommodate the water depth. Keeping your feet off the pool bottom, scissor your legs forward and backward from the hip. Move your arms and legs as if you were cross-country skiing.

- Concentrate on upper-body movements to maintain proper body balance.

4. Straight-leg Toe Touch

Start with your body in the vertical position. With your legs straight, bring each leg near the surface. Then, alternating left and right, reach for your toes with your opposite arm and bring the other arm behind you like a hurdler.

- Tighten your buttocks as you push each leg down; tighten your abdominals as you pull each leg up.

- Incorporate long body movements, and keep breathing comfortably. For endurance training, do this exercise at a consistent pace.

- Skip this exercise if you suffer from back pain.

Station II: Upper-Body Strengthening/Conditioning

(For increased resistance, use pull buoys or buoyant dumbbells.)

Benefits: increases muscle endurance and performance; tones and strengthens muscles; helps repair injured muscles

Intensity: moderate to hard

Duration: one minute each

1. Touch in Front/Touch in Back

With dumbbells submerged at your sides, bring them both together, touching in front of your body then touching in back.

2. Back-arm Extension

Begin with your arms held closely to your sides and elbows positioned four to five inches behind your body.

Flex and extend your arms forward and back at the elbow. Keep your hands cupped, wrists stiff, back straight and arms close to your sides.

- Keep your chest lifted and avoid leaning forward.

3. Cross-Country Ski

With dumbbells close to your sides, alternate swinging your arms back and forth, simulating the arm action of cross-country skiing.

- Don't let the dumbbells break the water's surface and keep them close to your sides.

- Maintain good posture.

4. Curls

With elbows bent and arms held tightly at your sides, alternate pulling the dumbbells down into the water with your arms. Vary the movement by gripping the dumbbells palm up or palm down.

- Each time you use dumbbells begin slowly, using small, controlled movements.
- Listen to your body and pace yourself accordingly. Gradually increase the speed of your movements as you become stronger and more comfortable in the water.

Station III: Intervals

Benefits: increases cardiovascular endurance and metabolic rate; burns fat

Intensity: hard to very hard (depending on your fitness level)

Duration: 45 seconds work, 15 seconds rest for each

1. Flutter Kick

Position your body as illustrated and kick vigorously forward and back.

- Start this movement from your hips and thighs.
- Keep your knees and ankles relaxed.
- Rest your hand against the side of the pool wall for greater balance.

2. Straight Toe-Touch

See **Station I, exercise 4**

3. Running

Position your body with your head, shoulders, hips and feet vertically aligned. Using a modified running/bicycle motion, move your legs and arms to simulate running.

- Double your speed to quadruple the resistance of this motion.

- Don't lean too far forward. Maintain an erect posture, keeping your shoulders back and hips in.

4. Tires

See **Station I, exercise 2**

Station IV: Lower-extremity Strengthening

Benefits: burns more calories at rest by increasing muscle mass; reduces stress and tension

Intensity: Hard to very hard, depending on fitness level

Duration: 45 seconds work, 15 seconds rest for each exercise

1. Sit Kicks

Sit as if in a straight back chair with your thighs stabilized. Alternating legs, kick out from the knee, then pull your heel back as if you are trying to kick your buttocks.

2. and 3. Abduction/Adduction

In a vertical position with your arms and legs straight and feet flexed, open and close your legs. Emphasize pushing out on abduction for one minute; emphasize pulling water in on adduction for one minute.

4. Heels Behind

Slanted on your side with your legs together, alternate bending your knees and kicking your heels to your buttocks.

For all of **Station IV**:

- Maintain correct body position.

- Make the movements smaller and faster.
- Use buoyant and resistant equipment to increase the intensity.
- Do not hold your breath.

Station V: Abdominals

Benefits: tightens the abdominal area

Intensity: moderate to hard

Duration: one minute each

1. Double-knee Crunch

Lie on your back with your hips submerged, your knees bent and your lower legs at the surface. Using your abdominal muscles, curl forward drawing your knees toward your chest. Extend your legs and repeat.

2. Double-knee Twist

While still on your back, put your legs together and bend your knees. Then, twist your knees to one side. Keeping your legs together, twist to the opposite side.

3. Jacknife

Again, lie on your back with your hips submerged and your lower legs at the water's surface, then drop your hips while reaching your arms past your toes. Lift your chest toward your knees.

4. Side Situps

Lie on your side with your knees drawn toward your chest. Focus on crunching in at your side as you pull both your upper and lower body in toward your waist. Change sides and repeat.

For all of **Station V:**

- Pull in your abdominal muscles and exhale during the contraction; squeeze your buttocks while releasing the movement.

- Try the moves in a vertical position if you experience any discomfort while lying on your back.

Warmdown (two minutes)

Since the body cools down so quickly in the water, keep your warmdown short to minimize the risk of muscle tightening. After finishing the last station, go right in to cross-country skiing for one minute. Make sure to go slowly and work through a full range of motion. Then do straight-leg 2 toe touches for 15 seconds. With your legs submerged and in the bent-knee position, straighten your right leg, then point and flex your ankles five times; circle to the right; circle to the left. Bring your leg down and repeat the set for your left leg. Finally, move your head from side-to-side for five to eight repetitions.

Noble's Rate of Perceived Exertion Scale

Number	Perceived	% of VO_2* Max. Exertion
1	Very easy	
2	Easy	45
3	Moderate	55
4	Somewhat hard	62
5	Hard	70
6		
7	Very hard	85
8		
9		
10	Very, very hard	100

*VO2 Max is the maximum amount of oxygen that can be taken in by your body, delivered to your muscles, and used.

Colleen Mogil is an actress and freelance writer living in West Hollywood, California.

Diahanne Bedortha, a water-exercise pioneer, has been teaching for more than 10 years.

Chapter 26

How Tennis Affects Your Body

How does playing tennis affect your aerobic capacity? Your anaerobic capacity? Your heart rate? Your overall health?

How do your muscles and joints react to the movements intrinsic to tennis? To the forces generated from hitting a tennis ball? Does tennis make you strong? Flexible? Injury-prone?

For the past four years, researchers at the Lexington Clinic Sports Medicine Center in Kentucky have attempted to answer these and other questions to determine the specific effects the sport of tennis has on the body. Conducted by Ben Kibler, M.D., medical director of the Lexington center and a member of the U.S. Tennis Association's sport science committee, and Jeff Chandler, Ed.D., the center's director of research and a certified strength and conditioning specialist, the research has been quite revealing.

It has shown what tennis can—and can't— do for you. It has helped determine the healthy—and not so healthy—effects of tennis participation. Such information will help you play better, avoid injuries and improve your overall fitness and health.

Tennis: Aerobic or anaerobic?

The demands of various sports and activities differ. When running a marathon, you primarily use your aerobic system, which carries oxygen to the muscles; when running a 100-meter sprint, you use your

---

Tennis, May, 1992.

anaerobic system, which employs energy stored within the muscles. Though several factors determine the exact metabolic demand of a tennis workout, it has been estimated that tennis is approximately 90 percent anaerobic and 10 percent aerobic.

The numbers make sense when you consider that, in a tennis match, you rest much more than you play. Figures calculated by Bill Jacobson, inventor of CompuTennis, computer training programs for tennis players, show that the rest/work ratio in today's pro game is at least 4/1, and is significantly higher on fast surfaces such as grass (see "The Nine-Minute Workout" page 362). As an amateur player, with no one watching the clock between points and games, you also spend more time catching your breath than chasing down lobs.

Thus, the nature of tennis—short bursts of energy followed by longer recovery periods—makes it primarily an anaerobic activity. Rarely do you have to maintain muscle movement long enough during a point for your aerobic system—which is engaged after one to two minutes of continuous activity— to kick in, even on clay courts.

Instead, you mainly rely on the anaerobic energy source of ATP (which, in this context, stands for adenosine triphosphate, not Association of Tennis Professionals). This chemical found in the muscles can be engaged for immediate use, but it only lasts about 10 seconds. Your body, however, naturally replenishes ATP between points, games and changeovers. Research shows that within 20 seconds, 50 percent of the depleted ATP is replenished; in 40 seconds, 75 percent is replenished; and in 60 seconds, 87 percent is replenished.

Playing tennis regularly works your anaerobic system, training it to operate more efficiently. The result? You will react quicker and run faster. Tennis also helps your body increase its anaerobic endurance capacity. That is, it will help you perform better during longer bursts of intense movement.

But the other side of the tennis coin—only 10 percent aerobic metabolic demands—naturally concerns many health-conscious players. They fear that tennis, as a primarily anaerobic activity, does not provide the cardio-respiratory benefits associated with aerobic exercise— long, continuous activity that increases the body's efficiency to move oxygen from the lungs to the blood, then to the heart and muscles. Research has shown that by working these four areas—lungs, blood, heart and muscles—you can reap numerous health benefits: increased blood flow, decreased blood pressure and decreased risk of cardiovascular disease.

Tennis does not provide the same cardio-respiratory benefits as long-distance running and bicycling. The key word here, though, is "same." Studies of elite junior tennis players conducted at the Lexington Clinic Sports Medicine Center found that the players did, in fact, score very high in cardio-respiratory endurance tests. "They're not as aerobically fit as marathoners", says Kibler, "but tennis players still benefit aerobically from their sport."

A growing body of data supports the Lexington Clinic findings, suggesting that repeated short bursts of energy, such as the work patterns in tennis, do provide significant aerobic benefits. The reasons? For one, the aerobic system has been found to work during recovery from intense exercise. When you catch your breath between hard-fought points, you actually engage the aerobic system.

Second, there are two components to increasing aerobic endurance. Playing tennis doesn't dramatically increase the use of oxygen by the muscles, but it does improve the ability by the heart to pump blood.

"Tennis is not a do-all, end-all:" says Kibler. "But for the big question—am I helping my cardiovascular fitness?—the overall answer is yes. You're stimulating the heart, you're making the heart work harder and you're improving your heart's ability to pump blood."

The amount of aerobic benefits you can gain from tennis will vary based on dosage (singles more than doubles, for example), the level of competition (serious competition more than hit-and-giggle matches), the initial fitness level of the player (the worse your physical condition, the more dramatic the aerobic effect) and the style of play (baseliners more than serve-and-volleyers).

Thus, as an intense anaerobic activity that also provides certain aerobic benefits, playing tennis provides many rewards associated with better fitness. Studies done at the Institute of Aerobics Research in Dallas found that physically fit men are 53 percent less at risk of premature death, and physically fit women are 98 percent less at risk of premature death than sedentary men and women. For example, the researchers found that physically fit men die four times less often from cancer and are less likely to die from cardiovascular disease than unfit men.

Playing tennis regularly will raise the percentage of beneficial HDL cholesterol and help reduce harmful LDL cholesterol. It also will lower blood pressure, and help you manage stress: Gallup surveys have shown that exercisers are more likely to be able to relax when under pressure.

Strength and Flexibility

Kibler adds an important warning to all this good news: "You may have a good heart from playing tennis," he says, "but you're not going to be able to continue playing if your shoulder is all screwed up."

The inherent nature of tennis—the twisting and turning, the starting and stopping— puts many demands on various parts of your body. When you combine the anatomical demands with the above-discussed metabolic demands, you can understand why tennis compares so favorably to other sports in developing all-around athletic ability (see "How Does Tennis Muscle Up?" page 362).

But playing tennis creates muscular imbalances that can lead to injury, making it essential to stretch and strengthen your body away from the tennis courts. Although every player's body is different, Kibler and Chandler have pinpointed four distinct areas of the anatomy that adapt unnaturally to the demands placed on them by tennis.

1. The back of the dominant or playing shoulder;

2. The inside and outside of the dominant elbow;

3. The lower back, especially on the side opposite the dominant arm;

4. The hip, especially on the side opposite the dominant arm.

These are, in a sense, the four weak links in a tennis player's body. Tennis develops muscles in these areas, but in such an unbalanced fashion that they become vulnerable spots for injuries. Also, while the body possesses many muscles that generate power to hit a tennis ball, it has relatively few muscles to absorb—or dispense—the stress that occurs during a tennis stroke.

The shoulder muscles, for example, rotate in several different directions to produce power for serves and ground strokes. But the glenoid or socket of the shoulder joint also must withstand forces estimated to be two times a person's body weight, and it's often ill-equipped to do that.

The forces exerted on the shoulder by a tennis stroke are just part of the complex kinetic chain of activity that starts with the planting of your feet and continues through to your racquet swing. While the excessive stress put on the elbow has been well-documented over the years, most tennis players are unaware that their sport also puts an inordinate amount of stress on the back and hips. These two areas not only serve as the center of rotation during all tennis strokes, but also as the key transfer link for the large forces generated by the legs to the shoulder and arm.

"The ultimate effects of all these forces placed on these four specific areas are decreased flexibility and strength," says Chandler.

In one Lexington Clinic study, researchers measured the flexibility of 139 non-tennis athletes to that of 86 elite junior tennis players. The tennis players were significantly tighter in several areas, specifically where the muscles were required to rotate excessively during movements required for tennis strokes. Another study found that tennis significantly strengthened some of a tennis player's shoulder muscles but not others.

These imbalances predispose tennis players to injury. You probably know a handful of players at your club who have suffered from rotator cuff injuries, tennis elbow and back ailments. Some tennis players have had to undergo hip replacements. For these reasons, Kibler and Chandler recommend that all tennis players employ a stretching and strengthening program to correct these deficits.

Although the pounding and twisting involved in tennis can pose potential problems, it should not be viewed simply as a negative effect of the sport. On the contrary, active participation in tennis certainly will prove to be more beneficial for your overall physical condition than inactivity. When you play tennis, you move practically all your muscles, stimulating blood flow and strengthening them through constant use.

Older women, especially, will benefit from the time spent on the courts. Playing tennis regularly delays bone loss and promotes bone formation in women most at risk of osteoporosis, a thinning of the bones that coincides with aging. It also eases leg fatigue and improves circulation so blood doesn't pool in leg veins, which causes varicose veins.

A Healthy Game

The research by Kibler and Chandler, which they will continue to pursue, certainly offers encouraging news for tennis players of all ages and abilities. It supports what many tennis players always have felt: The sport of tennis provides them with an invigorating workout that, if supplemented by strength and flexibility exercises to offset potential injuries, can reap healthy rewards for a lifetime. What more can one ask for from a game?

How Does Tennis Muscle Up?

	Flexibility	Strength	Speed	Anaerobic	Aerobic	
Tennis	3	3	4	4	4:	**18**
Basketball	3	3	4	4	4:	**18**
Pitching	4	3	2	4	4:	**17**
Sprinting	4	3	4	4	2:	**17**
Football	2	4	4	4	2:	**16**
Baseball	3	3	3	3	2:	**14**
Running	3	2	2	2	4:	**13**

Muscle tissue has five measurable characteristics basic to all athletic activity: flexibility, strength, speed, anaerobic endurance and aerobic endurance. This Lexington Clinic sports characterization chart shows that tennis can provide you with the potential to reap significant fitness benefits.

4: Essential to best performance.
3: Important to best performance.
2: Needed at a certain level, usually for injury prevention.
1: Needed at a minimal level.

The Nine-Minute Workout

If you missed the 1991 Wimbledon final between Boris Becker and Michael Stich, don't despair: You missed only nine minutes of actual playing! But you did miss hours of string repositioning and toweling off.

Statistician Bill Jacobson of CompuTennis says that today's power-based pro tennis makes the sport more a waiting game than a playing one. The average length of a point in the Becker/Stich serving contest was 2.6 seconds. This computed to three minutes and 42 seconds of actual play in an hour, only nine minutes during the entire two-hour, 31-minute match. "About 90 percent of the time on court is spent recovering from bursts of energy," concludes Jacobson, "not spending it."

When you compare the Stich/Becker match to the classic John McEnroe/Bjorn Borg 1980 Wimbledon final, where the two superstars were actually moving and hitting for 12 minutes per hour, you realize how much the men's game has evolved away from fitness and finesse to power and punch. The McEnroe/Borg numbers on grass from 12 years ago now compare only to duels on slower clay courts. In the 1991 French Open final, baseliners Jim Courier and Andre Agassi battled nearly 15 minutes each hour.

Clearly, in today's pro game, patience in only a high virtue *between* points.

Chapter 27

Walking for Exercise and Pleasure

Walking: An Exercise for All Ages

Walking is easily the most popular form of exercise. Other activities generate more conversation and media coverage, but none of them approaches walking in number of participants. Approximately half of the 165 million American adults (18 years of age and older) claim they exercise regularly, and the number who walk for exercise is increasing every year.

Walking is the only exercise in which the rate of participation does not decline in the middle and later years. In a national survey, the highest percentage of regular walkers (39.4%) for any group was found among men 65 years of age and older.

Unlike tennis, running, skiing, and other activities that have gained great popularity fairly recently, walking has been widely practiced as a recreational and fitness activity throughout recorded history. Classical and early English literature seems to have been written largely by men who were prodigious walkers, and Emerson and Thoreau helped carry on the tradition in America. Among American presidents, the most famous walkers included Jefferson, Lincoln, and Truman.

Walking today is riding a wave of popularity that draws its strength from a rediscovery of walking's utility, pleasures, and health-giving qualities. This chapter is for those who want to join that movement.

President's Council on Physical Fitness and Sports. GPO: 1994-155-072.

Walking: The Slower, Surer Way to Fitness

People walk for many reasons: for pleasure . . . to rid themselves of tensions . . . to find solitude . . . or to get from one place to another. Nearly everyone who walks regularly does so at least in part because of a conviction that it is good exercise.

Often dismissed in the past as being "too easy" to be taken seriously, walking recently has gained new respect as a means of improving physical fitness. Studies show that, when done briskly on a regular schedule, it can improve the body's ability to consume oxygen during exertion, lower the resting heart rate, reduce blood pressure, and increase the efficiency of the heart and lungs. It also helps burn excess calories.

Since obesity and high blood pressure are among the leading risk factors for heart attack and stroke, walking offers protection against two of our major killers.

Waiking burns approximately the same amount of calories per mile as does running, a fact particularly appealing to those who find it difficult to sustain the jarring effects of long distance jogging. Brisk walking one mile in 15 minutes burns just about the same number of calories as jogging an equal distance in 8½ minutes. In weight-bearing activities like walking, heavier individuals will burn more calories than lighter persons. For example, studies show that a 110-pound person burns about half as many calories as a 216-pound person walking at the same pace for the same distance.

Although increasing walking speed does not burn significantly more calories per mile, a more vigorous walking pace will produce more dramatic conditioning effects. When looking at the benefits to heart/lung endurance, how far one improves depends on his/her initial fitness level. Someone starting out in poor shape will benefit from a slow speed of walking whereby someone in better condition would need to walk faster and/or farther to improve. Recent studies show that there are also residual benefits to vigorous exercise. For a period of time after a dynamic workout, one's metabolism remains elevated above normal which results in additional calories burned.

In some weight-loss and conditioning studies, walking actually has proven to be more effective than running and other more highly-touted activities. That's because it's virtually injury-free and has the lowest dropout rate of any form of exercise.

Like other forms of exercise, walking appears to have a substantial psychological payoff. Beginning walkers almost invariably report that they feel better and sleep better, and that their mental outlook improves.

Walking also can exert a favorable influence on personal habits. For example, smokers who begin walking often cut down or quit. There are two reasons for this. One, it is difficult to exercise vigorously if you smoke, and two, better physical condition encourages a desire to improve other aspects of one's life.

In addition to the qualities it has in common with other activities, walking has several unique advantages. Some of these are:

Almost everyone can do it. You don't have to take lessons to learn how to walk. Probably all you need to do to become a serious walker is step up your pace and distance and walk more often.

You can do it almost anywhere. All you have to do to find a place to walk is step outside your door. Almost any sidewalk, street, road, trail! park, field, or shopping mall will do. The variety of settings available is one of the things that makes walking such a practical and pleasurable activity.

You can do it almost anytime. You don't have to find a partner or get a team together to walk, so you can set your own schedule. Weather doesn't pose the same problems and uncertainties that it does in many sports. Walking is not a seasonal activity, and you can do it in extreme temperatures that would rule out other activities.

It doesn't cost anything. You don't have to pay fees or join a private club to become a walker. The only equipment required is a sturdy, comfortable pair of shoes.

Walking for Physical Fitness

What makes a walk a workout? It's largely a matter of pace and distance. When you're walking for exercise, you don't saunter, stroll, or shuffle. Instead, you move out at a steady clip that is brisk enough to make your heart beat faster and cause you to breathe more deeply.

Here are some tips to help you develop an efficient walking style:

- Hold head erect and keep back straight and abdomen flat. Toes should point straight ahead and arms should swing loosely at sides.

- Land on the heel of the foot and roll forward to drive off the ball of the foot. Walking only on the ball of the foot, or in a flatfooted style, may cause fatigue and soreness.

- Take long, easy strides, but don't strain for distance. When walking up or down hills, or at a very rapid pace, lean forward slightly.

- Breathe deeply (with mouth open, if that is more comfortable).

What to Wear When Walking

A good pair of shoes is the only "special equipment" required by the walker. Any shoes that are comfortable, provide good support, and don't cause blisters or calluses will do, but here are some suggestions to help you make your selection:

- Good running shoes (the training models with heavy soles) are good walking shoes, as are some of the lighter trail and hiking boots and casual shoes with heavy rubber or crepe rubber soles.

- Whatever kind of shoe you select, it should have arch supports and should elevate the heel one-half to three-quarters of an inch above the sole of the foot.

- Choose a shoe with uppers made of materials that "breathe," such as leather or nylon mesh.

Weather will dictate the rest of your attire. As a general rule, you will want to wear lighter clothing than temperatures seem to indicate. Walking generates lots of body heat.

In cold weather, it's better to wear several layers of light clothing than one or two heavy layers. The extra layers help trap heat, and they are easy to shed if you get too warm. A wool watch cap or ski cap also will help trap body heat and provide protection for the head in very cold temperatures.

Walking Poses Few Health Risks

If you are free of serious health problems, you can start walking with confidence. Walking is not as strenuous as running, bicycling, or swimming and consequently involves almost no risk to health. Of course, this statement assumes that you will exercise good judgment and not try to exceed the limits of your condition.

Most physicians recommend annual physical examinations for persons over 40 or 45 years of age. Also, if you have high blood pressure or other cardiovascular problems, you should consult your physician before beginning any kind of exercise program.

Warmup and Conditioning Exercises

Walking is good exercise for the legs, heart, and lungs, but it is not a complete exercise program. Persons who limit themselves to walking tend to become stiff and inflexible, with short, tight muscles in the back and backs of the legs. They also may lack muscle tone and strength in the trunk and upper body. These conditions can lead to poor posture and chronic lower-back pain, a problem that partially cripples or disables thousands of middle-aged and older Americans.

The exercises that follow are designed to increase flexibility and strength and to serve as a "warm-up" for walking. Always do the exercises before walking.

Stretcher: Stand facing wall arms' length away. Lean forward and place palms of hands flat against wall, slightly below shoulder height. Keep back straight, heels firmly on floor, and slowly bend elbows until forehead touches wall. Tuck hips toward wall and hold position for 20 seconds. Repeat exercise with knees slightly flexed.

Reach and Bend: Stand erect with feet shoulder-width apart and arms extended over head. Reach as high as possible while keeping heels on floor and hold for 10 counts. Flex knees slightly and bend slowly at waist, touching floor between feet with fingers. Hold for 10 counts. (If you can't touch the floor, try to touch the tops of your shoes.) Repeat entire sequence 2 to 5 times.

Knee Pull: Lie flat on back with legs extended and arms at sides. Lock arms around legs just below knees and pull knees to chest, raising buttocks slightly off floor. Hold for 10 to 15 counts. (If you have knee problems, you may find it easier to lock arms behind knees.) Repeat exercise 3 to 5 times.

Situp: Several versions of the sit-up are listed in reverse order of difficulty (easiest one listed first, most difficult one last). Start with the sit-up that you can do three times without undue strain. When you are able to do 10 repetitions of the exercise without great difficulty, move on to a more difficult version.

- Lie flat on back with arms at sides, palms down, and knees slightly bent. Curl head forward until you can see past feet, hold for three counts, then lower to start position. Repeat exercise 3 to 10 times.

- Lie flat on back with arms at sides, palms down, and knees slightly bent. Roll forward until upper body is at 45-degree angle to floor, then return to starting position. Repeat exercise 3 to 10 times.

- Lie flat on back with arms at sides, palms down, and knees slightly bent. Roll forward to sitting position, then return to starting position. Repeat exercise 3 to 10 times.

- Lie flat on back with arms crossed on chest and knees slightly bent. Roll forward to sitting position, then return to starting position. Repeat exercise 3 to 10 times.

- Lie flat on back with hands laced in back of head and knees slightly bent. Roll forward to sitting position, then return to starting position. Repeat exercise 3 to 15 times.

How Far? . . . How Fast? . . . How Soon?

Now that you have decided to begin walking for exercise, you may be shocked at how poor your condition is. If at first you have difficulty in meeting the standards suggested here, don't be discouraged. You can systematically build your stamina and strength back to acceptable levels. Patience is the key to success. Some experts say that it takes a month of reconditioning to make up for each year of physical inactivity.

No one can tell you exactly how far or how fast to walk at the start, but you can determine the proper pace and distance by experimenting. We recommend that you begin by walking for 20 minutes at least four or five times a week at a pace that feels comfortable to you. If that proves to be too tiring, or too easy, reduce or lengthen your time accordingly.

Some very old people and some people who are ill begin by walking for one or two minutes, resting a minute, and repeating this cycle until they begin to be fatigued. Where you have to start isn't important; it's where you're going that counts.

As your condition improves, you should gradually increase your time and pace. After you have been walking for 20 minutes several days a week for one month, start walking 30 minutes per outing. Eventually, your goal should be to get to the place where you can comfortably walk three miles in 45 minutes, but there is no hurry about getting there.

The speed at which you walk is less important than the time you devote to it, although we recommend that you walk as briskly as your condition permits. It takes about 20 minutes for your body to begin realizing the "training effects" of sustained exercise.

The "talk test" can help you find the right pace. You should be able to carry on a conversation while walking. If you're too breathless to talk, you're going too fast.

The more often you walk, the faster you will improve. Three workouts a week are considered to be a "maintenance level" of exercise. More frequent workouts are required for swift improvement.

Listen to Your Body

Listen to your body when you walk. If you develop dizziness, pain, nausea, or any other unusual symptom, slow down or stop. If the problem persists, see your physician before walking again.

Don't try to compete with others when walking. Even individuals of similar age and build vary widely in their capacity for exercise. Your objective should be to steadily improve your own performance, not to walk farther or faster than someone else.

The most important thing is simply to set aside part of each day and walk. No matter what your age or condition, it's a practice that can make you healthier and happier.

Chapter 28

Weight Training: Putting a Lift in Your Workout

By Guyton Hornsby

Years ago, strength training was left to big, intimidating, muscular men down at the local gym. You remember these guys...they kicked sand on many of us at the beach. But times have changed. Local gyms have turned into glamorous health clubs and now men and women of all sizes can be found lifting barbells and pushing sophisticated resistance machines. (And no one kicks sand anymore.)

One reason is that people are beginning to realize that aerobic training is not enough to develop all aspects of physical fitness. They're learning that a comprehensive fitness program must also include exercise to develop muscle strength and endurance.

And as popularity has risen, so has research into and knowledge about the methods and effects of strength training. For years, people have known that lifting progressively heavier weights can make muscles stronger, but training methods are being more clearly defined. Different training methods can be used to produce very different results. The type of program that's best for you will depend on what you want to achieve.

There are a few things to consider before jumping into a weight training program. One of the most important steps is to check with your health-care team to make certain that weight training is good for you. (Weight training can be harmful for people with some com-

Diabetes Forecast: January, 1990. Used by Permission. (See editor's note at end of chapter.)

373

plications. For example, weight training may be harmful for someone with retinopathy, making the condition worse.)

If you're thinking about starting a weight training program, you probably have several questions. The following are the answers to some common questions people have about weight training.

What is Weight Training?

Weight training is a planned program whereby you develop muscular strength and endurance either by lifting free weights (barbells and dumbbells) or on a machine that provides resistance for your muscles to work against.

How Can Weight Training Help You?

Weight training can make you look and feel better, and work and play better. It also protects against injuries and improves health.

One of the most popular goals of weight training is building an attractive body. Competitive body builders spend many hours shaping massive muscles to achieve ideal proportions. Many other people want to have muscles that are toned, defined, and wellshaped. These goals are actually quite similar. The only difference in body building and general toning is in the magnitude of the change that is desired (just how big do you want that muscle?).

Physical appearance largely depends on body composition—the body's ratio of muscle to fat. Weight training is a good choice for improving body composition because it affects both muscle and fat. Building 2 pounds of muscle can increase metabolism by as much as 100 calories per day. In one year, this simple change can take off 10 pounds of fat. (You may not lose 10 pounds—you may lose 10 pounds of fat and shift that weight to 10 pounds of muscle, altering your body composition.)

Many people are afraid to train with weights because they don't want to build big muscles. Big muscles are not built by accident and are not built overnight. It takes tremendous genetic potential and years of specific training to become a champion bodybuilder. Very few people are gifted with the natural ability to make huge gains in muscle size.

Instead of being afraid of developing large muscles, people should be concerned about having too little muscle. As people grow older and become less active, muscles that are not used shrink in size. In shrinking, they lose power. This loss of muscle lowers the metabolic rate. If adjustments are not made in diet, the extra calories are stored as fat. Proper weight training can restore muscle size, prevent the drop in metabolism, and improve body composition.

Activities such as carrying groceries, lifting a suitcase, and climbing up stairs all take considerable muscle force. Stronger muscles allow people to perform their daily tasks with more energy and less effort. The capacity for work increases and muscles are more resistant to fatigue. "Work," as used here, means your body's ability to be active. Weight training can help you become more productive and can contribute to your enjoyment of life.

Stronger muscles also allow you to run faster, jump higher, move with agility, and play without tiring. Improved speed, power, flexibility, and muscular endurance can give you an edge in your sports activities. Stronger muscles can also make house cleaning, yard work, and Saturday morning errand-running less tiring.

Many sports overdevelop certain muscles, leaving other muscles relatively weak. For example, many runners have strong leg muscles, but their upper bodies are underdeveloped. Weight training allows you to select specific exercises to develop all major muscle groups and reduces the risk of injury. Stronger, balanced muscles are better able to protect the joints they cross.

Aerobic activities such as walking, jogging, and bicycling burn many calories and are important for improving heart and lung health. But adequate strength and endurance is required to perform repetitive muscle contractions, such as those involved in these activities.

Weight training can improve health in several other important ways. When muscles become stronger, physical work becomes easier, and the relative stress on the heart is reduced. Muscle contractions place tension on bones and increase their mineral content. This makes bones more dense and may be especially important in preventing osteoporosis, a disease associated with excessive bone loss. The same changes that make people look better—increased muscle and decreased fat—tend to make people healthier.

How Do Muscles Get Stronger?

Training can make muscles stronger in two basic ways: One, muscles can get bigger and two, the nervous system can learn to recruit muscles more effectively. Before a muscle contracts it must receive a message or impulse carried by the nervous system. A person trained by lifting weights is able to call on more individual muscle fibers, resulting in increased muscle recruitment and greater muscle force. Specific programs can improve strength either by increasing muscle size, by improving recruitment without large changes in size, or by increasing both muscle size and muscle recruitment.

Muscles become stronger only by working against heavier loads. As you get stronger, you need to increase the weight you lift to keep pace with improved fitness. For example, if you have been lifting 30 pounds for a period of time, you may need to increase that weight by 5 pounds to continue to improve.

The actual gains in strength, and the type of strength that is developed, will depend on how often, how hard, and how long you lift.

How often you train is up to you. However, muscles become stronger when they are exercised two to three times a week. Muscles need rest to develop properly. For most people, two days are enough for the muscles to recover. Experts often recommend that you NOT train every day because the muscle needs the rest.

You may choose to lift two or three days each week with 8 to 10 exercises that cover muscle groups over the entire body. If you plan to use more than 10 exercises, you probably would be better off using a split routine. For example, you might train the legs, shoulders, and abdomen on Mondays and Thursdays, and the chest, back, and arms on Tuesdays and Fridays. By splitting the workouts, you could train four or even six days a week, without training the same muscle group more than three times a week.

How hard you train is possibly the single most important aspect of training. The relative weight you want to train with will depend on what you want to accomplish. Training intensity (how much weight is on the bar) is frequently based on a percentage of the maximum weight you can lift one time for each different lift. This is called the one-repetition maximum or 1RM. Knowing your 1RM will help you determine how much weight to train with on the bench press, or any other lift. The amount of weight you choose to train with will depend on your goals.

For example, assume the maximum you can lift on the bench press is 80 pounds. 80 pounds would then be your 1RM for the bench press. Lifting very light weights of 40 to 60 percent of 1RM can develop good muscle endurance, but improvements in strength and size are minimal. At this level, if you use the bench press example of 80 pounds, you then would lift between 32 and 48 pounds.

Using moderate training loads of 70 to 80 percent of 1RM develops good muscle strength as well as endurance. (From the example, you'd then lift between 56 to 64 pounds.) If you lift these weights many times, muscle size will also improve. To develop strength (but not long-term endurance) lift heavy weights of 85 percent to 95 percent of 1RM. Doing this helps the nervous system learn how to effectively exert maximal force. (Here, you'd be training at weights between 68 and 76 pounds, if you used the bench press example above.)

It's not necessary or advisable to actually lift maximal weights unless you are a competitive weightlifter or powerlifter. It is far safer to determine lifting intensity by seeing how many times you can lift a weight that is comfortable for you to handle.

In general, very light weights (40 to 60 percent 1RM) can be lifted 20 to 40 times. Moderately heavy weights (70 to 80 percent 1RM) can be lifted 10 to 15 times, and very heavy weights (85 to 95 percent 1RM) can be lifted only two to six times.

How Long Should I Train?

The total time you spend lifting weights is a combination of the time you actually spend lifting the weights and the time you spend resting between lifts. How long you train will depend on what you are trying to accomplish. A general fitness program will probably take 20 to 30 minutes, while serious athletes may train from 45 minutes to two hours.

In strength training, it's more important to look at the volume of training rather than the total training time. Volume refers to the number of repetitions and sets of lifting that are performed. A repetition, or rep, is one complete movement or lift. A set is a group of repetitions. For example, if you were lifting a barbell overhead from the resting position (about shoulder height below your chin) to the top of the movement (arms fully extended, over your head) and then back to the resting position, that would be one rep. If you do this 20 times, that would be 20 reps.

The proper number of reps depends on the intensity you use and the number of sets you perform. If you perform only one set per exercise, it is best to select a weight that allows you to complete 8 to 12 reps. This will typically be about 80 percent of 1 RM. For this type of lifting, you should do as many reps as possible. When your strength increases to allow you to do more than 12 reaps, you should add more weight.

Single-set programs are good when you start a weight training program. However, if you want to continue to improve, you should move to multiple sets. Increasing the volume of lifting by doing multiple sets raises the potential to develop muscle fitness. Three to six sets are typically the standard to produce optimal gains.

Should I Always Train the Same Way?

Exercise scientists have found that muscle strength is developed best by programs of training that stimulate a variety of training responses. *Periodization* is a method of training that systematically changes the volume and intensity during different periods or "cycles."

A typical periodization program might include four cycles that are two to four weeks in length. In the first cycle, you develop good muscle size by lifting moderately heavy weights many times. During the second cycle, you improve muscle recruitment and strength by lifting heavier weights with fewer repetitions. In the third cycle you bring strength to a peak by lifting very heavy weights a few times. In the final cycle you don't lift weights at all, but rather have a period of active rest (do exercises such as walking and swimming) to provide your body with a physical and emotional break from weight training. Then you start the first cycle again.

Should I Use Free Weights or Machines?

When free weights (barbells and dumbbells) are lifted, the weight of the bar remains the same throughout the lift. A constant resistance can also be applied by a machine with a weight stack and cable or chain if it uses a pulley that is perfectly round. If the pulley is elliptical or off-center, the weight becomes lighter or heavier as the angle of movement changes. Variable resistance machines, such as Nautilus, use an off-center cam to change the weight as the leverage during exercise changes.

Muscles become stronger when they are overloaded by an appropriate resistance. It makes little difference whether the resistance is applied by a barbell or dumbbell, or a specialized machine. Some machine manufacturers make outlandish claims about the superiority of their machine over other training devices. There is little evidence that any one type of equipment is clearly more effective than another. The particular advantages and disadvantages of free weights or machines must be judged by each person based on his or her individual goals and preferences.

What Exercise Should I Do?

Strength training is very specific to the muscles that are used in the exercise program. To develop balanced strength, it is essential to select at least one exercise for each major muscle group. For general fitness, basic exercises should be done for the legs (quadriceps and hamstrings), chest, shoulders, back, arms (biceps and triceps), and abdomen.

There are virtually hundreds of exercises to choose from. However, most of these are simply variations of the basic exercises. In general, exercise should be arranged from the large muscle groups to the small muscle groups. The typical order is to start with the large muscles in the legs and hips, move to the muscles of the chest, backs shoulders, and arms, and end with the abdominals. There are other patterns and combinations for different goals, but this order seems to offer good results.

What About Safety?

Safety is one of the most important considerations in any successful fitness program. Safety begins with a comprehensive medical checkup. You should work closely with your physician and diabetes health-care team to avoid unnecessary risks. If possible, find a Certified Strength and Conditioning Specialist (C.S.C.S.) to help you develop a weight training program just for you.

Here are a few safety tips to remember:

- Always warm up. Before you begin lifting, perform a general warm-up of 5 to 10 minutes to increase body temperature and blood flow. You should also stretch and perform a specific warm-up for each lift using light to moderate weights.

- Know proper use of equipment. If you don't know, learn how to use and adjust all equipment properly before lifting.

- Breathe evenly. Holding your breath while you lift can cause blood pressures to reach abnormally high levels. Always continue breathing during lifts. Inhale as the weight is lowered and exhale as you push the weight up.

- Use a full range of motion. For each repetition, move the weight through its full range of motion. A muscle that performs only partial movements loses flexibility. However,

379

moving a muscle through maximum extension and flexion can increase flexibility.

- Use proper form. Improper form increases the risk of injury and reduces the effectiveness of the exercise. If a muscle is being isolated, the movement should be performed in a slow, controlled effort. If a lift is being performed to develop muscle power, explosive movements should be done in a coordinated effort with special attention to correct body alignment.

- Use safety equipment and spotters. When using free weights, a spotter can assist you if you are too fatigued to complete a lift. Collars (that hold the weights in place) should be used to secure weights when lifting barbells and dumbbells. Use safety racks when performing lifts such as squats or bench presses. Wear a lifting belt for all overhead lifts and for lifts that put pressure on the lower back.

- Always cool down. Never stop a workout abruptly. You should always spend time cooling down with an activity such as walking or cycling to allow the body to slowly readjust to a lower intensity.

- Monitor blood glucose. Anyone who takes insulin or oral agents to control diabetes should carefully monitor blood-glucose levels when doing any type of exercise. While glucose levels typically fall as a result of mild aerobic activity, very intense exercise, such as weight training, may not have the same effect.

While some people may see a fall in glucose, others may see an abnormal increase if lifting is extremely intense. Often there is a slight temporary increase in blood glucose, followed by a drop in blood glucose after the exercise is completed. This reduction in blood glucose may be rapid and prolonged for 24 to 48 hours. It is important for you to measure how your own body responds, and work with your healthcare team to keep diabetes in good control.

Always have some form of glucose with you when you are exercising. Also, it's advisable to let others around you and your spotters know that you have diabetes and what they should do if you have an insulin reaction.

Putting it All Together

People who have been lifting weights for years realize that muscle power is the basis for all physical activity. If you have not been active at all, strength training may be a good place to start. If you have been working on aerobic fitness, try to strike a balance with weight training to also develop adequate strength and muscular endurance. The key to total fitness is a balanced approach through proper exercise.

Guyton Hornsby is Wellness Center Director and Assistant Professor in the Department of Physical Education and Recreation at East Tennessee University. He is a Certified Strength and Conditioning Specialist and serves as Secretary on the American Diabetes Association Council on Exercise.

[*Editor's Note:* Because exercise is an important part of managing the symptoms of diabetes, the American Diabetes Association devotes a considerable amount of its resources to providing information regarding physical fitness activities. Much of this material represents some of the best introductory information to various physical activities available, and is therefore included in this section as a useful reference for all readers.]

Chapter 29

The New Yoga

By Daryn Eller

Every winter, Greg Hartwig, 43, leaves his home in Oakland, Calif., and with skis in hand heads to Aspen, Colo., for a week of vigorous skiing with his brother, a professional ski instructor. In years past
he prepared for the trip with weeks of intense running, cycling and
weightlifting. This year he decided to take a different route to fitness:
yoga. "For the first time, he had no problem with the altitude, and
his endurance didn't wane," says Rodney Yee, codirector of the Pied-
mont Yoga Studio in Oakland and Hartwig's instructor. "Instead of
burning out after three or four days, he was able to keep up with his
brother for the duration of the trip."

And you thought yoga was for wimps.

Not anymore. In fact, fitness-minded people are taking it up with
a fervor not seen since the advent of step aerobics. In part, that's because yoga—or at least the way it's taught—has changed in recent
years. To attract the mainstream crowd that might be put off by the
discipline's spiritual aspects, many teachers have dispensed with sitting cross-legged on the floor and chanting "om"; others have created
East-West hybrids of yoga and aerobics. And classes are now offered
in gleaming health clubs and aerobics studios—a far cry from the
cramped, incense-filled garrets of yore.

American Health, July/August, 1993.

But yoga's new, spiffed-up image is not the whole story. Its renewed popularity also reflects a shift in attitude about getting fit. Molly Fox, co-owner of Molly Fox Fitness Club in New York City, says people are looking for a slower, more mentally engaging workout, and yoga fits the bill. It reduces stress and improves strength, flexibility and self-awareness—benefits that carry over into other life pursuits.

You don't have to practice with unwavering devotion to reap the rewards, either. "Yoga can be a complete physical, mental and spiritual workout, or it can be a 15-minute-a-day enhancement for whatever else you do," says Yee, who appears in the video *The Yoga Practice Series*.

In fact, many of us already incorporate some form of yoga in our daily lives. The stretch runners often do before a jog—hands and feet on the ground, buttocks in the air—is almost the same as a yoga pose called Downward-Facing Dog. The side stretch commonly used in aerobics classes—done standing with legs wide apart—is a variation on the triangle, another yoga pose. (For some basic poses, see "A Yoga Sampler" below.))

But stretching in a yoga studio is different from typical workout stretches. "Yoga engages all the muscles of the body," says Sharon Gannon, codirector of the Jivamukti Yoga Center in New York City. For instance, when you do a yoga side stretch, you don't simply bend your arm and torso to the side: You actively reach to the side, with your leg muscles tightened and your feet pushing against the floor. That way, your legs get stronger too.

If this all sounds fairly taxing, it is. "Turn-of-the-century versions of yoga offered a watered-down version, easily managed by mostly older, female patrons," Gannon explains. "And for better or worse, that's what most Americans think of as yoga."

But hatha-yoga (a general term for the series of physical poses, or asanas, taught in most classes today) is quite rigorous. The thousands of positions, devised roughly 6,000 years ago, were meant to prepare the body for meditation. The yogis, or yoga practitioners, who created them believed that a fit body must be capable of sitting in one position for an extended period of time.

Granted, most newly converted enthusiasts—from stressed-out stockbrokers to professional athletes—aren't interested in marathon meditation sessions. They're hooked on the faster and more arduous yoga offshoots, such as "yogarobics," cropping up across the country. (For a rundown of the various schools of yoga, see "A Yoga Primer," below.) Even at its most intense, though, yoga differs from other vigorous activities. It involves exacting, deliberate movements that call for a high level of body awareness.

But as demanding as yoga can be, "it's not about doing impossible contortions," says Dr. Mary Schatz, author of the yoga book *Back Care Basics* (Rodmell Press, 1992) and medical staff president of Centennial Medical Center in Nashville, Tenn. "Beginners don't have to be especially agile." In fact, yoga demands as much strength as flexibility. Its sheer physicality challenges even those who consider themselves to be in great shape. Since it works every muscle group, weaknesses quickly become obvious, allowing you to target the areas on which you need to focus, according to Yee.

Don't confuse yoga's muscle-building benefits with those you'd get from weight training, however. When you lift weights, you're breaking down muscle tissue, which then repairs itself and becomes stronger and often bulkier than before. Yoga stresses the muscles enough to start the repair-and-strengthen cycle, but since you're stretching as you strengthen, muscles also get leaner.

As Yee so poetically puts it, each pose is a delicate balance between effort and surrender. (Hatha, in fact, stands for balance in Sanskrit, "ha" meaning sun, "tha," moon.) Back bends, for instance, stretch the front of the body and strengthen the back muscles as they hold the pose.

For athletes, this strength-agility mix is especially appealing. Runners who take yoga, for instance, can increase hip flexibility, which helps them take longer strides and cover more ground. At the same time, the poses build strength in runners' weaker upper bodies. And since yoga stretches and strengthens opposing muscle groups (say, the hamstrings and quadriceps), it also helps prevent muscle imbalances that can lead to injury.

Another plus: Yoga builds endurance. If Greg Hartwig's legs lasted longer on his most recent ski trip, it was probably because they had developed enough strength from the poses to stay in a bent, mogul-schussing position, run after run.

For all its physical demands, yoga is still very much a mental discipline, which has to do largely with breathing. As you move into a pose and hold it—for anywhere from 30 seconds to 30 minutes—you can't help but focus on your inhalations and exhalations. "Breathing is the link between body and mind," says Jake Jacobson, owner of The Center for Yoga in Los Angeles. "Slow it down and you relax; speed it up and you feel energized."

"Yoga is wonderful for harried, Type-A personalities," says Mara Carrico, who teaches yoga at the Shiley Sports and Health Center of the Scripps Clinic in La Jolla, Calif. Many of her students are cardiac patients referred to her by their doctors. "I teach them to use breathing as a tool. They learn how to achieve a calm state of mind."

As evidence grows that stress may play a role in heart disease, physicians have taken a new look at yoga's therapeutic effects. Dr. Dean Ornish, director of the Preventive Medicine Research Institute in Sausalito, Calif., and the leading proponent of a nonsurgical, nondrug approach to treating heart disease, devotes a chapter to yoga and meditation in Dr. Dean Ornish's *Program for Reversing Heart Disease* (Ballantine Books, 1992). "Yoga is one of the most powerful ways of managing stress," he says. In one study, conducted at the University of California at San Francisco, he found that patients with severe heart disease who participated in a program including yoga, moderate exercise, quitting smoking, a lowfat vegetarian diet and group support had a 91% reduction in chest pain within two weeks. "In a month," Ornish adds, "we measured improved blood flow to the heart; within a year, a reduction in blockages in the arteries." A control group showed an increase in chest pain and a worsening in artery blockages.

Athletes also benefit from yoga's emphasis on controlled breathing. At Seton Hall University in South Orange, NJ., Diana McNab, an adjunct professor of sports psychology, teaches "Zen and Yoga," a popular course among members of the men's and women's basketball, track and tennis teams. Many of them come to enhance physical flexibility, but they end up honing mental flexibility too, she says. Jocks who "choke" or get psyched out can learn to use focused breathing when it counts most—in competition. And this emphasis can give weekend exercisers the extra oomph they need to keep from quitting.

There's also some evidence that yoga's spiritual aspects are gaining wider acceptance. Jivamukti's Gannon recalls being warned to "tone down the chanting or you'll alienate the market." But if her packed classes are any indication, students seem to relish the chanting and meditation as much as they do the more rigorous posing.

Perhaps the ultimate attraction is that yoga, which in Sanskrit means union, brings people together. Unlike in aerobics classes, where students jostle for choice spots near the mirror, there's a sense of camaraderie in most yoga studios. "The poses teach you to reach away from the center of your body so that your muscles extend outward and nothing is compressed," explains Gannon. "It makes sense that opening up physically leads to an emotional release as well." That may be ancient wisdom, but in the '90s, the idea of striving to connect with others seems thoroughly up-to-date.

A Yoga Sampler

These six yoga poses both stretch and strengthen the body: some also help promote balance. As a rule of thumb, inhale as you prepare for a pose, then exhale as your body moves into place. "Try to hold the position for as long as you can continue to breathe evenly," says Sharon Gannon, codirector of the Jivamukti Yoga Center in New York City. If that's only a few seconds, don't be discouraged—it takes time to build up yoga-specific strength. The poses can be done on their own three times a week or as a cooldown after an aerobic workout.

Standing Pose

Warrior Pose *stretches the back, chest and arms; tones the inner thighs; strengthens the quadriceps.*

Stand with your left foot about three feet in front of your right. Turn your right foot out (toes to the right) so that the arch is perpendicular to your left foot. Keep your weight on the outside of your right (back) foot. With your hips facing forward and your right leg straight, bend your left knee, keeping it directly over your left ankle. Raise your arms straight over your head till your palms meet, keeping your shoulders down and relaxed and your upper body elongated. Hold the position, breathing evenly. Repeat with your right leg forward.

Forward and Backward Bends

Downward-Facing Dog *lengthens and strengthens the legs, arms and back; stretches the front and back of the body.*

Get on your hands and knees, arms directly below your shoulders. Exhale, straightening your legs and lifting your buttocks so your body forms an inverted "V". Think of your hands and feet as anchors as you stretch away from the floor. (Try to keep your heels down.) Feel your arms lifting up off your wrists and your legs lifting up off your ankles. Hold the position, breathing evenly. Inhale and move directly into the pose below.

Upward-Facing Dog *lengthens and stretches the spine.*

Walk your arms forward until your legs are lengthened and parallel to the ground. Your toes should be flexed. Inhale and contract your buttocks and abdominal muscles, straightening your arms and lifting your upper body so that you're supported by your hands and toes. Exhale, pressing your hands and toes down and stretching upward through the crown of your head. Hold the position. breathing evenly.

Standing Pose

Free Pose *stretches the inner thighs; strengthens the arms and legs.*

Stand erect, with your weight evenly distributed. Press your palms together in front of your chest. Inhale and turn your right foot out, placing your right heel at the arch of your left foot. As you exhale, bend your right leg and grasp your right ankle with your right hand, placing your foot as high on your left inner thigh as possible. To steady yourself, press your raised foot and left thigh firmly together and balance your weight evenly on the inner and outer edges of your standing foot. Hold, breathing evenly, and press your palms together. Repeat on the other side.

Sitting Pose

Spinal Twist *stretches and strengthens the back.*

Sit with your right leg straight in front of you and your left foot flat on the floor. Inhale and lift your torso, placing your left hand behind you for support. Place your right elbow against the outside of your left knee. Exhale and slowly twist to the left, pressing your elbow against your knee and contracting the muscles of your straight leg. Hold, breathing evenly. Repeat on the other side.

Relaxation Pose

Child's Pose *relaxes the entire body.*

Kneel on the ground. Bring your chest down to your knees and lower your buttocks so that you're sitting on your calves. Place your forehead on the ground in front of your knees and try to keep your buttocks on your heels. Turn your palms up and relax your arms, resting them next to your legs. Hold the position, breathing evenly.

A Yoga Primer

Since every yoga class is different and there's no national accreditation for teachers, finding a program that suits you may take some trial and error. You can get an idea of what to expect, however, if you know which school of yoga is being taught. Below is a guide to the types you're likely to encounter.

Iyengar: Some of the more vigorous yoga classes now offered are based in the Iyengar tradition, which emphasizes posture and precision. Iyengar also uses props to facilitate certain moves: A rolled-up towel placed beneath the upper back stretches the chest; straps slipped under the soles of the feet and grasped at both ends draw the legs close to the upper body, deepening a hamstring stretch.

Kundalini: Fairly fast-paced, Kundalini involves inhaling and exhaling rapidly while holding a pose. Adherents claim that it stimulates the body's center of energy at the base of the spine. In lay terms, the combination of rapid breathing and sustained posing raises body temperature, builds endurance and makes for a bracing workout.

Ashtanga: The only aerobic form of pure yoga, Ashtanga practitioners move continuously from pose to pose as they breathe rhythmically. "It keeps the heart rate up to the same extent as other cardiovascular activities," says Mara Carrico, a yoga teacher who is also a student of this method and who shed 15 pounds over a year from taking Ashtanga classes .

Jivamukti: With instructors in New York City, Seattle and San Francisco, Jivamukti draws on more traditional Indian roots. Classes are physically challenging but also include more spiritual elements, such as chanting. "Breathing and physical poses are emphasized equally," explains Sharon Gannon, codirector of the Jivamukti Yoga Center in New York City. "The movements are flowing. One pose follows another—like a dance."

Yogarobics: This combination of aerobics, dance and yoga created by fitness instructor Larry Lane of Goodbody's Fitness Clinic in Dallas is also taught at several other studios around the country. Kinder to the body than more frenzied aerobics classes—it's low-impact, the music is soothing and everyone is shoeless—the cardiovascular benefits it delivers are similar. Urban Yoga, which draws crowds at Crunch Fitness, and La Nouvelle Yoga, taught at the Atrium Club, both in New York City, are two similar aerobics-yoga hybrids.

Daryn Eller is a New York City-based freelance writer specializing in fitness and health.

Chapter 30

Exercise in Everyday Life

Chapter Contents

Section 30.1

Staying in Shape With Garden Exercise

Source: *Flower and Garden, June/July, 1993.*

By Jeffrey P. Restuccio

The typical impression of gardening is that it's a good way to relax, enjoy the outdoors and grow fresh vegetables. The fact that gardening can be enjoyed so many ways is a plus for anyone who wants to change his or her body type but has been unable to do so. If your goal is strength, endurance and low body weight, spend an extra half hour each day digging, weeding or doing push-ups.

Anyone starting an exercise program should first consult a physician. While you're at the physician's office, please show your doctor this article. I've learned that gardening is popular with doctors; however, most of them have never thought of it as a comprehensive fitness lifestyle. Using the techniques in this article, gardening can be included with jogging, walking, swimming and other aerobic exercises.

Research has shown that raising the pulse rate for at least 20 minutes in the morning will raise metabolism for several hours thereafter. Light gardening exercises—mulching, cultivating and harvesting—done half an hour before eating or about 40 minutes after eating, can burn extra calories.

If you're like most gardeners, you'll garden as long as it takes to get the job done. For optimal health benefits, however, gardening should be broken into two- and three-hour periods rather than marathons. Space out activity during the week. Workouts should ideally be at least every other day. It's important to allow at least 30 minutes a few times a week for each garden workout. A 30 minute workout should be brisk, with a conscious effort to warm up, increase your heart rate and properly cool down afterward.

Before you start, take a few moments to write down your exercise and fitness goals. If you've been inactive and you're a novice gardener, start a small garden—just one or two 4 x 8 foot beds. You should always enjoy exercising in the garden. If you find yourself mumbling and grumbling, then it's time to reassess your gardening and fitness objectives.

If you already exercise more than seven hours a week, view gardening exercise as a cross-training program. Use weeding to stretch leg muscles. Turn the compost to strengthen arms and legs. Use the perennial flower bed as a focal point for rest and relaxation.

As an exercise program, gardening assumes the same pattern of stretching, warm-up, exertion and cool-down as an aerobic exercise class. The main difference is that you'll be exercising in your garden instead of the gym.

Always drink plenty of *water* both during and after all gardening exercise. Plants need water and so do you. It's best to drink water before gardening; don't wait until you're thirsty.

It's important to stretch and warm up your muscles before garden exercise. Don't overexert yourself the first couple of days if you've been inactive most of the winter. Stretch both before and after gardening.

Dress in comfortable, loose clothing. Breathe in and out deeply several times. Stand straight, with arms stretched out in front of you, bend at the waist, and touch the ground. Hold your legs straight, but don't lock your knees. Stretch thoroughly, moving your hands first to your right foot and then to your left foot. Slightly bend your knees and repeat the motion. Straighten your legs and spread them out to the sides a little more. Pay attention to your breathing as you stretch. Breathe out. Relax. Breathe in and stretch a little further as you breathe out. Repeat this sequence of motions several times.

Stand straight with your legs bent slightly at the knee. Hold a rake handle over your head. Bend at the waist and twist your body first toward your left foot and then toward your right foot. Hold the rake handle over your head and stand straight; twist your torso side to side a dozen times.

Sit down and spread your legs wide. stretch your hands forward and down to the ground. Move your legs out as far as they will go; breathe out and first touch your left foot and then your right foot. Repeat this motion.

Stand straight with your feet about feet apart. Keep your legs straight. Touch the ground with your hands. bend your legs at the knee and continue to stretch and touch the ground. With your hands on the ground, straighten your legs. Spread your legs to the side a little more and continue. Combine stretching with light gardening exercises. Stand and step forward with your left leg, bending the knee as far down as you can, keeping your right leg straight behind you with the knee almost touching the ground. Weed or cultivate with a hand tool for about ten seconds. Stand up and continue, alternating legs. Continue lunging, stretching and weeding until you feel well stretched.

Weeding is now a pleasant, 20- to 30-minute aerobic exercise for arms and legs. Always bend at the knees, never the waist. While hand weeding, spread your legs and bend at the knees. Weed for about 20 seconds. Still in the wide stance, straighten your legs. Spread them out wide, bend your knees and keep weeding. Continue with this sequence. It will take time for this activity to feel comfortable.

Next weed with one knee down behind you, your other leg in front of you, knee bent, foot on the ground. Weed in this position for about 20 seconds. Stand up and alternate legs. (You may want to carry a foam garden mat to place under your bent knee.)

Now squat with your feet flat on the ground, bending at both knees with your elbows resting on the inside of your legs. Weed in this position about 20 seconds, stand up and repeat. You may not be able to do this routine until you've gained a degree of flexibility. Keep at it. It will take months of stretching every day to increase and maintain flexibility.

Alternate between six weeding positions: standing straight, lunge and weed, down on one knee, squatting with both legs, both knees down, and sitting and weeding.

If bending on one or both knees is uncomfortable, sit and weed or stand straight using a long-handled tool. For maximum aerobic benefit, maintain a steady rhythm and alternate your grip. Don't worry about what the neighbors say; gardening exercise may took funny, but health and well-being is a serious matter.

When using a wheelbarrow or garden cart, keep your back straight and lift with your legs. If you are using a basket, always squat with your feet flat (if you can) when picking it up.

Whether you use a hoe, rake or other long-handled tool, the technique is the same:

- Keep your back straight.

- Spread your legs in a wide, bent-knee stance.

- Alternate your grip.

- Think in terms of sets and repetitions rather than counting actual movements.

- Breathe in and out in a steady rhythm.

When you've completed your gardening exercise, take time to cool down. Walk around the garden at a leisurely pace. Rest, have a drink of your favorite beverage and enjoy the flowers, butterflies, birds and other sights and sounds of the garden.

For some people, gardening will be a cross-training activity to their primary exercise program or sport. Gardening can also serve as an alternative to competitive sports for those who prefer to compete against themselves and the vagaries of nature. It's ideal for those who seek more qualitative and spiritual rewards from their lifestyle. Gardening is truly an activity for everyone, in which young and old, rich and poor, quick and slow, big and small can be on the same plying field.

The techniques and concepts presented in this article define the gardening process to achieve optimal flexibility, aerobic and muscle-toning benefits. Adopt the ones you like and don't be afraid to invent your own.

Just remember:

- Stretch thoroughly, both before and after gardening.

- Remember to breathe in and out; stretch and relax your body as you exercise and garden.

- Warm up, exercise and cool down just as you would with any other aerobic exercise.

- Use your legs, not your back!

- Use the positions that are comfortable for you and try others as your body becomes flexible and limber.

- Space out workouts in the garden at least every other day or alternate with other exercise activities.

- Enjoy exercising in the garden.

Jeffrey Restuccio is an author who formed Balance of nature Publishing to promote the concept of fitness and gardening. This article is an excerpt from his book, Fitness the Dynamic Gardening Way: a Health and Wellness Lifestyle.

Section 30.2

The House and Garden Workout.

Five exercises to help get you through the many small challenges of daily living—whether hoisting a case of beer or hauling a load of firewood

Source: *Men's Health*, September 1994.

P. Myatt Murphy

Weight training. Aerobics. Weekends on the tennis court. You thought you were in pretty good shape. Then you helped a buddy move into his new house and woke up the next day with every muscle in your body throbbing in unison. You've discovered the difference between the gym and real life.

Regardless of how fit you are, there are certain responsibilities of being male that require some specialized strength and flexibility. Things like lugging a sofa up a flight of stairs, or hoisting the kids' new swingset out of the trunk of a car. That's where real-life training comes in: "You could be in great shape as a runner, but then reach down to pick up a tool or just to tie your shoe and throw out your back," says Jo Coetzee, M.D., exercise research physician at the Cooper Institute for Aerobic Research. So add these exercises to your regular gym routine. Next time your partner decides to rearrange the living room, you'll be ready to hoist that day- bed without winding up confined to it.

The 24-Bottle Pick-Up

(Upright rows develop the muscles of the middle back and shoulders needed for lifting, say, a case of beer out of your trunk.)

Stand straight, feet shoulder-width apart, with a dumbbell in each hand. Let your arms hang straight down in front of you so each dumbbell rests on your upper thighs, palms facing your body. Slowly draw the weights up toward your chin, keeping your hands close to your body and letting your elbows extend outward. At the top of the movement, your hands should rest under your chin and your elbows should be slightly higher (up around your ears). Hold for a moment, then slowly return to the starting position. Do two sets of 10 to 12 repetitions.

The "Daddy's Home" Back Bracer

(Leg crisscrosses build the muscles of the lower back, used in picking increasingly heavy objects off the floor.)

Sit on the floor with your legs extended in front of you, slightly bent at the knee. Keeping your hands on the floor and your knees bent, lift your feet a few inches off the floor. Now cross your left foot over your right, keeping about half an inch of space between the two. Hold for a moment, then reverse your feet, crossing your right foot over your left. Do two sets of 12 to 15 repetitions.

The "Who Said Anything About an Elevator?" Flex

(Flat bench leg lifts strengthen the abdominal and hip flexor muscles, both of which are stressed when carrying a heavy piece of furniture up a flight of stairs.)

Sit on the end of a flat exercise bench. Reach down and grab the sides of the bench for support. Lean back until your back is flat against the bench, but with neck and shoulders raised slightly. Extend your legs parallel to the floor. With knees slightly bent, raise your legs until they form a right angle to your body. Hold for a count of one and slowly lower them until they are at a 45-degree angle, halfway to the bench. Do two sets of 10 to 12 lifts.

The Lawn-Boy Twist

(Reverse trunk twists strengthen the oblique abdominals — muscles used in raking leaves, pushing the lawn mower and other push/pull activities.)

Lie on your back on the floor with your arms straight out to the sides, palms down. Bend your knees and place your feet flat on the floor. With your legs and feet together, slowly lower them to the left until your left thigh touches the floor. Hold for a moment, then raise your legs back to the starting position and repeat the exercise to your right side. Do 15 to 20 repetitions.

The No-Choke Pull-Start

(Two-arm dumbbell tows isolate the latissimus muscles of the upper back, used for sharp pulling motions like starting a stubborn lawn mower or snow blower.)

Stand with a dumbbell in each hand, then bend at the waist, placing your forehead against a chair seat or table so your back is almost parallel to the floor. (Cushion your head by putting a folded towel on the table or chair.) Your knees should be straight but just out of lock position, and both arms should be hanging freely. Now raise both hands slowly up until the dumbbell touch the sides of your chest. Hold for a count of one, then slowly lower the weights to the starting position. Do 8 to 12 repetitions.

Chapter 31

Presidential Sports Award

A Program of the President's Council on Physical Fitness and Sports Administered by the Amateur Athletic Union

The Challenge

A strong, vital America depends on physically fit Americans. Can we depend on you!

The Presidential Sports Award program was developed by the President's Council on Physical Fitness & Sports in 1972 in conjunction with national sports organizations and associations. Its purpose is to motivate all Americans to become more physically active throughout life, and emphasizes regular exercise rather than outstanding performance. The program is administered by the Amateur Athletic Union (AAU).

The challenge of the Presidential Sports Award is to make a commitment to fitness through active and regular participation in sports and fitness activities. Earning the award means that you have put in time and effort to meet the challenge of personal fitness. The Award recognizes this achievement, and the fact that you are part of a nationwide effort toward a healthier, more vital America. We hope that you encourage your family, friends, teammates, and fellow employees to join in earning the Award.

Anyone age six (6) or older is eligible to participate in the Presidential Sports Award program. However, the completed fitness log(s) of all participants between the ages of 6-13 must be signed and veri-

---

President's Council on Physical Fitness and Sports.

fied by an adult. In addition, it is especially important that participants over the age of 40 who have not been active on a regular basis undergo a thorough medical examination before undertaking any physical activity program. It is very important that all participants take necessary steps to make their activity enjoyable and safe. Unfortunately, unintentional injuries can occur even when proper safety precautions are taken. For example a helmet should be as common . for a bicycler as for a football player, racquetball players and shooters should wear appropriate eye protection and walkers, joggers, runners, and bicyclists should make sure that they are visible to motorists.

According to the United States Public Health Service, unintentional injuries rank fourth among the leading causes of death in the U.S. and constitute the first cause of years of potential life lost before age 65. Therefore. whenever necessary—PUT A LID ON IT!

The Award

You can earn the award in any one of the sports fitness activities listed in this brochure, and you can earn as many Awards in as many categories as you like. Any individual age six (6) years of age or older is eligible to participate.

To earn the award:

1. Select your sport or fitness activity (or several).

2. Keep a record of your participation on the fitness log (if you need additional fitness logs, please make copies or attach separate sheets of paper).

3. When you have fulfilled the qualifying standards, send the completed and signed fitness log and $6 per award for United States and APO/FPO delivery ($8 in Canada, $10 for all other countries—U.S. currency only) to:

> Presidential Sports Award
> P.O. Box 68207
> Indianapolis, IN 46268-0207

4. The fitness log(s) of all participants age 13 or younger must be signed and verified by an adult.

Please allow up to six weeks for delivery. For additional information concerning the program, or for questions concerning your order, call (317) 872-2900, extension 22 or 51.

Your Award Consists of the Following Five Items:

1. A certificate of achievement from President Clinton, personalized with your name and suitable for framing.

2. A letter of congratulations from the Chairman of the President's Council, suitable for framing.

3. A blazer patch (embroidered emblem) signifying the sport or fitness activity in which you earn your award.

4. A sports bag identification tag, imprinted with the award logo.

5. A shoe pocket, which attaches to shoe strings and is designed to hold identification, money, keys, etc., while you work out.

Note: To receive additional emblems, add $3 to the award total for each additional emblem ordered and be sure to designate the category desired.

New! Family Fitness Award

In addition to the standard award packet described, family members who participate in the program and earn awards together will receive an embroidered strip which reads "Family Fitness" and is designed to fit just above the award emblem. Family Fitness strips will be awarded each time a minimum of one parent/guardian and one child apply to receive awards at the same time and meet the program criteria. Each family member will receive one strip. There is no additional cost to receive the Family Fitness strip.

Qualifying Standards

Now Available for Ages 6 and Up

1. For maximum benefit, the criteria for each activity should be fulfilled within a four-month period. Exceptions will be made only for such things as (but not limited to) injury, ill-

ness, change of season, or individual medical history, and must be briefly explained when the participant applies to receive an award.

2.   Individuals who participate in a variety of categories within a four-month period, but not enough to earn an award in any one category, should log their activity under either the Cross Training or Sports/ Fitness categories. If requested, those who meet the requirements for Sports/Fitness can choose to receive an award for the category in which the majority of the 50 hours is accumulated.

Aerobic Dance

1.   Participate in a minimum of 50 hours of aerobics, aerobic dance, step aerobics, dance exercise, or similar activity.

2.   Credit no more than one (1) hour per day and four (4) hours per week to the total.

3.   It is recommended that one hour of activity include a 5-10 minute warm up, 20-30 minutes of aerobic activity within your target heart rate range, 10-15 minutes of strengthening exercises and a 5-10 minute cool down.

Archery

1.   Shoot a minimum of 3,000 arrows with no more than 90 arrows credited to the total per day.

2.   Minimum target distance is 15 yards. In field or roving archery, there should be 14 different targets, each at 15 or more yards.

Backpacking

1.   Backpack a minimum of 50 hours with no more than three (3) hours credited to the total per day.

2.   Weight of pack must be at least 10 percent of body weight.

Badminton

1.   Play badminton a minimum of 50 hours with no more than two (2) hours credited to the total per day.

2.   Play must include a minimum of 125 total games with no more than five (5) games credited to the total per day.

Baseball

1.   Play baseball and/or practice baseball skills a minimum of 50 hours with no more than one (1) hour credited to the total per day.

2.   At least 15 of the 50 hours must be in an organized league or part of an organized baseball competition.

Basketball

1.   Play basketball and/or practice basketball skills a minimum of 50 hours with no more than one (1) hour credited to the total per day.

2.   At least 15 of the 50 hours must be in an organized league or part of an organized basketball competition.

Baton Twirling

1.   Practice twirling skills and/or compete in baton twirling a minimum of 50 hours with no more than two (2) hours credited to the total per day.

2.   Practice must include work in at least two of the recognized events (one baton, two baton, three baton, strut, dance twirl, group twirling).

3.   Participate in at least three (3) organized competitions.

Bicycling

1.   On a bicycle with more than five gears, bicycle a minimum of 600 miles with no more than 12 miles credited to the total per day.

2.   On a bicycle with five or fewer gears bicycle a minimum of 400 miles with no more than eight (8) miles credited to the total per day.

3.   On a stationary bicycle, bicycle a minimum of 25 hours with no more than 30 minutes of bicycling within your target heart rate range credited to the total per day.

Bowling

1. Bowl a minimum of 150 games with no more than six (6) games credited to the total per day.

2. The total of 150 games must be bowled on not less than 34 different days.

Canoe-Kayak

1. Paddle a minimum of 200 miles with no more than seven (7) miles credited to the total per day.

Cheerleading

1. Cheerlead, or practice cheerleading, a minimum of 50 hours with no more than one (1) hour credited to the total per day.

2. At least 15 of the 50 hours must be accumulated during organized games or competitions.

Cross Training

1. Complete at least one-half of the requirements for two different categories of this program simultaneously.

2. Activities should develop cardiorespiratory endurance, muscle strength and endurance, and flexibility.

Dance

1. Dance a minimum of 50 hours in Ballroom, Square, Folk, Round, pattern, Clogging, Country Western, or Dance Combination with no more than one and one-half (1 ½) hours credited to the total per day.

Disc Sports

1. Practice flying disc skills a minimum of 50 hours with no more than two (2) hours credited to the total per day.

2. Practice must include work in at least three of the recognized events distance, accuracy, self-caught flight, double disc court, golf, freestyle, discathlon, ultimate, or guts.

Equitation

1. Ride horseback or train horses a minimum of 50 hours with no more than one and one-half (1 ½) hours credited to the total per day.

Fencing

1. Practice fencing skills a minimum of 50 hours with no more than two (2) hours credited to the total per day.

2. At least 30 of the 50 hours must be under the supervision of an instructor or during competition.

Field Hockey

1. Play field hockey and/or practice field hockey skills a minimum of 50 hours with no more than one (1) hour credited to the total per day.

2. At least 15 of the 50 hours must be in organized league or tournament play.

Figure Skating

1. Skate a minimum of 50 hours with no more than one and one-half (1½) hours credited to the total per day.

2. Skating should include at least one of the following elements:

   a) figure-eight work (patch), b) free skating, c) ice dancing, or d) precision skating.

Football

1. Play football and/or practice football skills a minimum of 50 hours with no more than one (1) hour credited to the total per day.

2. At least 15 of the 50 hours must be in an organized league or part of an organized football competition.

Golf

1. Play or practice golf a minimum of 100 hours with no more than three (3) hours credited to the total per day.

2. No motorized carts may be used.

3. At least 15 rounds (18 holes) must be played as part of the 100-hour requirement.

Gymnastics

1. Practice gymnastic skills and/or compete in gymnastics a minimum of 50 hours with no more than two (2) hours credited to the total per day.

2. Practice must include work in at least one-half of the recognized events (two of four for women and girls; three of six for men and boys).

3. Participate in at least three (3) organized competitions.

Handball

1. Play handball a minimum of 50 hours with no more than one and one-half (1½) hours credited to the total per day.

2. Total must include at least 25 matches (2 of 3 games) of singles and/or doubles.

Horseshoe Pitching

1. Pitch horseshoes a minimum of 50 hours with no more than two (2) hours credited to the total per day.

2. Sanctioned league or tournament games may be used; 100 sanctioned games required.

3. If a combination of practice time and official games are used, credit one-half (1/2) hour for each sanctioned game (more than two hours can be credited if participating in a sanctioned tournament).

Ice Hockey

1. Play ice hockey and/or practice ice hockey skills a minimum of 50 hours with no more than one (1) hour credited to the total per day.

2. At least 15 of the 50 hours must be in an organized league or part of an organized ice hockey competition.

Ice Skating

1. Skate a minimum of 50 hours with no more than one and one-half (1½) hours credited to the total per day.

Jogging

1. Jog a minimum of 125 miles with no more than two and one-half (2½) miles credited to the total per day.

Judo

1. Practice judo skills a minimum of 50 hours with no more than one (1) hour credited to the total per day.

2. At least 30 of the 50 hours must be under the supervision of a qualified instructor.

Karate

1. Practice karate skills a minimum of 50 hours with no more than one (1) hour credited to the total per day.

2. At least 30 of the 50 hours must be under the supervision of a qualified instructor.

Lacrosse

1. Play lacrosse and/or practice lacrosse skills a minimum of 50 hours with no more than one (1) hour credited to the total per day.

2. At least 15 of the 50 hours must be in organized league or tournament play.

Lawn Bowling

1. Participate in a minimum of forty games in either social intraclub interclub, or Division events, with no more than three (3) games credited to the total per day.

2. These may be singles (18 points) or pairs, triples, fours, games of no less than 12 ends.

3. These games must be played in no less than 45 days and within the maximum of 120 days.

Marathon

1. Run a minimum of 40 miles per week for at least two months.

2. Weekly mileage should not be increased more than 10% over the previous week. A longer training run must be done at least every 10 days at a distance of at least 15 miles for two months once mileage level is at 40 miles a week.

3. At the end of a four-month cycle, complete a TAC-sanctioned marathon of 26.2 miles.

Martial Arts

(For all martial arts other than Judo, Karate, and Tae Kwon Do)

1. Practice martial arts skills a minimum of 50 hours with no more than one (1) hour credited to the total per day.

2. At least 30 of the 50 hours must be under the supervision of a qualified instructor.

Orienteering

1. Practice orienteering skills a minimum of 50 hours with no more than two (2) hours credited to the total per day.

2. Participate in at least three (3) organized orienteering events and locate all checkpoints within the allotted time.

Pistol

1. Fire a minimum of 2,000 rounds with no more than 100 rounds credited to the total per day.

2. Minimum target distances are 33 feet for air pistol, 50 feet to 50 yards for .22 rimfire pistol, and 25-50 yards for centerfire pistol.

Racquetball

1. Play racquetball a minimum of 50 hours with no more than one and one-half (1½) hours credited to the total per day.

2. Total must include at least 25 matches (2 of 3 games) of singles and/or doubles.

Rifle

1. Fire a minimum of 2,000 rounds with no more than 100 rounds credited to the total per day.

2. Minimum target distances are 33 feet for air rifle 50 feet to 100 yards for 22 rimfire rifle. and 100 yards for centerfire rifle.

Roller Skating

1. Roller skate a minimum of 50 hours with no more than one and one-half (1½) hours credited to the total per day.

Rope Skipping

1. Skip rope a minimum of 25 hours with no more than 30 minutes credited to the total per day.

2. Rope skipping can be done in single or double dutch ropes.

Rowing

1. Boat-Row a minimum of 50 miles with no more than one and one-half (1½) miles credited to the total per day.

2. Wherry-Row a minimum of 100 miles with no more than three (3) miles credited to the total per day.

3. Shell-Row a minimum of 120 miles with no more than three and one-half (3½) miles credited to the total per day.

Rugby

1. Play rugby, practice rugby skills, or condition for rugby a minimum of 50 hours with no more than two (2) hours of rugby or one (1) hour of conditioning credited to the total per day.

2. Conditioning may include participation in any of the eligible activities of this program, or in any exercise activities listed under the Sports/Fitness category.

Running

1. Run a minimum of 200 miles.

2. Run continuously at least three (3) miles during each outing. No more than five (5) miles may be credited to the total per day (longer runs are not discouraged, but miles counted toward the 200-mile total must be spread over at least 40 outings).

3. Average time must be nine (9) minutes or less per mile (27 minutes for 3 miles, 45 minutes for 5 miles, etc.). Exceptions to this time requirement due to injury or age must be noted.

Sailing

1. Sail a minimum of 50 hours (practice and competition) with no more than two and one-half (2½) hours credited to the total per day.

Scuba-Skin

1. Skin or scuba dive, or train for diving, a minimum of 50 hours with no more than three (3) hours of total diving time credited to the total per day.

2. Total time must include at least 15 logged dives on 15 separate dates under the Safe Diving Standards of one of the following groups: National Association of Skin Diving Schools, National Association of Underwater Instructors, the National YMCA, Professional Association of Diving Instructors, or the Underwater Society of America.

Skeet-Trap

1. Fire a minimum of 800 standard trap or skeet targets or sporting clays with no more than 50 targets credited to the total per day.

2. All shooting events must be under safe, regulated conditions.

Alpine Skiing

1. Ski, or train for skiing, a minimum of 50 hours with no more than three (3) hours of actual skiing time or 30 minutes of training on a ski-training apparatus credited to the total per day.

Nordic Skiing

1. Ski a minimum of 150 miles with no more than 10 miles credited to the total per day.

2. Comparable mileage accumulated on a workout apparatus may be credited to the total.

Snowshoeing

1. Snowshoe a minimum of 50 hours with no more than four (4) hours per outing credited to the total per day.

Soccer

1. Play soccer and/or practice soccer skills a minimum of 50 hours with no more than one (1) hour credited to the total per day.

2. At least 15 of the 50 hours must be in an organized league or part of an organized soccer competition.

Softball

1. Play softball and/or practice softball skills a minimum of 50 hours with no more than one (1) hour credited to the total per day.

2. At least 15 of the 50 hours must be in an organized league or part of an organized softball competition.

Sports/Fitness

1. Participate in a minimum of 50 hours in exercise activities, or in a combination of exercise and sports activities, with no more than one (1) hour credited to the total per day.

2. Exercise activity may consist of aerobics; aquadynamics; calisthenics; exercise or conditioning classes; fitness dancing; rope jumping; workouts on apparatus including stationary bicycles, rowing machines, and treadmills; or a combination of any or all of these activities.

3. Sports activity may include participation in one or more of the sports in which the Presidential Sports Award is offered, or other sports such as Diving, Water Polo, etc.

411

Squash

1. Play squash a minimum of 50 hours with no more than one and one-half (1½) hours credited to the total per day.

2. Total must include at least 25 matches (3 of 5 games) of singles and/or doubles.

Swimming

1. Swim a minimum of 25 miles (44,000 yards) with no more than three-fourths (3/4) of a mile (1,320 yards) credited to the total per day.

T'ai Chi

1. Participate in a minimum of 50 hours of T'ai Chi Chuan following the standards set forth by the American T'ai Chi Association.

2. Credit no more than one (1) hour per day and five (5) hours per week to the total.

3. It is recommended that one hour of activity include: 10-15 minutes of warm-up (including flexibility and strengthening), 20-30 minutes of T'ai Chi within your target heart-rate range, and a 15-minute cool down period.

Table Tennis

1. Play table tennis a minimum of 50 hours with no more than one and one-half (1½) hours credited to the total per day.

2. At least 10 of the 50 hours must be in league, tournament, club ladder, or round-robin play.

Tae Kwon Do

1. Practice tae kwon do skills a minimum of 50 hours with no more than one (1) hour credited to the total per day.

2. At least 30 of the 50 hours must be under the supervision of a qualified instructor.

Tennis

1. Play tennis a minimum of 50 hours with no more than one and one-half (1½) hours credited to the total per day.

2.   Total must include at least 25 sets of singles and/or doubles (tie-break rules may apply).

Track And Field

1.   Compete in and/or practice track and field events a minimum of 50 hours with no more than one (1) hour credited to the total per day.

2.   At least 10 of the 50 hours must be accumulated during organized meets.

Triathlon

1.   Run a minimum of 10 miles per week for at least two months. Participants must run a minimum of three days per week.

2.   Bike a minimum of 35 miles per week for at least two months. Individuals must bike a minimum of two days per week.

3.   Swim a minimum of 1 miles per week for at least two months. Individuals must swim a minimum of two days per week.

4.   Add no more than 10 percent to the distances for each sport each week. The individual should be completing three times the distance in their training mileage per week than the spring distance event in which they intend to compete up to one week prior to the event. One week prior to the event, training would be reduced to 1 times the distance of the event the athlete intends to compete (called tapering).

5.   A minimum of one and maximum of two sports should be practiced at least four days per week. One to two days of rest each week is recommended for recovery time.

6.   At least one workout per week should include a swim/bike or bike/run workout that includes performing the sports back to back but would include practicing the transition of going from one sport to another (called a "brick").

7.   At the end of the four-month period, compete in a Triathlon Federation/USA sanctioned sprint distance event (approximately a 1/2-mile swim, 12-mile bike, and 3.1 -mile run).

VolksSports

1. Train for, or participate in, a minimum of 50 hours in organized volkssport or volksmarch events with no more than two (2) hours credited to the total per day.

2. Exercise activity may consist of running, walking, cycling, climbing hiking, skiing, or any combination of similar activities that promote healthful physical activity.

3. For longer duration events, additional hours may be credited toward earning other awards.

Volleyball

1. Play volleyball, practice volleyball skills, or condition for volleyball a minimum of 50 hours with no more than two (2) hours of volleyball or one (1) hour of conditioning credited to the total per day.

2. Conditioning may include participation in any of the eligible activities of this program, or in any of the exercise activities listed under the Sports/Fitness category.

Endurance Walking

1. Walk a minimum of 225 miles, combining training walks and endurance walks.

2. Training walks must be a minimum of (1) hour in duration. At least three must be completed each week and the mileage should be credited to the 225-mile total.

3. Endurance walks must be continuous for at least five (5) miles. At least five of the outings must be 10 miles long and one must be 15 miles long during the time the 225 miles is being completed. No more than one 10-mile or 15-mile walk can be credited to the total each week.

Fitness Walking

1. Walk a minimum of 125 miles with no more than two and one-half (2½) miles credited to the total per day.

2. Each walk must be continuous, without pauses for rest, and the pace must be at least four (4) m.p.h. (15 minutes per mile).

Race Walking

1.   Race walk a minimum of 200 miles.

2.   Race walk continuously at least three (3) miles during each outing. No more than five (5) miles in any one day may be counted toward the total. The miles counted toward the 200-mile total must be spread over at least 40 outings.

3.   Average time must be 12 minutes or less per mile.

4.   Follow the basic rules of race walking—keep one foot on the ground at all times and keep the supporting leg straight as it comes under the body.

5.   At least two of the outings must be judged events.

Water Exercise

1.   Participate in a minimum of 50 hours of water exercise.

2.   Credit no more than one (1) hour per day and four (4) hours per week to the total.

3.   It is recommended that one hour of activity include a 5-10 minute warm up, 20-30 minutes of water exercise activity within your target heart-rate range, 10-15 minutes of strengthening exercises and a 5-10 minute cool down.

Water Skiing

1.   Water ski a minimum of 50 hours with no more than three (3) hours of total skiing activity credited to the total per day.

Weight Training

1.   Train with weights a minimum of 50 hours with no more than one (1) hour credited to the total per day.

2.   A workout must include at least eight separate weight/strength training exercises. Workouts should be balanced so that each body part is exercised during each cycle (daily, weekly, etc.). Each exercise should be performed in multiple sets, six to 15 times.

Wrestling

1. Wrestle or practice wrestling skills a minimum of 50 hours with no more than one (1) hour credited to the total per day.

2. At least 15 of the 50 hours must be in an organized league or part of an organized wrestling competition.

Chapter 32

Equipment and Facilities

Chapter Contents

Section 32.1

A to Z Guide to Athletic Footwear

Source: *Diabetes Self-Management,* May/June, 1992.

By Becky K. Papas

Compression-molded EVA. Encaps. Grids. Hydroflow. Stable air. These days, you're likely to bump into this high-tech vocabulary at, of all places, your local athletic-shoe store. If you're not familiar with these terms, you're not alone. And while you don't have to become fluent in this language, it is important that you understand something about the needs of your feet and about the footwear choices that are currently available to you. After all, exercise is an essential part of a diabetes self-management program, and the right pair of sneakers is crucial to a safe and comfortable workout— especially for people with peripheral neuropathy.

It's not easy to keep up with the latest trends. We've come a long way since the days of a few sneaker companies manufacturing a handful of models. Specialization has given rise to specific footwear for each activity; at the same time, the cross-trainers sweeping the market may have us heading back to a one-shoe-for-all-seasons approach. To make matters worse, competition between shoe manufacturers almost guarantees that many shoe models will be revamped or even eliminated within a year's time. So even after you find a shoe that works well for you, you may have to begin the hunt all over again next time around.

This article will help you avoid the dizzying confusion of the athletic-shoe store maze. Emerging victorious from the shoestore is not as simple as buying the most expensive sneaker on the market; this strategy may even defy good foot-sense in some cases. Rather, shopping for the perfect sneaker means considering your personal exercise goals, your unique gait, and your own ideas about comfort. Of course, it also means finding the shoes that offer the best fit. To keep this article to a manageable length, we have focused on running shoes and walking shoes, the most popular exercise footwear.

Why Exercise?

Among the many good reasons for people with diabetes to exercise, the most important is that it lowers blood sugar levels. In addition, it can help you to lose weight, improves circulation, and provides cardiovascular protection by improving cholesterol levels, lowering blood pressure, and improving heart function. All of these benefits can be gained through aerobic exercise; that is, any activity that uses large muscles for a continuous period long enough to sustain an elevated heart rate.

In deciding what exercise to do, take into account your life-style, workout goals, and medical conditions. Consult your physician before beginning any new exercise program, particularly if you are more than 35 years old or have any diabetes complications. If you're just starting out, begin gradually at a level you know you can handle. Don't overextend yourself. For instance, if running is too strenuous, try walking, which can be just as effective. In fact, more people than ever are taking to the streets in walking shoes. And the trend is not apt to lose momentum. A study published in *Journal of the American Medical Association* found that women who walked at a strolling, three-mile-an-hour pace, five days a week, raised their levels of high-density lipoprotein cholesterol, the type of cholesterol that is associated with lowered heart disease risk. For people with diabetes, who are already at increased risk for heart disease, these study results are the latest reminder to take exercise seriously.

Understanding the Mechanics

No matter what exercise you fancy, you need a shoe that allows you to perform it safely and comfortably. But to make the correct footwear choice, you must know a little about how your feet work, and what happens when you walk or run on them.

The foot, made up of 26 bones and 20 muscles, has two distinct but complementary functions. The design of the foot allows it to be loose enough to conform to any type of surface, even or uneven, while holding your leg—and the rest of your body—upright. At the same time, it remains rigid enough to lift your body and to step forward.

During fitness walking or running your foot becomes longer and wider wherever it touches the ground. But too much pressure on these areas can be harmful, causing callus build-up, blister formation, or even certain joint or muscle problems. So fitness shoes are designed

419

to distribute body weight evenly over a broad surface area. Your shoes should also hold your feet in a proper alignment and effectively absorb shock; this is especially important for people who have diminished sensation in their feet and who are therefore at increased risk for foot problems that result from mechanical dysfunction.

During normal walking, the body's weight is transferred from the heel, the first point of impact, along the outer edge of the foot to the ball and across to the big toe. But most people display one of two different variations of this gait, either overpronation or oversupination.

Overpronation occurs when the foot collapses under pressure ("flat foot") and rolls too far inward. This forces the inner border of the foot to bear the brunt of the weight during walking or running. *Oversupination* is less common and is caused when a stiff, high arch forces the outer portion of the foot to bear all of the body's weight. These conditions, which podiatrists and foot specialists believe are either inherited or arise during fetal development, open up the whole foot to muscle or bone problems and the weight-bearing areas in particular to calluses, blisters, or even ulcerations of the skin.

Still, not everyone with overpronating or oversupinating feet needs a shoe "fix." If you have no complications and experience no pain during exercise, you can wear any type of well-fitting athletic shoe. However, if you begin to feel pain or to develop neuropathy (which may deaden pain sensations that announce foot problems) or vascular disease (which increases the risk of infection from skin irritations), you'll need a shoe with ample cushioning—to minimize friction against the skin—and extra support.

For the most part, running and walking shoes are similarly constructed. However, running shoes have additional features to accommodate the greater impact that running imposes on the feet; a runner's foot must withstand pressure equal to about three times the body's weight. In addition, running styles differ; some people land on the balls of their feet, while others display more of a heel-to-toe-roll. So running shoes are most heavily cushioned in these two areas. Running shoes must also have a roomy, round *toe box,* so toes are not pinched when the foot is flexed, and a rigid *heel counter* (the cup around the heel) to stabilize the foot.

Because a walker strikes the ground heel-first then pushes off with the toes, walking shoes have a firm heel counter, a flexible forefoot that bends easily at the ball of the foot, and longitudinal stability. To make sure the shoe is stable enough, try to twist it; an adequately rigid shoe will not give.

What to Look For

With this basic knowledge underfoot, consider the following three factors when shopping for a fitness shoe, particularly if you are a runner: how many miles per week you plan to run (or walk), your gait, and your body weight. For example, a runner who weighs more than 170 pounds or who plans to run between 50 and 60 miles a week needs a very stable, well-cushioned shoe. Overpronators should also choose a more stable shoe, with soles that are straight along both sides. Features that add stability to a shoe include:

- a stiff or extended heel counter;

- a *board last* or *combination last*. (The last is the base of the shoe around which the rest is built.) A board last is made by gluing the upper to stiff cardboard, resulting in a very stable shoe. The combination last has cardboard at the heel while the rest of the shoe is *slip-lasted* (sewn together and glued to the sole); this gives stability to the rear-foot and flexibility to the forefoot.

- a midsole made from compression-molded EVA (ethylene vinyl acetate)—a styrofoam-like material—or polyurethane, or a combination of these two materials.

- footframes, and

- a higher back tab.

(For an extended discussion about the different parts of a shoe, see "Anatomy of a Shoe" on page 425).

On the other hand, if you plan to run only a couple of times a week or if you are very slim, you can wear a lightweight shoe made with a standard EVA midsole and without many additional features. A more flexible shoe is probably a better choice in this case, because more rigid shoes make bending the foot difficult, which can lead to muscle pain in the casual or thin runner. Oversupinators should also choose a more flexible shoe that is semicurved or curved inward along the arch, depending on the degree of supination. Walking shoes usually come in semicurved models only.

Feet with bunions, corns, or hammertoes may be more comfortable in shoes with extra-wide widths (available from New Balance shoes). Weak ankles need a wide platform and a flared heel. And foot special-

421

ists agree that for people with peripheral neuropathy and vascular disease, the governing principle is that more cushioning is better. A combination-lasted or board-lasted shoe with a compression-molded EVA midsole is a better choice than a softer, more flexible slip-lasted shoe with a sheet EVA midsole because it provides better heel control.

Not every expert believes that shoes should be sports-specific In fact, running shoes are sometimes recommended for walkers, especially women who weigh under 125 pounds, because they are lighter. In addition, the extra cushioning in running shoes tends to raise the heels, which cuts the likelihood of injury in women who normally wear high-heeled shoes.

The top-selling cross-trainer (also known as sports-trainer), the most popular athletic shoe on the market today, also defies the sports-specific principle of shoe-buying. But its basic midsole makes it a bad choice for those who run more than six miles per week. However, a gripping sole and good lateral support make the cross-trainer a good choice for tennis and other court games.

Fits for a King

Once you have analyzed your needs to determine the general shoe design that you are shopping for, go to the store to try on the appropriate models. Remember that the number-one concern is that the sneakers fit comfortably. But other criteria are important to keep in mind as well:

- Shoes should match the shape of your foot. They should be wide where your foot is wide and narrow where your foot is narrow.

- Your feet expand as you run, so try on shoes when your feet are slightly larger, for instance, at the end of the day or after walking or standing for an extended period. Your feet are widest and longest at these times.

- Don't forget to try on both shoes in a pair. One foot is usually bigger than the other.

- Stand up and walk around in the shoes. Shoes should feel comfortable from the moment you put them on. This is especially important with fitness shoes made from synthetic fibers; they will not stretch over time the way leather does.

- While standing in the shoes, feel for your longest toe. It should be 1/2 inch or about one thumb-width from the end of the shoe.

- Bring any orthotic devices you use to make sure they fit in the shoes you're trying on.

- Wear the type of socks that you wear when you exercise.

Foot Faults

Whether your athletic shoes are brand-new or you have had them for a while, be on the lookout for any of the following warning signs. They indicate that your shoes do not fit properly, have worn out, or do not provide adequate support:

- Heel or arch pain usually indicates that the cushioning has worn down. It can also be a sign of a flat foot that is not being corrected by the shoes. If you think you have a flat foot problem. consult your podiatrist.

- Lower back pain is a sign of overpronation, flat feet, or shoes that have worn down in the heel counter, all of which need to be addressed by your podiatrist.

- Bleeding under the toenails usually means that your shoes do not fit properly—specifically, that the toe box is too short.

- Blisters also are the result of poorly fitting shoes. Put Vaseline petroleum jelly on the "hot spots" to minimize friction. If the problem continues, you may need to buy a different pair of shoes.

- *Bunions* (swelling of the joint where the foot and big toe meet) and *corns* (hard lumps on the skin of the toe) can be irritated by spots on the inside of the shoe Try stretching out the toe box, making it wider (for bunions) or higher (for corns). If the front part of the shoe's arch is causing the irritation, you can cut it out, if you don't need the support.

- *Calluses* (thickened areas of skin) indicate friction or movement inside the shoe. You can buy insoles that fit inside your shoes and minimize movement. Insoles come in many shapes and sizes, and are made from a variety of materials such as neoprene, nylon, and sometimes polyurethane.

If adding insoles does not do the trick, you may need to use custom-built devices known as *orthotics,* (usually prescribed by a doctor) that can stabilize the foot, as well as support or align the bones in the foot, thus preventing friction. However, orthotics are usually reserved for people with serious foot problems such as severely flat feet, a muscular or skeletal defect, *plantar fasciitis* (an inflammation of the sole), previous ulceration, or surgery to relieve pressure that led to ulceration.

- Many of the friction-related conditions described above, if left untreated, can lead to ulceration. One way to avoid this problem is to change your shoes every three to four hours. This simple maneuver relieves pressure points against the skin and irritations caused by the stitching, creases, folds, or other unique features of a particular shoe's construction. It's an especially good idea to switch shoes if you have a bunion or a prominent bump that is easily irritated. Each time you take off a pair of shoes, take the opportunity to examine your feet for abrasions, blisters, foreign bodies, and injured skin.

Fine-Tuning Your Shoe

Over time, even the best pair of shoes may need an adjustment or two. Whatever it takes to make your shoe more comfortable, a cobbler can do it. They pad sore bunions, corns, and blisters by incorporating additional pieces of foam in the uppers (the top part of the shoe). They can insert a partial lift in the midsole (if the midsole can be removed) or make other adjustments to help you with a walking imbalance. And if your uppers need to be rebuilt to accommodate extra-large orthotics, they can do that, too. Expect these repairs to cost from $5 to more than $40.

But even with the best care, shoes will not last forever. When they just don't have the spring anymore—or if the heel counters or uppers are no longer vertical—they should be replaced. Running shoes may last up to 700 miles; that can encompass up to six months of regular workouts. Walking shoes last a little longer: If you're walking 10-15 miles each week, you may have to replace your shoes after about nine months.

It's a good idea to rotate two pairs of running shoes every three to five workouts to prolong the life of the shoe. This allows the EVA midsole, which compresses easily, to spring back. Of course, outfitting your feet with two pairs of shoes can get expensive. So you may want to buy your sneakers from a catalog company, which can save you as much as 20% of the retail price.

Sole Searching

It's hard enough to take the first step of a running or walking regimen. But it's much harder when you put your feet in a poorly fitting pair of running shoes. Ill-fitting shoes have a habit of ending up buried in a closet, leaving you on the couch, skipping another workout. So take the time to find the pair of shoes that are just right for you. No purchase will ever pay off as dramatically in the long run—or any other run for that matter.

Anatomy of a Shoe

Midsole

The part of the sole between the insole and the outsole. It is the part of a shoe most responsible for shock absorption and the first part to wear out. Midsoles are made from one or more of the following materials:

- sheet or standard EVA (ethylene vinyl acetate), a light, styrofoam-like material with great cushioning properties but little durability;

- polyurethane, a synthetic foam that is denser, heavier, and more durable—but less shock absorbent—than standard EVA;

- compression-molded EVA, which is denser and more durable than sheet EVA but more shock absorbent than polyurethane. Many running midsoles are made with a combination of these materials. Often, denser materials are used under the heel and the forefoot, and lighter materials under the arch. On the other hand, midsoles for many walking shoes and some running shoes are made exclusively of sheet EVA.

425

These can be replaced more easily than midsoles made of combined EVA and/or polyurethane materials.

Upper

The rest of the shoe above the sole Uppers are made from leather, synthetic materials, or a combination of both. Podiatrists often recommend leather uppers because synthetic materials are more likely to promote fungal or bacterial growth inside the shoe. Many walking shoe models are still being made with leather uppers.

Heel Counter

The rigid cuplike piece at the rearfoot (back of the shoe) that holds the heel firmly in place. Running shoes have more rigid heel counters than walking shoes.

Footrames

Thin strips of firm material that extend the top of the midsole or wrap around the rearfoot, framing the lower heel or rearfoot for additional stability.

Outsole

The part of the shoe that comes in contact with the ground. At the heel, outsoles are usually made of dense carbon rubber; the rest is lighter blown rubber. However, some soles are made completely from one or the other material.

Last

The foundation to which the uppers are attached. There are three types of lasts, easily identifiable once you lift the insole. A *board last* is a stiff piece of cardboard that runs the length of the shoe. It offers little flexibility. A *slip last* is sewn, without support, and glued to the insole It offers increased flexibility. A *combination last,* as the name implies, is a cross between the two other types, with cardboard at the heel attached to a slip last that reaches to the toe. The combination offers both heel support and forefoot flexibility.

Tongue

The padded strip beneath the laces. A loop on the tongue, through which the laces are drawn, can prevent the tongue from shifting to the side. Some podiatrists recommend lacing your shoes in a straight-across, ladder pattern, instead of a zigzag pattern, to ensure adequate circulation.

Becky Papas is a free-lance writer living in New York City.

Section 32.2

Fitness Equipment

Source: *Consumers Digest,* November/December 1994.

The fitness boom, which for a time seemed to be fading has bounced back stronger than ever. For reasons of health, pleasure, and to feel and look better, more people than ever are giving their bodies the gift of exercise. A 1994 American Sports Data study found that the number of Americans who engaged in at least one fitness activity 100 times or more per year increased 3.9 percent from 42.2 million in 1992 to 43.9 million in 1993. The boom is reflected in increased purchases of equipment for home exercise, with 1994 sales expected to top 1993's $1.7 billion. More manufacturers are entering the field, resulting in more models for you to consider, meaning more confusion but competitive prices.

To help you sort through the options, we looked at five types of aerobic home-exercise equipment—stationary bicycles/ergometers (including the recumbent variations), treadmills, cross-country ski simulators, rowers and stair climbers/steppers.

How To Shop

For help in finding the machine that matches your needs, talk to someone at a specialty fitness-equipment store. There, for the most part, salespersons are knowledgeable about the products. Most specialty stores encourage hands-on testing, essential to ensuring comfort, fit and long-term enjoyment. In fact, go shopping dressed to exercise. Plan to spend some time on the equipment. You can tell a lot about a machine by how it feels. Is it comfortable, smooth and quiet? Some specialty stores will even let you rent with the option to purchase. And, if you are new to aerobic exercise or have a health condition, be sure to check with your personal physician before buying anything. If you haven't yet decided what type of machine you'd like to buy, you might be interested in a poll we took of 18 fitness experts, in regard to the five types of equipment evaluated here. On a scale of 1 to 10, for physical fitness, they ranked rowers (6.8) first, then ski simulators (6.7), treadmills (5.9), stationary bicycles (5.5) and stair steppers/climbers (5.5). For user friendliness, they ranked bicycles (8.0) first, then rowers (7.2), skiers (6.3), stair steppers/climbers (5.8) and treadmills (5.7). But you're the expert in regard to your needs and preferences.

Treadmills

Treadmills are gaining rapidly in popularity; in fact, in some specialty stores they are outselling other equipment 10 to one, despite prices that range from $400 to more than $6,000. The motorized "mill" must work hard without slowing or breaking down, which accounts for the high cost of most models. Motorized treadmills propel a belt (track) along at variable speeds to resemble your own walking or running gait. When you walk or run on the belt, you are pushing the belt against the deck with the full force of your weight (or more when you are jogging/running because you land with a downward force of two to four times your body weight).

Therefore, look for a motor rating of 1.5 to 2 horsepower of continuous duty, especially if you weigh 180 pounds or more. Continuous duty is the constant speed the machine can bear weight for long periods of time. Beware substitute labels such as "treadmill duty" or "peak horsepower" that list a higher horsepower than the treadmill has with weight loads. However, because almost all treadmills on the market are powered by a motor from one or the other of two very reliable manufacturers (Baldor and Pacific Scientific), motor quality is uniformly good. More important is the integration of the motor and the rest of the parts. Those who service treadmills say that the electronics are more likely than the motor to need repair or replacement. Ask if the electronic components of the treadmill are made in the U.S.

Parts for imported electronics are hard to find. If you haven't used a treadmill before, let someone show you how to do so without falling.

What you need to pay for a treadmill is directly related to your weight and manner of use. Economy-range models priced from $400 to $1,500 are a good buy for lightweight (150 pounds or less) walkers only. Good products in this price range include ProForm's 920 and CrossWalk, which sell below $500. The Marathon 5K also ranked well in our tests, although there is some question about durability in the field.

Medium-priced treadmills cost between $1,500 and $3,000; this range allows jogging, but if you weigh 180 pounds or more you should probably refrain from running on them. In addition to our Best Buy, we also liked the Spirit ST200 Programmable, the Precor 9.2, the True 400 and Pace Master.

In the over-$3,000 "premium" category you'll find state-of-the-art machines that are built to last, designed for the serious athlete or the person who must have the very best. The prices are staggering, but many perform well, such as the Star Trac 1200, Lifestrider and True 500.

Our Best Buys reflect all three levels of equipment. However, we did not evaluate nonmotorized treadmills because of the following drawbacks: They aren't designed to handle either jogging, running or fast walking; they tend not to permit a normal walking movement; and they are too demanding for the unfit and those unaccustomed to exercise.

When shopping for a treadmill, get satisfactory answers to this checklist:

- Is there a shutoff switch that slows the belt gradually?
- Does the belt run smoothly and quietly?
- Does the belt drag, moan or stop when you plant your feet at low and high speeds?
- Does it absorb foot shock comfortably?
- Is the belt big enough for your size?
- Are readouts clear?
- Are roller bearings sealed?
- Does the control panel use a dial (rheostat) or a more-precise touch pad for speed control?
- Will the dealer deliver and install? What is the warranty? Are replacement parts available?

Stair Climbers/Steppers

Stair climbers—also called "steppers"—are still popular. The Fitness Products Council says that 1 million more Americans started using climbers last year, and the trend is expected to continue. There are two basic types of stair climbers/steppers. "Dependent" climbers, in which the two pedals are linked so that when one pedal drops, the other rises, are generally the most stable and easiest to master. The other, "independent," type tends to be more popular. The two steps are not linked, making each leg depend on its own power to move the step. Quality-wise, there's little difference, so choice depends on personal preference.

Resistance is obtained by many methods. The lower-priced (under $200) steppers generally use air-pressure shock absorbers and are not recommended because they tend to heat up fast and break the cylinder, which can't be repaired. Better units employ Gabriel or Monroe liquid-filled hydraulic shocks, which are smoother, quieter and longer-lasting. Other models are driven by a chain, belt or cable, and most are programmable. A quality machine of this type costs between $1,000 and $2,000. (In this price range, our pick is the Tectrix Personal Climber, but the Stairmaster 4000 PT is also quite good. Its drawbacks are noisy operation and a $2,195 price.) Belts and cables are generally quieter and smoother than chains. Try a variety of models until you find the one you like best. When shopping, follow this checklist:

- Does it feel stable when stepping, especially after increasing speed?
- Is your body properly aligned?
- Are various hand positions possible?
- Is it quiet?

Stationary Cycles

The stationary bike continues to improve and diversify. Upright positions are now complemented by fully recumbent and semirecumbent types which have a bucket seat and pedals more in front—rather than directly underneath. Semirecumbent seats are easier to get into and out of—an advantage especially for the elderly or for those with previous injuries. Both types are good for those with low back pain and/or high blood pressure.

For uprights or recumbents, resistance mechanisms vary—from a flywheel to air resistance to eddy-current models. Flywheels are weighted wheels turned by the pedals. Make sure the wheel weighs 35 to 50 pounds as the heavier the wheel, the smoother and more consistent the pedal motion. Flywheels use either a belt for tension (which wraps around the outside) or brake shoes. The belt is preferred because it has a more equal draw, is easier to tighten and to replace when worn. In addition, the belt lasts longer than brake pedals because it has more surface to absorb the wear.

Air-resistant models use a fan-blade wheel. The harder you pedal, the more air is brought in and more resistance is created. Finally, the eddy-current system, computer controlled, uses a thin flywheel between the two magnets. As the magnets draw closer, there is more resistance. The advantage? No touching parts, and therefore no friction to wear them out.

For basic, quality upright bikes without the computer glitz, look to pay about $300. Medium-priced models add more features for between $300 and $750, although you will pay more for the best-quality exercise bikes. Consider these factors when shopping:

- Is the seat comfortable and easily adjustable, and do the handlebars adjust easily?

- Does the bike wobble as you increase speed? Is pedaling smooth, without dragging?

- Are toe clips/straps available?

- Is it quiet?

Rowers

Rowers are less popular today than they once were, but many users still find that the machines provide a great total-body workout. Test the rower to see if the action is comfortable, smooth and quiet. Rowing exerts considerable pressure on the lower back, so if you have a history of back pain, proceed with caution and follow the directions of the manufacturer carefully. Wind-resistance models, such as the Concept II, cost $700 to $800 and use either a chain or a cable to drive a fanwheel. The chains are very durable but require light maintenance which can be messy. They also tend to be a bit noisier than cables. Be sure to compare other attributes such as the comfort of the seat.

The WaterRower offers another type of resistance. A round tank holds up to five gallons of water. A blade turns through the water when you pull back on the handle, creating more resistance the faster you go. It produces a pleasant sound, simulating oars pulling against water.

Cross-Country Skiers

The name NordicTrack is synonymous with cross-country ski machines, although there are other quality ski companies. Options range from the type of arm mechanisms such as poles or ropes, to the type of foot resistance available. With a shuffle-type skier, your feet move back and forth on two pads in skate-like fashion. These are generally less expensive and easier to learn than machines that more-accurately simulate cross-country skiing. In addition, the shuffle-type takes less space as there are no protruding skis.

The ski-type connects a boot to skis that move back and forth. Some feel this has a less-balanced feel. Others think the motion most realistically imitates the sport. Most ski-types use a flywheel-type "clutch" for resistance, which feels smooth and natural. Some use a nylon belt and rollers instead. You should compare the bases to see which has the sturdier design. The ski arms can be dependent—linked together with one automatically moving back as the other is pulled forward, or independent—you must push each one back in place. Some have an up-and-down movement. It's a matter of personal preference.

Cross-country machines require a different type of coordination than other equipment, and some people find them difficult to learn. We recommend that you allow 15 minutes or so of practice before rejecting this type of equipment. Start with just a leg movement. Add the arm movement after you feel confident. One common mistake people make is to lean into the hip pad, causing instability and lower-back discomfort, rather than pressing against it with a straight back. Once you are practiced, it is exceptional exercise, especially since it works both the upper and lower body. If you find the movement requires too much concentration, however, you probably won't use it. Some evaluators praise the medium-price Fitness Master 340 and the premium-price Precor 515e and Tunturi XC560, and all are worth a look. But NordicTrack really rules this market.

Best Buys In Fitness Equipment

Treadmills

[P] **Trotter 525** (List $4,195; Best Price $3,795). This state-of-the-art home treadmill includes a wide variety of programmed workouts, and can store up to 10 of them. Its combination of dot-matrix and digital displays is user-friendly. It has a smooth, cushioned running surface and an open front to accommodate long striders. Powered by a durable two hp (continuous duty) motor, it has a speed range of one to 10 mph and an incline range of zero to 12 percent.

[M] **Cybex Q20ci** (List $2,495; Best Price $2,295). The sharp and snappy Q20ci provides what Cybex calls a "controlled-impact" system. The suspension system provides impact cushioning at every point on the deck surface. A low-profile motor hood extends the usable running surface. The zero to 11 mph speed adjustment and zero to 12 percent motorized incline are suitable for most potential buyers. The control board displays speed, time, distance, pace, calories and elevation. The unit has a five-year warranty, including labor, on all major components, and a lifetime guarantee on structural parts.

[E] **Trimline 2200** (List $950, Best Price $799). This offers a 0-10 mph speed and zero to 10 percent elevation. The panel shows the length of workout in seconds, minutes and miles. The machine is for walking—jogging and running are not recommended. At both high and low speeds, the belt stopped when we planted our feet firmly.

Stair Steppers/Climbers

[P] **Tectrix Personal Climber** (List $2,250; Best Price $1,979). This attractive, smooth, quiet and well-made climber, from a reputable company features independent step action and self-leveling footpads. Programming is great, with choices of manual, custom, race, peak and interval training offered on an imposing display panel. There is precise speed control across 29 climbing speeds ranging from 10 to 150 feet per minute.

[M] **BMI Summit 6100** (List $499; Best Price $449). A true climber, the Summit provides ladder-like action, somewhat like rock-climbing. You reach over your head for the handgrips with motion that

433

alternates with your feet, insuring a complete body workout. The digital display tells load. tempo, calories, steps and time. It should be noted that the chain is a bit noisy, and the height of the machine could be a problem in a low-ceiling room.

[E] Tunturi Tri-Stepper 500 (List $249; Best Price $199). An independent stepper that maximizes calorie burn, this machine has a tripod design that makes for stability and eliminates vibration. The contoured handlebars promote good posture and are comfortably padded. The wide pedals minimize slippage, and an electronic meter displays time, steps and calories expended.

Upright Stationary Bikes

[P] Lifecycle 6500HR (List $1,595; Best Price $1,495). The fact that this cycle generates its own electricity for digital displays means that you can place it anywhere. Also noteworthy is the heart-rate sensor, built right into the handgrips. Programming is motivating and fun with six programs, including one that simulates the racing and gear-shifting action of a 12-speed bike. Among the many features is a display of a target heart-rate zone, rpm, mph, calories per hour, total miles ridden, elapsed time, stopwatch and fitness test. A shell helps protect all components from dirt, dust and moisture. For less than half the price, the **Lifecycle 3500** (Best Price $629)—with the optional software program, Exertainment—allows you to compete while riding.

[P] Spinnaker 3000 CE (List $1,595; Best Price NA). The manufacturer claims that this very attractive machine duplicates the feel and conditioning effects of outdoor bicycle riding. Our panel of biking consumers agreed. The bike features a drivetrain mechanism that converts air pressure into resistance to provide a smooth, comfortable ride. Motivational conditioning programs include two user-controlled, self-paced workouts, three training-interval programs and three racing programs.

[M] Schwinn Air Dyne Pro (List $699; Best Price NA). This is the original and best-known dual-action (works the arms also) air-resistance bike. The air-resistance wheel provides a cooling breeze during the workout. Attractive and solidly built by a reputable company—now under new ownership—its only drawback (for some us-

434

ers) is that the arms and pedals are permanently linked. Strong dealer support is a real advantage.

[E] Tunturi TEE (List $249; Best Price $199). If you don't need all the extras, this sturdy, comfortable machine is an excellent buy. It accurately measures calories burned, uses a 40-pound steel flywheel with felt brake and a 100 percent carbon-steel frame. The bike also has a cushioned SofGel seat. Pedals conform to the feet, and handlebars and seat adjust easily. A panel displays speed, rpm, time, distance and a 60-minute countdown.

Recumbent Stationary Bikes

[P] Lifecycle 5500 (List $1,995; Best Price $1,795). The semirecumbent seat position of this bike provides stability and comfort for reading while exercising. There are 13 different levels of pedal resistance. Programs include a hill profile in an interval-training format with visual displays of the terrain coming up. A random program accesses over a million combinations of hills and valleys at the varying pedal speeds. A three-year warranty is provided.

[M] Schwinn C1230 (List $899; Best Price NA). Rated as the most user-friendly by our evaluators, this comfortable, slightly noisy semirecumbent bike is a workhorse. It has an easy-to-read display panel that gives you time, rpm, speed, calories and distance. It also has various programs, including manual, intense, summit, hills plateau and triathlon.

[E] Precor Mode I (List $399; Best Price $350). This was the only fully recumbent bike selected. Although the seat can be hard to adjust, it is comfortably contoured to firmly support your lower back while positioning your body to work all muscle groups in the legs and buttocks. Pedal resistance can be changed while pedaling, and the 40-lb. flywheel gives a smooth, quiet workout.

Rowers

[P] WaterRower (List $1,499; Best Price $1,295) This is an impressive-looking machine with nicely finished woods, but its great appeal is the soothing sound of rowing through water, accomplished by using a water tank with blades turning inside. The basic model comes only with a countdown clock. An optional programmable computer shows speed, time, distance and strokes per minute and can be connected to your home computer to compile a running log of your progress.

[M] Concept II Model C (List $700; Best Price NA). The first rower that felt like sculling, this is a long-standing favorite in the field, now featuring a new seat and a versatile flex-foot. The chain-driven pulley system can be a bit noisy. The monorail detaches easily for storage. The display panel provides a timer, stroke output, strokes per minute, and total workout. A wind damper increases the range of resistance options.

Cross-Country Ski Simulators

[P] NordicTrack Pro (Best Price $600). The wide front frame of this solid-oak-and-steel model provides added stability for very vigorous workouts. The front elevation adjustment can be set at six positions and the hip pad adjusted to fit different users. Back wheels make it easy to move, and it folds for storage. Electronics measure distance, time and speed.

[M] NordicTrack Challenger (Best Price $340). A great basic model with ski-type action for a realistic cross-country ski motion, the Challenger employs a flywheel and one-way clutch mechanism. Numbered lower-body and adjustable upper-body resistance settings help tailor your workout, while cord-pulley action for the arms helps assure total body conditioning. A simple design and attractive black-varnish finish make this unit appealing to the eye, as well.

[E] ProForm 570XC (List $179; Best Price $150). For beginners, this is a nice machine. Its easy-to-read, well-positioned console displays time, speed, distance and calories used. The ski pedals move smoothly on the ski rails and a resistance dial allows for adjustment of tension on ski-pole movement. The incline of the ski rails can be lowered or raised, as the user wishes.

For More Information

Treadmills: Cybex, 206/821-8233; Trimline Hebb Industries, 903/534-3832; Trotter, 800/671-6544.

Stair Steppers/Climbers: BMI, 800/321-9838; Tectrix, 800/767-8082; Tunturi, 800/827-8717.

Stationary Bicycles: LifeCycle, 800/877-3867; Precor, 800/4PRECOR; Schwinn, 708/231-5340; Spinnaker, 800/635-2936; Tunturi 800/827-8717.

Rowers: Concept II, 800/245-5616; WaterRower, 800/852-2210.

Skiers: NordicTrack, 800/328-5888; ProForm, 800/727-9777.

Section 32.3

How To Choose A Health Club

Source: *Diabetes Self-Management,* March/April, 1992.

by Richard M. Weil, M.Ed., C.D.E.

You have probably been told more times than you care to remember about the benefits of exercise—better blood glucose control, maintained weight control, improved muscular condition, and protection against cardiovascular discs—but starting or staying on an exercise program is often easier said than done.

If you have found it difficult or inconvenient to work out at home, maybe a change of scenery would help. Consider trying a place with a lot more structure, some variety, and individual instruction—a health club.

Whatever type of club you're interested in—serious "pumping iron" gyms, women's weight-loss clubs, aerobic dance studios, or full-service facilities that offer everything including massages, sauna rooms, suntan beds, and even organized ski trips—there's a workout spot to fill your need. But making the right choice can mean the difference between getting yourself into shape and wasting your time and money. So take the time to evaluate the clubs in your area to determine which one is right for you. The following information shows you how.

Taking The First Step

To get started, visit several clubs in your neighborhood for an idea of the services available Talk to anyone you know who belongs to a club; members can often give you information that you might not learn during a club visit. Drop in on a club during the hours that you will be most likely to go. Be prepared for some crowds, especially during peak hours (before and after work and around lunchtime). If you plan to exercise at these times, look for a club with enough equipment to handle the traffic.

As you begin to narrow down your choices, revisit those clubs still in the running At most clubs, a salesperson will take you on a 10- to 15-minute tour, but be prepared for a tough sales pitch afterward. Don't be badgered into signing anything until you are ready; a "to-day only" special price might be tempting, but chances are that the club will extend the price offer if you ask..

What to Look For

Here's a checklist of things to think about and to look for as you search for the "perfect" health club:

Equipment

Cardiovascular conditioning—exercise that lowers blood glucose levels, increases insulin sensitivity, reduces the risks of heart disease, and maintains good circulation—should be a primary exercise goal for people with diabetes. To maximize cardiovascular conditioning look for a club that offers a full range of training equipment designed to give you an aerobic workout (exercise that causes an elevated heart rate). Such a range of equipment might include treadmills, station-ary bikes, rowing machines, stairclimbers, and ski machines If you have circulatory problems or neuropathy, look for airdynes and/or re-cumbent bikes, these are modified stationary bikes that allow you to exercise vigorously without the leg or foot pain you might experience with some other equipment. Swimming is also an excellent aerobic activity that doesn't tax your feet If you're interested in weight train-ing which provides some aerobic benefit, increased muscle tone and strength, and increased circulation, look; for an array of free weights (barbells and dumbbells) and weight-lifting machines.

If you find yourself consistently waiting a long time for equipment, perhaps you can arrange to use the gym during off-peak hours. Your doctor should be able to help you accommodate an alternative exercise schedule by adjusting your insulin regimen and your food intake.

Don't let all the different brands of equipment overwhelm you. Almost all commercial exercise equipment manufactured these days is designed for both safety and efficiency. So whether the equipment is Nautilus, Universal, or another brand, you'll get an adequate workout.

Location

If the club isn't nearby, you probably won't go very often. Even world-class facilities are worthless if you never use them. Find a club that is not more than a 20- to 25-minute drive or a 10-minute walk from your home or place of business.

Business Hours

Make sure that the club is open during hours that are convenient for you. Check the weekend schedule, which is often different from weekday hours, as well as holiday closings.

Cleanliness

Inspect the locker rooms, showers, bathroom stalls, sauna and steamrooms, and whirlpool facilities. A dirty club is not only unsanitary, but a sure sign of inattention to detail, and it probably reflects how the club is run in general.

Workout Area

The club should have enough floor space so that you don't feel cramped, especially during busy times. Long waits for workout machines can be discouraging so if, you must exercise during a club's busy times, be sure it has enough equipment to handle the traffic. See that there is also an area where you can comfortably stretch before and after your workout.

Staff

A personal trainer who oversees your every move may be too much to ask for, but it is not unreasonable to expect to have a staff member available at all times to give you suggestions for exercise adjustments and upgrades. A health club should have enough staff on hand to cover all areas of the exercise floor.

Don't be afraid to ask for staff credentials. The best health clubs are staffed by fitness instructors certified by the American College of Sports Medicine. Likewise, a club's dance instructors should be certified by either the International Dance and Exercise Association or the Aerobics and Fitness Association of America. Certification does not guarantee that an instructor is terrific, but it does reflect the commitment and management standards of the club.

A certified fitness instructor is qualified to evaluate your fitness level, prescribe exercise, monitor your blood pressure during exercise if your doctor has requested it, and demonstrate proper exercise techniques. Some fitness instructors are certified exercise specialists or exercise physiologists who, if you're lucky, will have experience with people who have diabetes. Most of the better gyms have them on staff. But even if your gym has these instructors on hand, it's important that you know how exercise affects your blood sugar. Before beginning any exercise program, discuss it with your physician or diabetes educator. Then make the health-club staff aware of your diabetes and make sure that they know how to recognize and treat hypoglycemia And always have fast-acting carbohydrate with you for emergencies.

Specialty classes

Some people like to get a good workout without using any equipment. Aerobics and dance classes, for instance, can give you as much cardiovascular conditioning as you need. Other classes, such as, yoga or stretch and tone, while not aerobic, can help maintain flexibility, increase strength, and relieve stress. Although diabetes related problems such as leg pain or loss of balance may make some of the more rigorous classes inappropriate, stretch-and-tone classes (in which most of the time is spent on the floor) are nice substitutes. If you have retinopathy, avoid exercises that put your head below the level of your heart or that force you to strain, thus raising your blood pressure. And if you have any kind of complication, make sure you ask your doctor about exercise limitations.

Medical Clearance

Most health clubs require a physician's medical clearance before permitting you to start an exercise program; some will even ask you to take a stress test. If your doctor feels that a stress test is unnecessary, ask him or her to write a letter to the club fitness manager clearing you.

Exercise Prescription

Some clubs offer a fitness evaluation and exercise orientation before you start. The evaluation should include a test of your aerobic capacity, as well as your flexibility, strength, and body-fat percentage. With this information, and your input regarding fitness goals, the club can help you devise an efficient exercise program and keep track of your progress over time. This service may carry an additional charge (usually less than $100). Occasionally, a physical therapist is also available for a fee to evaluate your posture, spine, or other orthopedic problems. Again, ask about credentials because these fitness coordinators are not always knowledgeable about diabetes. When a specialist or exercise physiologist is on the premises, he or she should be the one to prescribe your exercise program and oversee your progress.

Sauna Facilities

Dry saunas, steamrooms, and whirl pool baths are all just rewards for a hard workout. In most cases, people with diabetes can enjoy any of these in moderation (10-15 minutes). However, if you have high blood pressure, you may have to avoid the heat (ask your doctor). In addition, if you have a loss of sensation in hands, legs, or feet, be especially careful not to burn yourself in these facilities. In these areas especially, make sure that facilities are clean and well maintained. Also make sure that there is a staff member on hand who has been certified by the department of health to operate these facilities and who can spot potential problems. This is required by law.

Record Keeping

Some clubs insist that you keep a record of your attendance and workouts on a club form. This is a good way for you and the staff to keep tabs on your progress. Keeping records also helps to keep you motivated.

Social Activities

Health clubs are a good way to make new friends. Don't be shy about asking if the club offers parties, ski trips, volleyball tournaments, or other group activities.

Closing The Deal

Once you have made up your mind to sign the contract, read it carefully. It must state the following:

- your right to cancel the contract within three days after you sign it;

- if you move more than 25 miles from the club and no affiliated club or similar club will honor your contract, then you are no longer responsible for fees;

- if you become disabled, you can either extend your membership for the length of time you were disabled or you can cancel your membership.

It's a good idea to take the contract home and read it before signing, especially if you have any doubts. Try to find out who owns the club and how long the club has been in existence. Ask if there have been any renovations or if any are planned. The last thing you want to do is to hand your money over to a club on the verge of closing its doors.

If the club is part of a citywide or nationwide chain, or if it is a member of a sports organization such as the International Racquetball and Squash Association (IRSA), ask if you are entitled to use affiliated clubs in other cities. This service can be valuable if you travel frequently. In some cases, the participating club may charge a guest fee (usually about $15).

A health-club membership is likely to run anywhere from $150 to $2000 a year. Keep in mind that a clean, well-maintained, and service-oriented club is expensive to operate. A club that offers a lifetime membership at a ridiculously low price is likely to be so crowded, dirty, or poorly maintained that you may rarely use it. You get what you pay for in the health club industry.

Additional fees can add up. so be prepared for them. Some clubs charge for towels, lockers, and special services like massage. Make sure you're an are of all extra fees before you sign the contract. Clubs often charge a one time initiation fee that can range from $100 to $500. Try negotiating this fee or spreading it out over several payments. Most clubs also have some sort of guest fee, usually $5 to $15 per day. Ask for some free guest passes when you sign up.

Your method of payment will be up to you and the club. Of course, collecting the annual fee right away is management's preferred choice. Better for you, however, is an installment plan that authorizes the club to charge your credit card each month or to electronically transfer monthly payments directly from your checking account This way you don't pay a large initial sum (although the club will usually ask for the first one or two months up front), you can cancel your membership at any time without losing money, and you have time to try the club without committing the full price. The disadvantage is that the monthly fee spread out over a year will add up to more than the lump-sum price.

Types of Memberships

How much your membership costs will depend on the type of plan you choose. A standard yearly membership usually entitles you to all the services of the club at any time and is often accompanied by one or two free months if you pay all at once. On the other hand, quarterly membership or another type of limited-visit membership may be a better choice if you need the use of the club just for the summer, or if you want to try it out before signing up for a longer period. A quarterly membership costs more than a quarter of a yearly membership, but you can usually convert it to a yearly one for a small fee. Some clubs offer reduced rates for members who plan to use the club only during off-peak hours, usually between 9:00 AM and 11:30 AM and 1:00 PM and 4:00 PM.

Ace of Clubs

The competition between health clubs is stiff. That's good news for the consumer because the more interested the club is in keeping you as a long time member, the more likely it is to offer special attention. The equipment, instruction, and the range of services are of a higher quality than they were 10 years ago. This also means better choices for you. You can afford to be more demanding in this market, so take your time and make the choice that fits your needs.

Richard M. Weil, M.Ed., C.D.E., an exercise physiologist, is a consultant to the Diabetes Treatment Center at The New York Eye and Ear Infirmary, and to Park Avenue Diabetes Care in New York City.

Part Five

Recent Research in Fitness

Chapter 33

The Health Benefits of Physical Activity

In 1990, *Healthy People 2000* was released by Dr. Louis Sullivan, Secretary, Department of Health and Human Services. The document elaborated national health promotion and disease prevention goals for the year 2000. A central goal of the document is to increase the span of healthy life for Americans. While improved treatment of disease to prevent premature death is an important concern, *Healthy People 2000* emphasizes the importance of prevention of illness/disease, especially lifestyle or chronic illnesses that have become the leading sources of death in our society. But perhaps most important of all, the goals focus on efforts to promote a quality of life and a sense of well-being associated with good health. Dr. Michael McGinnis, Director of the Office of Disease Prevention and Health Promotion, recently made the following statement.

> ...it is not through happenstance that the physical activity
> category is the first priority area of the *Healthy People 2000*
> effort. Physical activity is related to the health of all Ameri-
> cans. It has the ability to reduce directly the risk of several
> major chronic diseases as well as to catalyze positive
> changes with respect to other risk factors of these diseases.
> Dr. William Foege, former Director of the Centers for Dis-
> ease Control, suggests that physical activity may provide
> the shortcut we in public health have been seeking for the

Physical Activity And Fitness Research Digest, Series 1, No.1, February 1993.

control of chronic diseases, much like immunization has facilitated progress against infectious diseases (McGinnis, 1992, p. S196).

The inclusion of physical activity as an important lifestyle for promoting good health is now clear. But for those interested in the health benefits of physical activity, it is not easy to find a single source that summarizes these benefits. For this reason, we have attempted to provide a simple summary of the benefits in three sections: disease prevention and treatment; health promotion; and physical fitness development. Six principal sources are used for this summary. Readers are encouraged to consult these references and their sources for more complete details.

Disease Prevention and Treatment

Prior to 1940, the leading killers in the United States were infectious diseases. Improvement in public health practices, implementation of personal and public health education, and vaccines have greatly reduced the incidence of these diseases. As indicated in the early statement by Dr. Foege, "chronic diseases" are now our major health concerns. These chronic diseases are often referred to as "lifestyle diseases" because changes in lifestyle, including increased activity and fitness, can reduce the threat of early death and the incidence of disease. Table 1 lists several of the diseases for which regular physical activity can reduce risk, either of getting the disease or of dying from it. Also illustrated in Table 1 (below) are some of the possible reasons why exercise reduces risk of these diseases.

In spite of the fact that deaths from heart disease have decreased in recent years, it is still the leading cause of death. Studies by Paffenbarger and colleagues (1989) as well as others have clearly shown that those who do regular physical activity are at less risk of dying from this major killer. Physically inactive people have almost twice the risk of developing heart disease as active people (Powell et al., 1987). In fact, the American Heart Association (Fletcher et al., 1992) has recently classified inactivity (sedentary living) as a primary risk factor for heart disease comparable to high blood pressure, high blood cholesterol and cigarette smoking. Both stroke (lack of blood flow and oxygen to the brain) and peripheral vascular disease (lack of blood flow and oxygen to the limbs) have been shown (Haskell et al., 1992) to be associated with sedentary living for many of the same reasons why inactivity is related to heart disease (see Table 1). High blood pressure or hypertension is a condition that predisposes people to other health risks such as heart disease and diabetes. Regular exercise has been shown to reduce blood pressure among those who have high levels though, by itself, exercise cannot normalize high blood pressure for most people (Haskell et al., 1992).

In the introduction of the Physical Activity and Fitness section of *Healthy People 2000* (Public Health Service, p. 94), it is noted that physical activity can help to prevent and manage non-insulin-dependent diabetes and osteoporosis. Recent evidence also has shown that inactive people have a higher incidence of colon and breast cancer than active people. While the evidence is less than complete, one researcher reached the following conclusion based on a review of recent research.

> Given the consistency in the direction and magnitude of the findings regarding colon cancer . . . the evidence supports the conclusion that activity is protective against colon cancer. Although that protective effect may be small, the attributable risk of colon cancer associated with inactivity may be quite high given the prevalence of inactivity in Western societies. (Sternfeld, 1992, p. 1195)

It is generally conceded that regular muscle fitness and flexibility exercise can aid in improving posture. Together, exercise and good posture can have a positive effect on back problems as evidenced by less risk of back pain. In a recent review, Plowman (1992) noted that while we do not yet know the exact amounts of muscle strength, muscle endurance, and flexibility necessary to reduce the risk of back pain, there is support for the notion that poor scores on these fitness measures are predictive of low back pain.

The potential benefits of regular physical activity in reducing obesity are well documented. Regular exercise expends calories that can result in reduced fat storage in the body's fat cells. At the same time, exercise designed to build muscle fitness increases lean body tissue (muscle), which can result in a lesser relative percentage of fat in the body and a higher resting metabolism. Getting obese Americans to adopt regular exercise that would help them achieve normal levels of body fatness is not as successful as we might hope. Nevertheless, physical activity has great potential for reducing the incidence of obesity in our society (Epstein et al., 1990).

Depression is a major medical problem that causes much pain and suffering. The number of bed days and disabilities associated with

Table 1. Physical Activity and Major Lifestyle Diseases

Disease	Physical Activity Benefit
Heart Disease	-Healthy heart muscle • lower resting heart rate • more blood pumped with each beat • reduced blood pressure in submaximal work -Healthy arteries • less atherosclerosis (deposits in arteries) • higher HDL ("good" cholesterol) • better blood fat profile (fewer "bad" fats) • decreased platelet and less fibrin (related to atherosclerosis) • better blood flow -Better working capacity • fewer demands during work • greater ability to meet work demands
Stroke	-Healthy arteries (see above) • lower blood pressure
Peripheral	-Improved working capacity
Vascular Disease	-Higher HDL • Better blood fat profile
High Blood Pressure	-Reduction in blood pressure among those with high levels. -Reduction in body fatness (associated with high blood pressure)
Diabetes (non-insulin)	-Reduced body fatness (may relieve symptoms of adult onset diabetes) -Better carbohydrate metabolism (improved insulin sensitivity)
Cancer	-Less risk of colon cancer (better transit time of food?)

Obesity	-Increases lean body mass
	-Decreases body fat percentage
	-Less central fat distribution
Depression	-Relief from some symptoms
Back Pain	-Increased muscle strength and endurance
	-Improved flexibility
	-Improved posture
Osteoporosis	-Greater bone density as a result of stressing long bones

depression is greater than that for the eight major chronic health conditions (Public Health Service, 1990). A recent position statement of the International Society of Sport Psychology (1992) states that studies on depressed patients reveal that aerobic exercises are as effective as different forms of psychotherapy. In addition, the Society summarizes by saying: "Exercise can have beneficial emotional effects across all ages and for both sexes."

Health Promotion

The previous section dealt primarily with disease. Of course, disease treatment and prevention are critical to good health in our society. Nevertheless, it is widely acknowledged that optimal health is much more than freedom from disease. The challenge of *Healthy People 2000* (Public Health Service, 1990) illustrates this point.

> The health of people is measured by more than death rates. Good health comes from reducing unnecessary suffering, illness, and disability. It comes as well from an improved quality of life. Health is thus best measured by citizens' sense of well-being (p. 6).

Prevention of disease is a high priority and regular physical activity has been shown to help prevent the conditions discussed in the preceding sections. But what of high-quality living and a sense of well being? Many of these are quite subjective. Corbin and Lindsey (1990) summarize some of the perceived benefits of exercise based on subjective feelings of people responding to national surveys. Some of the

451

reported benefits are supported by scientific evidence, including a reduction in stress levels and in symptoms of depression (International Society for Sports Psychology, 1992), improved appearance, and increased working capacity. Other benefits such as improved sleep habits, greater ability to enjoy leisure, improved general sense of well-being, and improved self-esteem are less easy to document. Nevertheless, what people think is true influences their quality of life and the results of national opinion polls show that many Americans have positive feelings about the benefits they receive from regular exercise (Corbin and Lindsey, 1990). Among older adults, regular physical activity has been shown to increase independent functioning, increase the ability to drive a car, and improve social interactions (Corbin and Lindsey, 1990). There is similar evidence to show that physical activity can positively influence other health-related behaviors (Blair, 1985). One recent survey, for example, showed that regular exercisers were 50% more likely to quit smoking; 40% more likely to eat less red meat; 30% more likely to cut down on caffeine; 250% more likely to eat low calorie foods and drinks, 200% more likely to lose weight, and 25% more likely to cut down on salt and sugar than non-exercisers (Harris & Gurin, 1985).

Physical activity's contribution to quality of life and a personal sense of well-being is more difficult to document than its contribution to prevention and treatment of disease. In the long run, however, it may be equally important if the national goal of lengthening healthy life is to be achieved. It is doubtful that most Americans would favor an extended life if "quality of life" was lacking. The evidence suggests that humans were designed to be physically active and that physical activity has great potential for enhancing quality of life and sense of well-being. Additional research is necessary to determine the full extent of activity's contribution to these important variables.

Physical Fitness

There is no doubt that regular physical activity builds physical fitness. Previous issues of this *Digest* written by H. Harrison Clarke clearly document this fact. What has become increasingly clear in recent years is that physical activity and physical fitness, as evidenced by performance on fitness tests, are independent but related phenomena. Likewise, physical fitness is associated with good health. For example, Blair et al. (1989) have shown that those with "good" levels of fitness have less heart disease risk than those with "low" levels of fitness. The previously cited review by Plowman (1992) suggests that muscle fitness is necessary to prevent back pain. Others have pointed out the importance of fitness to injury prevention (McGinnis, 1992). Body fatness, often considered a health-related component of physical fitness, is associated with medical problems of various kinds.

Fitness, as measured by fitness tests, is NOT solely related to regular physical activity. As noted in Figure 1, there are many other factors that contribute to physical fitness. Among children, fitness scores are influenced by chronological age and maturation (physiological age). In some cases, children and adolescents who are inactive have higher fitness scores than younger or more active peers (Pangrazi & Corbin, 1990; Pate, Dowda, & Ross, 1990). Bouchard and colleagues (1992) have demonstrated that heredity plays a significant role in a person's ability to improve fitness as a result of exercise (this will be discussed in more detail in an upcoming issue of the *Digest*). Some people respond to training more favorably than others, so it is possible that regular exercisers could sometimes have lower fitness performance levels than those who are sedentary. Of course, other factors such as nutrition, learned skills, and environment also play a role in fitness performances.

There is little doubt that good physical fitness is associated with reduced risk of disease. Further, it can be stated that good fitness helps people function effectively, look better, and have the ability to enjoy their free time. But evidence exists to support other important statements about physical fitness.

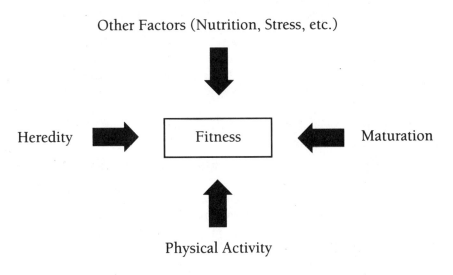

- Physical fitness, as measured by fitness tests, is not as meaningful to good health as physical fitness that results from regular physical activity as part of the normal lifestyle.

- Physical fitness, as measured by fitness tests, will ultimately improve as the result of regular exercise to the extent that hereditary predispositions allow. The amount and rate of change in fitness will take longer for some to achieve than for others.

- Physical fitness is associated with good health but is not the same as good health. Regular physical activity has positive benefits for both good health and adequate physical fitness.

- For good health benefits to result, it is important NOT to be in a low fit category. On the other hand, high levels of fitness test performance do NOT seem to be necessary for attaining health benefits. All people with regular physical activity have the potential to achieve adequate levels of fitness that are associated with good health.

Summary

In recent years, much has been learned about regular physical activity and physical fitness. Many of the health benefits of exercise and physical fitness are now well documented. Other potential benefits require much more research. In the meantime, the following quotes seem to best summarize our knowledge.

From leading researchers Paffenbarger and Hyde (1980):

> Evidence mounts that the relationship between exercise and good health is more than circumstantial. If some questions are not yet answered, they are far less important than those that have been.

From Edward Cooper during a news conference for the American Heart Association, July 1, 1992:

> Now I'd like to say to those who are not engaged in "exercise training" that any physical activity is better than none. According to our panel, housework, gardening, shuffleboard— anything that causes us to move—is beneficial. Maybe you don't have time or ability to attain "cardiovascular fitness,"

that is, to enable your heart to function at its most efficient level...maybe you don't have the money to join a health club or buy a bicycle...still there are activities you can perform as a part of your daily life that will benefit your heart. I encourage you to make activity a part of your routine every day—just as much a part of your day as brushing your teeth or enjoying breakfast.

John Dryden, spoken several hundred years ago, as cited by Paffenbarger and Hyde (1980):

Better to hunt in fields, for health unbought, than fee the doctor for nauseous draught; the wise, for cure, on exercise depend; God never made his work for man to mend.

References

Blair, S.N. (1985) Relationship between exercise or physical activity and other health behaviors. *Public Health Reports.* 100, 172-180.

Blair, S. N., Kohl, H.W., Paffenbarger, R.S., Clarke, D.G., Cooper, K.H. & Gibbons, L.W. (1989) *Journal of the American Medical Association.* 262, 2395-2401.

Bouchard, C., Dionne, F.T., Simoneau, J., Er Boulay, M.R. (1992) Genetics of aerobic performances. In J.O. Holloszy, (Ed.) *Exercise and Sport Sciences Reviews*: Vol. 20 (pp. 27-58). Baltimore: Williams and Wilkins.

Corbin, C.B. & Lindsey, R. (1990) *Concepts of Physical Fitness.* (7th ed.). Dubuque, IA: Wm. C. Brown Co.

Epstein, L.H., McCurley, M., Wing, R.R., Valoski, A. (1990) Five-year follow-up of family-based behavioral treatments for childhood obesity. *Journal of Consulting Clinical Psychology.* 58, 661-664.

Fletcher, G.F., Blair, S.N., Blumenthal, J., Caspersen, C., Chaitman, B., Epstein, S., Falls, H., Froelicher, E., Froelicher, V., and Pina, I. (1992) Statement on exercise: Benefits and recommendations for physical activity for all Americans. Circulation. 86, 2726-2730.

Harris, T. G. & Gurin, J. (1985) Look who's getting it all together. *American Health*. 4 (2), 42-47.

Haskell, W.L., Leon, A.S., Caspersen, C., Froelicher, V. F., Hagberg, J. M., Harlan, W., Holloszy, J.O., Regensteiner, J.G., Thompson, P.D., Washburn, R.A., & Wilson, P. W. F. (1992) Cardiovascular benefits and assessment of physical activity and physical fitness in adults. *Medicine and Science in Sports and Exercise*. 24, S201-S220.

International Society of Sport Psychology. (1992) Physical activity and psychological benefits. *Physician and Sportsmedicine*. 20, 179-184.

McGinnis, J.M. (1992) The public health burden of a sedentary lifestyle. *Medicine and Science in Sports and Exercise*. 24, S196-S200.

Paffenbarger, R. S. & Hyde, R.T. (1980) Exercise as protection against heart attack. *New England Journal of Medicine*. 302, 1026-1027.

Paffenbarger, R.S., Hyde, R., Wing, A.L., & Hsieh, C. (1986) Physical activity, all-cause mortality, and longevity of college alumni. 314, 605-614.

Pangrazi, R.P. & Corbin, C.B. (1990) Age as a factor relating to physical fitness test performance. *Research Quarterly for Exercise and Sport*. 61, 410-414.

Pate, R.R., Dowda, M. & Ross, J.G. (1990) Association between physical activity and physical fitness of children. *American Journal of Diseases in Children*. 144, 1123-1129.

Powell, K.E., Thompson, K.D., Caspersen, C.J., & Kendrick, J.S. (1987) Physical activity and the incidence of coronary heart disease. *Annual Review of Public Health*. 8, 253-287.

Public Health Service. (1990) *Healthy People 2000*. Washington, D.C.: U.S. Government Printing Office.

Sternfeld, B. (1992) Cancer and the protective effect of physical activity: The epidemiological evidence. *Medicine and Science in Sports and Exercise*. 24, 1195-1209.

Chapter 34

Physical Activity and Intrinsic Motivation

Introduction: Theory Development

Over the past 20 years, we have accumulated considerable evidence to document the health benefits of physical activity (see Chapter 33). Researchers have established with a fair degree of confidence just how much physical activity is necessary to produce fitness improvement and benefits to health (ACSM, 1990). Given this rather clear picture of how to obtain desirable benefits, an obvious question is why do less than one quarter of the population engage in light-to-moderate physical activity? The answer to this question is found largely in the realm of psychology—specifically in the area of motivation. The task of this issue is to review current knowledge and to translate it into suggestions for enhancing physical activity. Specific guidelines for fostering intrinsic motivation toward physical activity are outlined in the final section.

Motivational studies have long focused on factors that initiate, influence and modify behavior. Early theories dealt essentially with the deterministic aspects of those factors; focusing on instinctual drives (e.g., Freud, 1923/1962), physiological drives (e.g., Hull, 1943), or environmental influences (e.g., Skinner, 1953, 1971). Although these theories had (and still have) considerable value, their apparent view of people as passive beings that are pushed and pulled around by their physiology or environment has given rise to concern and criticism. A different point of view was published as a monograph by

Physical Activity And Fitness Research Digest, Series 1, No. 2, May 1993.

(White, 1959) who proposed that people are driven by a need to be competent, or effective in mastering all aspects of our environment. He suggested that when attempts to master the challenges of our surroundings were successful, the result was positive—a "feeling of efficacy" (p. 329)—which, in turn, served to intrinsically motivate further behavior. White's monograph led to a wealth of study on intrinsic motivation, and in that respect it can be seen as the foundation of subsequent studies that are described below.

Refinements of the Theory

A major development of White's (1959) monograph is represented by the addition of a formal statement of cognitive evaluation theory (Deci, 1975; Deci & Ryan, 1985). Cognitive evaluation theory states that intrinsic motivation is driven by an innate need for competence and self-determination in dealing with one's surroundings. The intrinsic rewards for the behaviors motivated by this need are satisfying feelings of competence and autonomy, positive emotions such as enjoyment and excitement, and possibly the sensation of flow (complete absorption in the activity). These feelings, in turn, serve to maintain or increase a person's intrinsic motivation for the particular behavior.

In a nutshell (according to the theory), an individual's desire to pursue a particular activity depends upon whether his or her feelings of competence, autonomy, and positive affect persist over time. Conversely, if an individual begins to perceive him or herself as incompetent at the activity and/or under external control to do it, then his or her intrinsic motivation is undermined. The outcome is then either a state of extrinsic motivation (the activity might continue dependent on the continuance of external rewards and/or coercion), or a state of amotivation (further activity unlikely because the perceptions of incompetence lead to a sense of futility).

A wealth of studies in general psychology have supported the validity of cognitive evaluation theory. Many studies have clearly shown that when individuals receive information that undermines their sense of competence and/or perception of self-determined choice, their intrinsic motivation declines. Readers who wish to comprehensively review that research are referred to Deci and Ryan (1985). However, of immediate interest to this paper is an overview of the ways in which intrinsic motivation is enhanced—or undermined—in the field of sport, exercise, and other physical activities.

Intrinsic Motivation in Sports, and Exercise

Common sense alone tells us that participation in many sports and physical activities can lead to feelings of autonomy and competence and may produce joy, excitement, thrills, and other satisfying emotions. In that respect it is easy to see that physical activities may be inherently intrinsically motivating. On the other hand, some people say that they would not participate unless there was a material payoff, or unless they were coerced. Others declare that attempting physical challenges leaves them feeling incompetent and humiliated, anxious or pressured. Thus, if we wish to help people reap the benefits of participation and avoid the motivational pitfalls, it is necessary to understand the processes that may lead to specific perceptual outcomes.

Persistence at exercise is related to the motivational constructs described above and has research support. For example, young athletes cite "fun" as a primary reason for participating in sports (Gill, Gross, & Huddleston, 1983; Scanlan & Lewthwaite, 1986). Further examination has shown that this feeling of fun depends on experiencing the intrinsic satisfactions of skill improvement, personal accomplishment, and excitement—rather than being a result of extrinsic factors such as winning, getting rewards, or pleasing others (Wankel & Kreisel, 1985; Wankel & Sefton, 1989). Similar findings have also been related by Gould (1987) in a review of the reasons why children drop out of sports, and by Brustad (1988) from a study of affective outcomes of competitive youth sport.

However, as researchers know well, circumstantial support for the use of a theory of motivation to a particular area (in this case physical activity) is not enough to make a case for its value. The theory should also hold up under experimental testing. In particular, manipulations of people's perceptions of competence and control should produce changes in their intrinsic motivation. Unfortunately, there is not the volume of evidence in the physical activity setting as there is in general and educational psychology, but several studies do show support for the hypotheses predicted by intrinsic motivation theory.

For example, Orlick and Mosher (1978) hypothesized that an extrinsic reward (a trophy) for performance on a stabilometer (balance board) would be perceived by children as controlling—and thus their intrinsic motivation for what is generally an interesting and challenging physical task would be undermined. The hypothesis was supported: When given a free choice period, the children whose earlier participation was for a trophy showed a decrease in the time they spent voluntarily playing on the stabilometer compared to the children who had no expectation of a reward.

In another study of performance at a stabilometer task, Rudisill (1989) hypothesized that training children to understand that their performance improvement was personally controllable (i.e., dependent on practice and effort) would improve their subsequent performance—and would also lead them to persist longer at mastery attempts—even in the face of perceived failure. Again, the results of the experimental manipulation supported the hypothesis that perceptions of personal control enhance intrinsic motivation.

Taking research outside the laboratory, Thompson and Wankel (1980) manipulated the perception of exercise choice of adult women who had recently enrolled in a health club. After an initial meeting to discuss activity preferences, the women were randomly allocated to either a perceived choice or a perceived no choice condition. The initial activity preferences were actually used as the basis for all of the women's programs. However, the women in the no-choice group were led to believe that they had been assigned a standard program determined by the instructor. Six weeks later the attendance of the women in the perceived choice group was higher, and they also expressed a greater intention to continue exercising at the health club.

Experimental manipulations designed to affect perceptions of competence at physical activities have also been shown to change intrinsic motivation in line with the predictions of the theory. As before, some studies have employed a stabilometer. For example, Weinberg and Jackson gave subjects bogus success or failure feedback for their balancing ability by telling them that they had either exceeded the 82nd percentile ("...very good..."), or they had fallen below the 18th percentile ("...not very good..."). In line with intrinsic motivation theory, success feedback enhanced interest and enjoyment, and reduced boredom with the task—and failure feedback had the opposite effect.

Using a similar type of protocol and a stabilometer task, Vallerand and Reid (1984, 1988) manipulated feedback by making verbal comments to subjects suggesting that they were doing either well or poorly. Like Weinberg and Jackson (1979) the results showed that success feedback led to enhanced intrinsic motivation while lack of success feedback reduced it. Additionally, a more in-depth analysis of the results allowed the experimenters to show that it was not the effect of the feedback per se, but rather it was the effect of feedback on the subjects' perceptions of competence that moderated changes in intrinsic motivation. In other words, this study showed that it was not the feedback itself so much as the meaning of the feedback to the subjects that produced the motivational outcome.

Wishing to see if similar results would be obtained from manipulations of feedback in a youth physical fitness testing situation, Whitehead and Corbin (1991) set up an experiment in a junior high school using a shuttle run-type fitness test (the Illinois Agility Run). Bogus high or low percentile feedback was given to randomly determined groups, and the results replicated the Vallerand and Reid (1984, 1988) findings. Again, apparently high percentile scores raised intrinsic motivation and low percentile scores lowered it—and as before, the motivational outcomes were mediated by the subjects' perceptions of competence at the task rather than directly changed by the feedback itself.

The Individuality of Perceptions

So far, and in its simplest form, the theoretical model of motivation has been presented as follows: Our intrinsic need to be competent or effective motivates mastery behaviors. If the attempts are self-determined and successful, then intrinsic motivation is maintained or enhanced. If not, intrinsic motivation is undermined and may be replaced by extrinsic motivation or amotivation. However, as several of the studies above have shown (e.g., Thompson & Wankel, 1980; Vallerand & Reid, 1984; Whitehead & Corbin, 1991) this is an over-simplification. It is a person's perception of events that counts. A person's motivation will depend on their personal cognitive evaluation (through intuition and appraisal) of their success and autonomy in any particular situation. Given that point, it is obviously important to try to understand factors that lead to individual differences before the theory can be translated into guidelines for motivational enhancement (see Table 1).

A primary concern is the need for an understanding of differences in the ways in which individuals form perceptions of competence. There appear to be three main ways (or orientations) in which individuals judge their competence. Those with a competitive orientation tend to compare their abilities or performance to those of their peers. Those with a cooperative orientation tend to look for social approval while involved in group activities. Those with a individualistic orientation tend to focus more on their individual improvement and task mastery (Ames and Ames, 1984). Logically, an obvious potential problem with a competitive orientation is that it leads to perceptions of winning and losing that are dependent on who beats whom, or where a person ranks in a hierarchy (e.g., a percentile table). In contrast, a cooperative, or more particularly, an individualistic orientation would seem to hold more hope of personal success because improvement under those conditions almost inevitably results from effort and practice.

This logic has been supported by research in sport and fitness settings. For example, Marsh and Peart (1988) randomly assigned eighth grade girls to fitness classes that either stressed competition or cooperation. Results showed that the cooperative program led to enhanced perceptions of physical competence. Similarly, Lloyd and Fox (1992) studied adolescent girls in a fitness program. They found that putting the focus on an individualistic orientation led to improvements in enjoyment and motivation compared to the outcomes of a competitively focused environment. The logic also held in a sport setting: Seifriz, Duda, and Chi (1992) found that when high school basketball players perceived an individual mastery-oriented climate in their practice sessions they experienced more enjoyment, and had higher intrinsic motivation compared to those players who perceived practice as a more competitive performance-oriented environment.

Also of immediate concern is the need to appreciate how events may be perceived as controlling. The previously mentioned Thompson and Wankel (1980) study showed that the perception of choice can be modified and other studies have revealed that the context in which potentially controlling events occur makes a difference. For example, Ryan (1980) found some sport specificity in whether athletes perceived sport scholarships as affirmations of their competence (thus supporting intrinsic motivation), or as extrinsically controlling (thus undermining intrinsic motivation). Specifically, athletes in the sport of football (where scholarships were common at that time) were more likely to perceive the scholarships as controlling than were wrestlers or female athletes (for whom scholarships were rare in the late 1970s).

Other research has shown several other factors that may or may not be perceived as controlling depending on the social context and informational emphasis. For example, competition, performance awards, and coaching styles can produce alternative outcomes. Unfortunately, space limitations preclude a detailed citation of individual studies here, but it may be sufficient to say that a common determining factor of an extrinsic focus is whether an individual senses an external pressure to perform or behave in a particular way. Readers who wish to look further at research on those topics are encouraged to read the review by Vallerand, Deci, and Ryan (1987). Suggestions for practitioners may be found in pages 2 and 3 of this chapter.

Table 1: Applying Theory to Practice

The following recommendations represent an attempt to logically translate the theoretical exposition into guidelines for promoting motivation in practical situations. Note that although these guidelines are presented as a series of DO's and DON'Ts, they are not meant to be coercing or controlling. The reader has the choice of which to accept!

DO try to emphasize individual mastery.

Since the foundation of intrinsic motivation is said to stem from a need to be effective it makes sense to begin with a recommendation for promoting competence perceptions. For example, when giving feedback to an exerciser or sport participant in a coaching or teaching situation, try to reinforce the personal progress that has been made (e.g., "You're really starting to get the hang of that backhand stroke."). Also, sweeten bitter medicine by prefacing comments with a competence-promoting introduction (e.g., "If you want to make that good shot great—why not try to...").

DON'T overemphasize peer comparisons of performance.

This is an alternative form of the previous recommendation. Peer comparisons inevitably do the greatest motivational damage to those who need encouragement the most—those with low ability. Teachers, coaches and fitness leaders should consider the perceptions that are created by their grading plans, or other evaluation procedures. In particular, since children's fitness test scores are determined to a considerable degree by genetics and level of maturation, the use of rankings, curves, or percentile tables for evaluation is questionable. What counts is an active lifestyle—so why not find a plan that reinforces mastery of the learning and participation process? (see Fox & Biddle, 1988 for an exposition on this point).

A footnote to this part: Since comments (like those above) about the use of percentiles have sometimes been interpreted as a blanket castigation, a clarification is merited. Although the use of percentiles for individual evaluation is questioned, this is because (by definition) it forces peer comparison—and consequently, it promotes competitive competence-seeking orientations. In contrast, the calculation of percentile scores to follow national fitness changes over time would be an example of a highly appropriate use of comparative data.

Table 1: Applying Theory to Practice (cont.)

DO promote perceptions of choice.

A second conceptual area for recommendations is concerned with the other fundamental aspect of intrinsic motivation—perceptions of control. In many ways translating this guideline into action involves awareness of the connotations of words and phrases. For example, consider the meaning of the term "exercise prescription." This language certainly doesn't suggest choice. On the other hand, this does not mean that exercise leaders and teachers have to let participants do whatever they want! A perception of choice can be fostered—even within fairly narrow guidelines providing reasons are given for constraints. Thus an exercise leader might be advised to explain which activities, equipment, facilities, etc., are appropriate for a client's current fitness level—but then a choice should be allowed from within that range.

DON'T undermine an intrinsic focus by misusing extrinsic rewards.

This guideline is a different way of expressing recommendations concerning perceptions of control. If the answer to the question: "Why are we doing this exercise, skill, fitness test, sport, etc.?"—is "Because it's for a payment/trophy/reward," or "Because you have to do it," then the focus is moved to external regulation. In that case the behavior will most likely cease when the extrinsic motivator is won, lost, or removed. This does not mean all forms of awards are harmful. It depends on how they are perceived. Because of a growing appreciation of this point, recently disseminated youth fitness programs have emphasized individual competence attainment by using recognition (of exercise participation and mastery) schemes, rather than employing the extrinsically focused traditional awards that are solely dependent on fitness test results (Fitness Canada, 1992; *Prudential FITNESSGRAM,* 1992).

DO promote the intrinsic fun and excitement of exercise.

Fortunately, this is easy to do because many physical activities are naturally intrinsically motivating—so long as we keep them that way by attention to the other guidelines.

DON'T turn exercise into a bore or a chore.

To use an analogy: Rather than a bland repetitive "diet" of a physical activity, think of a "menu" in which taste is enhanced by variety, new "recipes," and the "sugar and spice" of fun, excitement, and thrills (Whitehead, 1989). In the same vein, it should be remembered that health-related fitness is a construct that is adult-oriented (Malina, 1991). This is not meant as a criticism of health-related fitness itself. The point (particularly when dealing with children) is that we should not over-shadow the play value inherent in physical activity with an overbearing view of its potential as a "medicine."

DO promote a sense of purpose by teaching the value of physical activity to health, optimal function, and quality of life.

This recommendation is designed to highlight the motivational value of cognitive learning. Even if many forms of exercise do not produce the in-trinsic rewards of excitement, pleasure, etc., knowledge of the benefits of exercise may promote a sense of purpose for choosing to do it. It may also require the development of cognitive skills such as fitness self-evaluation and problem-solving (Corbin, 1987). Research on the out-comes of conceptually-based fitness classes does support the premise that learning fitness knowledge and skills promotes activity in the future (Slava, Laurie, & Corbin, 1984).

DON'T create amotivation by spreading fitness misinformation.

While this might seem painfully obvious, the sobering reality is that many people believe in ineffective or dangerous methods of weight manage-ment (e.g., fad diets, spot reducing, sauna suits), and many others are hoodwinked into paying for quack methods of fitness improvement such as passive exercise or unproven dietary supplements (Gauthier, 1987; Jarvis, 1992; Lightsey & Attaway, 1992). Unfortunately, the likely motiva-tional penalty for the continued failure that results from the use of ineffec-tive or useless products and methods is amotivation. True fitness professionals are thus urged to make every effort to disseminate knowl-edge that is derived from good science and experience.

Summary

This paper argues that intrinsic motivation is one key element in promoting active healthy lifestyles. Figure 1, "The Stairway to Intrin-sic Motivation," provides a visual summary of the various stages of personal motivation. The wise use of the guidelines presented in the preceding pages will help people move from a state of amotivation, through external or extrinsic motivation, to autonomous personalized and integrated behavior characterized as intrinsically motivated behavior. Theory suggests that personal competence and control are essential to the development of intrinsic motivation. Fortunately, a wide variety of sports and physical activities are available, and these provide many opportunities for self-chosen optimal challenges that can help **all people** to achieve intrinsic motivation characterized by autonomy and mastery. By their very nature most physical activities are intrinsically appealing because of the fun, excitement, and thrills that result from them.

References

Ames A., & Ames, R. (1984). Goal structures and motivation. *The Elementary School Journal*, 85(1), 40-52.

Banister, D., & Fransella, F. (1980). *Inquiring man: The psychology of personal constructs*. New York: Penguin.

Brustad, R.J. (1988). Affective outcomes in competitive youth sport: The influence of intrapersonal and socialization factors. *Journal of Sport and Exercise Psychology*, 10, 307-321.

Corbin, C..B. (1987). Physical fitness in the K-12 curriculum: Some defensible solutions to perennial problems. *JOPERD*, 58(7), 49-54.

Deci, E.L. (1975). *Intrinsic motivation*. New York: Plenum.

Deci, E.L., & Ryan, R.M. (1985). *Intrinsic motivation and self-determination in human behavior*. New York: Plenum.

Department of Health and Human Services. (1990). *Healthy people 2000. National health promotion and disease prevention objectives*. Washington, DC: Author.

Fitness Canada. (1992). *The Canadian Active Living Challenge*. Ottawa: Government of Canada.

Fox, K.R., & Biddle, S.J.H. (1988). The use of fitness tests: Educational and psychological considerations. *JOPERD*, 59(2), 47-53.

Freud, S. (1923/62). *The ego and the id*. New York: Norton.

Gauthier, M.M. (1987). Continuous passive motion: The no-exercise exercise. *The Physician and Sports Medicine,* 15(8),142-148.

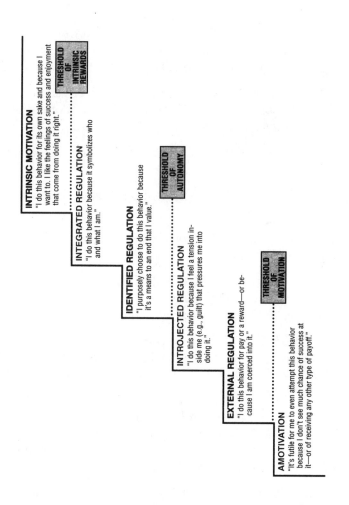

INTRINSIC MOTIVATION
"I do this behavior for its own sake and because I want to. I like the feelings of success and enjoyment that come from doing it right."

THRESHOLD OF INTRINSIC REWARDS

INTEGRATED REGULATION
"I do this behavior because it symbolizes who and what I am."

IDENTIFIED REGULATION
"I purposely choose to do this behavior because it's a means to an end that I value."

THRESHOLD OF AUTONOMY

INTROJECTED REGULATION
"I do this behavior because I feel a tension inside me (e.g., guilt) that pressures me into doing it."

EXTERNAL REGULATION
"I do this behavior for pay or a reward—or because I am coerced into it."

THRESHOLD OF MOTIVATION

AMOTIVATION
"It's futile for me to even attempt this behavior because I don't see much chance of success at it—or of receiving any other type of payoff."

The different types of motivation are from Vallerand and Reid (1990), and Vallerand and Bissonnette (1992). The examples of cognitive self-statements in the figure are based upon their descriptions. The arrangement of the types into a stairway, and the inclusion of the three thresholds is the work of the author of this paper.

467

Gill, D.L., Gross, J.B., & Huddleston, S. (1985). Participation motivation in youth sports. *International Journal of Sport Psychology,* 14,1-14.

Gould, D. (1987). Understanding attrition in children's sport. In D. Gould, & M.R. Weiss (Eds.), *Advances in pediatric sport sciences* (Vol. 2, pp. 61-85).Champaign, IL: Human Kinetics Publishers.

Harter, S. (1981). A new self-report scale of intrinsic versus extrinsic orientation in the classroom: Motivational and informational components. *Developmental Psychology,* 17, 300-312.

Hull, C.L. (1943). *Principles of behavior.* New York: Appleton-Century-Crofts.

Jarvis, W.T. (1992). Quackery: A national scandal. *Clinical Chemistry,* 38, 1574-1586.

Kelly, G.A. (1955). *The psychology of personal constructs* (vols. 1 & 2). New York: Norton.

Lightsey, D.M., & Attaway, J.R. (1992). Deceptive tactics used in marketing purported ergogenic aids. *National Strength and Conditioning Association Journal,* 14(2), 26-31.

Lloyd, J., & Fox, K.R. (1992). Achievement goals and motivation to exercise in adolescent girls: A preliminary intervention study. *British Journal of Physical Education Research Supplement,* 11(Summer), 12-16.

Malina, R.M. (1991). Fitness and performance: Adult health and the culture of youth. In R.J. Park & H.M. Eckert (Eds.), The Academy Papers: Vol. 24. *New possibilities, new paradigms* (pp. 30-38). Champaign, IL: Human Kinetics Publishers.

Marsh, H.W., & Peart, N.D. (1988). Competitive and cooperative physical fitness training programs for girls: Effects on physical fitness and multidimensional self-concepts. *Journal of Sport and Exercise Psychology,* 10. 390-407.

Orlick, T.D., & Mosher, R. (1978). Extrinsic rewards and participant motivation in a sport related task. *International Journal of Sport Psychology,* 9, 27-39.

Prudential FITNESSGRAM. (1992 flier). The Prudential FITNESSGRAM recognition system & program materials. Dallas, TX: Cooper Institute for Aerobics Research.

Rudisill, M.E. (1989). Influence of perceived competence and causal dimension orientation on expectations, persistence, and performance during perceived failure. *Research Quarterly for Exercise and Sport,* 60, 166-175.

Ryan, E.D. (1980). Attribution, intrinsic motivation, and athletics: A replication and extension. In C.H. Nadeau, W.R. Halliwell, K.M. Newell, & G.C. Roberts (Eds.),*Psychology of motor behavior and sport* (pp. 19-26). Champaign, IL: Human Kinetics Publishers.

Scanlan, T.K., & Lewthwaite, R. (1986). Social psychological aspects of competition for male youth sport participants: IV. Predictors of enjoyment. *Journal of Sport Psychology,* 8, 25-35.

Seifriz, J.J., Duda, J.L., & Chi, L. (1992).The relationship of perceived motivational climate to intrinsic motivation and beliefs about success in basketball. *Journal of Sport and Exercise Psychology,* 14, 375-391.

Skinner, B.F. (1953). *Science and human behavior.* New York: Macmillan.

Skinner, B.F. (1971). *Beyond freedom and dignity.* New York: Penguin.

Slava, S., Laurie, D.R., & Corbin, C.B. (1984). Long-term effects of aconceptual physical education program. *Research Quarterly for Exercise and Sport,* 55, 161-168.

Thompson, C.E., & Wankel, L.M. (1980). The effects of perceived activity choice upon frequency of exercise behavior. *Journal of Applied Social Psychology,* 10, 436-443.

Vallerand, R.J., & Bissonnette, R. (1992). Intrinsic, extrinsic, and amotivational styles as predictors of behavior: A prospective study. *Journal of Personality,* 60, 599-620.

Vallerand, R.J., & Reid, G. (1984). On the causal effects of perceived competence on intrinsic motivation: A test of cognitive evaluation theory. *Journal of Sport Psychology,* 6, 94-102.

Vallerand, R.J ., & Reid, G. (1990). Motivation and special populations: Theory, research, and implications regarding motor behavior. In G. Reid (Ed.), *Problems in movement control* (pp. 159-197).Elsevier Science Publishers.

Vallerand, R.J., Deci, E.L., & Ryan, R.M. (1987). Intrinsic motivation in sport. In K.B. Pandolf (Ed.), *Exercise and sport science reviews* (Vol. 15, pp. 387-425). New York: Macmillan Publishing Company.

Vallerand, R.M., & Reid, G. (1988). On the relative effects of positive and negative verbal feedback on males' and females' intrinsic motivation. *Canadian Journal of Behavioral Sciences*, 20, 239-250.

Wankel, L.M., & Kreisel, P.S.J. (1985). Factors underlying enjoyment of youth sports: Sport and age group comparisons. *Journal of Sport Psychology*, 7, 51-64.

Wankel, L.M., & Sefton, J.M. (1989). A season-long investigation of fun in youth sports. *Journal of Sport and Exercise Psychology*, 11, 355-366.

Weinberg, R.S., & Jackson, A. (1979). Competition and extrinsic rewards: Effect on intrinsic motivation and attribution. *Research Quarterly*, 50, 494-502.

Weiss, M.R., Bredemeier, B.J., & Shewchuk, R.M. (1985).An intrinsic/extrinsic motivation scale for the youth sport setting: A confirmatory factor analysis. *Journal of Sport Psychology*, 7, 75-91.

White, R.W. (1959). Motivation reconsidered: The concept of competence. *Psychological Review*, 66, 279-333.

Whitehead, J.R. (1989). Fitness assessment results—some concepts and analogies. *JOPERD*, 60(6), 39-43.

Whitehead, J.R., & Corbin, C.B. (1991). Youth fitness testing: The effect of percentile-based evaluative feedback on intrinsic motivation. *Research Quarterly for Exercise and Sport*, 62, 225-231.

Chapter 35

Physical Fitness and Healthy Low Back Function

Introduction:

The initial issue of the *Physical Activity and Fitness Research Digest* (see Chapter 33) gave a general overview of the benefits of physical activity and how those benefits related to major lifestyle diseases and the Healthy People 2000 promotion and disease prevention priorities. This issue focuses on physical activity, physical fitness, healthy back function and low back pain.

The following key points are discussed in detail in this article:

- At some time in their lives, 60-80% of all individuals experience low back pain. The condition is disabling to 1-5% of this population.

- To have a healthy, well-functioning back, flexible lumbar muscles, hamstrings, and hip flexors and strong fatigue-resistant abdominal and back extensor muscles are necessary.

- The Healthy People 2000 goals aim to decrease disability from chronic disabling disease and to increase the proportion of the population who regularly perform activities to enhance muscular strength, endurance, and flexibility. In terms of low back health, the latter goal may be one way of achieving the former goal.

Physical Activity and Fitness Research Digest, Series 1, No. 3, August 1993.

- Exercises to maintain or increase muscular function in the low back region are presented in Table 1.

- The anatomical logic (presented in Table 2) linking low back health and physical activity is stronger than the research evidence at this time.

Studies (see body of text) support the fact that individuals who have suffered low back pain (LBP) have weaker, more fatigable, and less flexible muscles in the trunk region even after the acute pain episode has subsided than do those who are pain free. Continued weakness, low endurance and restricted range of movement appear to be contributing factors to recurrent LBP. The ability to predict first-time LBP from muscular strength, endurance or flexibility values has not been established. Likewise, a direct relationship between LBP and cardiovascular or body composition fitness has not been established. On the other hand, with one exception which is noted in the following text, the studies reviewed have not shown that high levels of any of these fitness components are in any way linked as causal factors to LBP. Therefore, it appears prudent at this point to continue recommending a specific program of truncal muscular fitness as a part of a comprehensive physical fitness activity program. This recommendation is in accordance with the Healthy People 2000 goal, which states the aim of increasing to at least 40 percent the proportion of the population 6 years old and above who regularly perform physical activities that enhance and maintain muscular strength, muscular endurance, and flexibility (Public Health Service, 1990). A comprehensive program would, of course, utilize the entire body and, along with the trunk region, stress upper arm and shoulder girdle areas. While baseline data suggests that the goal is close to being met for high school students, for the total population the 1991 estimate is that only 16% are involved in such programs.

For the trunk and low back region, it is imperative that the neuromuscular program go beyond traditional sit-ups for abdominal strength (actually, partial curls should be substituted for sit-ups) and modified hurdler's stretches for hamstring flexibility. The exercise program should be designed to include all five major anatomical areas and abilities listed in Table 1 without overemphasizing lumbar flexibility. Ignoring any element in the whole may lead to imbalances. Table 1 presents suggested flexibility and muscular strength/endurance exercises for the five identified areas with a progression from relatively easy to reasonably hard. Individual selections can be made from this chart for each area. Even if these components have not been shown irrevocably to be protective against the development of LBP, truncal muscular strength, endurance and flexibility are important aspects of a healthy, fully functioning, fit body.

The Problem

The incidence of low back pain has been and continues to be consistently high. At some time in their lives, 60-80% of all individuals experience back pain. Both sexes are affected equally. Most cases occur between the ages of 25 and 60 years, but no age is completely immune. Approximately 12-26% of children and adolescents are LBP sufferers. Fortunately, most LBP is acute and, with or without treatment of any kind, resolves itself within three days to six weeks. After six weeks to a year, the condition is considered to be chronic. For the 1-5% so afflicted, the condition is disabling. This statistic speaks directly to the Healthy People 2000 priority of reducing disability from chronic disease, for while LBP is not the most prevalent disabling disease in the U.S., it is one of the many (Public Health Service, 1990). The psychological, social and physical costs to individuals cannot begin to be calculated. The medical, insurance and business/industry costs have been estimated into the billions of dollars per year (Cailliet, 1988; Plowman, 1992).

Most cases of acute LBP arise spontaneously from no known cause. Without knowing the exact cause, or causes of, LBP, it is difficult to determine risk factors which might predispose an individual to LBP. Among the possible risk factors most commonly linked with LBP is a lack of physical fitness. Indeed, LBP has often been labeled as a hypokinetic disease, that is, as a disease caused by and/or associated with a lack of exercise (Kraus and Raab, 1961).

The Theoretical Link Between Physical Activity, Physical Fitness and LBP

The theoretical link between physical activity, physical fitness and LBP is largely based on functional anatomy. Anatomically, back pain is primarily located in the lumbosacral region of the back which normally forms a lordotic curve. Twenty-four vertebrae comprise the entire spine. Effective functioning of the back requires coordination of all of the vertebra, the pelvis, the hip and thigh joints, and the

Table 1. Suggested Exercises for Various Fitness Levels.

Neuromuscular Fitness Components	Low	Moderate	High
a. Lumbar mobility*	*Knee To Chest* In supine lying position bring one orboth knees to the chest, grasping the leg, under the thigh(s), raise and lower head slowly.	*"Mad Cat"* Kneeling on all fours alternate head up with sway back and head tucked with rounded back.	*Crossed Leg Flexion* Sitting position with knees flexed and ankles crossed. Slowly bend forward until head approaches floor.
b. Hamstring flexibility*	*Modified Hurdler's Stretch* Sit with one leg straight, the otherleg flexed. Move the flexed knee to the side and bend forward.	*PNF Supine Position* Place jump rope around foot or anklewith leg raised as straight as possible. Contract against rope, relax and pull leg straighter. Repeat.	*Standing Stretch* Stand with oneleg placed on a support at about 90° hip flexion. Keeping back straight with shoulders back, flex forward.
c. Hip flexor flexibility*	*Hip Extension* Stand with pelvis in neutral position. Extend leg backward at hip.	*Lying Stretch* Lie on table with knees over the edge and back flat. Pulling one leg to thechest (hands on thigh) stretches the opposite hip.	*Standing Stretch* Stand in forward backward stride position. Bend front knee and thrust back hip forward. Keep front knee over ankle.

d. Abdominal strength/ endurance

Pelvic Tilt
In supine lying or standing position—press pelvis to floor or wall.

Partial Curl (crunch)
Hook lying position, feet not held, tilt pelvis, curl up, sliding hands at side 3-4 1/2 inches.

Oblique Curl
Lying on side— twist trunk and curl up reaching for top leg with opposite arm.

e. Back extensor strength/endurance

Hyperextension - 1
Lying in prone position with hands at thighs. Keep neck and chin in neutral position and raise shoulders off floor.

Hyperextension - 2
Lying in prone position with arms and hands extended forward. Keep neck and chin in neutral position and raise shoulders off floor.

Hyperextension - 3
Lying in prone position on a table or bench with body supported and stabilized from top of pelvis down. Flex waist to 90° and extend to several inches above level.

* Move into stretch positions slowly and hold for 10-60 seconds.
** Repeat controlled movements 5-25 times.

muscles, fascia and ligaments which originate and insert on these bones. Such coordination is task-specific, but to be normal it should be completed with minimal and equalized stresses within the spine (Cailliet, 1988; Gracovetsky, 1990).

Table 2 presents the theoretical relationships between all of the components of health-related physical fitness and healthy and unhealthy functioning of the low back. It can be seen that there is a strong anatomical rationale for all components of fitness. The actual research-based support is not as strong as the anatomical relationships.

The Research Link Between Physical Activity, Physical Fitness and Low Back Pain

Studies which have attempted to determine the relationship between physical activity and/or fitness and low back function or pain/injury are of two primary types. The first are retrospective studies. In a retrospective study, the relationship between the activity or fitness component and LBP is examined, or an attempt is made to distinguish between those who do and do not have low back pain based on the activity or fitness score. Retrospective studies must be interpreted cautiously since there are at least three possible confounding problems. First, activity or fitness measures in individuals already suffering from LBP may represent less than maximal effort due to real or feared pain. Second, physical activity is generally spontaneously decreased in individuals suffering from LBP, with the result that scores may reflect detraining as much as LBP per se. Third, these studies statistically establish just relationships (some of which may be statistically significant but not practically meaningful) and not cause and effect.

The second type of study is prospective. Prospective studies are longitudinal studies which test either normal individuals with no history of LBP, individuals with a history of LBP, or both, and then wait a specified time to see who develops LBP. The initial activity or fitness variables are then statistically analyzed to determine which, if any, had the most predictive value for the development of LBP. Perspective studies are obviously more valuable but they are also harder to conduct.

Throughout this section it has been emphasized that either physical activity or physical fitness can be used to determine the linkage with low back health or pain. In point of fact, very few studies have even attempted to relate physical activity per se in non-athletic populations with LBP. Those which have examined activity are weak in design and contradictory in outcome, precluding any meaningful comments or conclusions. The biggest difficulty is the inconsistent classification of physical activity and a primary reliance on frequency of participation to the exclusion of duration and intensity (Plowman, 1992). Even the most direct study by Porter, Adams, and Hutton (1989), which found a significant positive relation between spinal motion segment compressive strength and physical activity in young men killed in motorcycle accidents, relied only on a sports history obtained from the next of kin. Thus, no exercise prescription guidelines specific for low back health can be documented from the literature. This is a fertile area for research.

The rest of this report will concentrate on the linkage between physical fitness and low back health or pain. Some specific studies will be mentioned for illustrative purposes, but the primary emphasis will be on general consensus. For a more in-depth presentation of the research literature, the reader is referred to Plowman (1992). Complete references are also provided there.

Cardiovascular Fitness and LBP

As stated in Table 2, a properly functioning cardiovascular system is necessary for disc nourishment and to slow disc degeneration. The exact relationship with total body cardiovascular fitness has received little attention. Only two retrospective studies have measured cardiovascular fitness, and neither established a definitive linkage with low back function (Plowman, 1992).

Likewise, only two prospective studies have designs specific enough to draw conclusions from, but unfortunately the conclusions that must be drawn are in opposition to each other. The first study was completed on fire fighters by Cady, Thomas, and Karwasky (1985). Cardiovascular condition was assessed by physical working capacity (PWC). The 20 fire fighters with the lowest PWC incurred much higher low back injury costs than the 20 with the highest PWC, showing a beneficial effect. The second study is the study with the stronger design. It was conducted by Battie et al. (1989). Maximal oxygen consumption (VO_2max) was predicted from a submaximal treadmill test on over 2400 Boeing airplane employees. VO_2max was not found

Table 2. Theoretical Relationship Between Physical Fitness Components and Health"/Unhealthy Low Back/Spinal Function.

Physical Fitness Component	Normal Anatomical Function in Low Back-Healthy	Dysfunction	Results of Dysfunction-Unhealthy
Cardiovascular-Respiratory Endurance	Discs obtain nutrients and dispose of wastes by absorption from adjacent blood supply.	Poor circulation, low CVR endurance	May speed up disc degeneration.
Body Composition	High musculature allows for proper functioning as outlined below and provides mechanical loading on the vertebrae for maintenance of bone mass.	High % body fat content	Increases the weight the spine must support; may lead to increased pressure on discs or other vertebral structures.
Neuromuscular:			
a. Lumbar flexibility	Allows the lumbar curve to almost be reversed in forward flexion.	Inflexible	Disrupts forward and lateral movement; places excessive stretch on hamstrings leading to low back and hamstring pain.

Factor		
b. Hamstring flexibility	Allows anterior rotation (tilt) of the pelvis in forward flexion and posterior rotation in sitting position.	Inflexible	Restricts anterior pelvic rotation and exaggerates posterior tilt; both cause increased disc compression; excessive stretching causes strain and pain.
c. Hip flexor flexibility	Allows achievement of neutral pelvic position.	Inflexible	Exaggerates anterior pelvic tilt if not counteracted by strong abdominal muscles, thereby increasing disc compression.
d. Abdominal strength/endurance	Maintains pelvic position; reinforces back extensor fascia and pulls it laterally on forward flexion providing support.	Weak, easily fatigued	Allows abnormal pelvic tilt; increases strain on back extensor muscles.
e. Back extensor strength/endurance	Provides stability for spine; maintains erect posture; controls forward flexion.	Weak, easily fatigued	Increases loading on spine; causes increased disc compression.

to be predictive of the 228 back problems which occurred in these employees over the subsequent 4 years.

There is no evidence that a highly fit cardiovascular system is detrimental in any way, but the evidence of benefit is minimal. This is another area which requires further research.

Body Composition and LBP

The skeletal system in general and the spine in particular are the primary supporting structures of the body. As pointed out in Table 2, if the weight the spine supports is largely muscular and the muscles are both strong and flexible, healthy functioning should result. However, if a large portion of the body mass is fat, this adds excess weight and pressure on the discs without any positive assistance. The few studies which have utilized body mass index (WT/HT2) as an indication of body composition have shown split results. No studies have been done on LBP in which body composition has been directly assessed by a laboratory criterion measure such as underwater weighing (Plowman, 1992).

Neuromuscular Fitness and LBP

The most important components of fitness in relation to healthy functioning of the low back are muscular strength, muscular endurance and flexibility. It is necessary that each separate muscle group possess both strength/endurance and flexibility, and that anatomically opposing muscle groups are balanced in strength/endurance and flexibility. The goal in relation to the low back region is that the vertebra will be kept in proper alignment without excessive disc pressure throughout the full range of possible motions. In addition, the pelvis must freely rotate both posteriorly and anteriorly without strain on the muscles or fascia. Table 2 presents the specific actions of the back, hip, abdominal and hamstring muscles and what can theoretically happen if these muscles are allowed to become weak, easily fatigued and/or inflexible.

The research evidence shows that regardless of the testing mode (that is, whether the test is one of static or dynamic function), individuals with low back pain exhibit lower strength values of both the abdominals and back extensor groups than do individuals without LBP. Only two studies looked at trunk extensor endurance specifically, but both of these found that individuals with LBP severe enough to

480

limit function had scores lower than those without such limitations (Plowman, 1992).

Perhaps the most interesting studies in this area are those utilizing electromyographic (EMG) analysis of back extensor fatigue. In each of the three studies (DeVries, 1968; Roy, DeLuca, and Casavant, 1989; Roy et al., 1990), 80-100% of those with LBP showed increased electrical activity during sustained static muscle contraction. While these were not intended to be prospective studies, in one case an individual who showed high EMG activity but no history of LBP developed LBP the following year. Retrospective studies of low back pain and hamstring flexibility have shown the same trend. That is, that there is a significant relationship between tightness in those muscle groups and LBP (Plowman, 1992).

Prospective studies of neuromuscular fitness are neither as numerous nor as definitive as the retrospective ones. Only one strength/endurance study found any variable predictive of first-time low back pain, and this showed the predictive variable to be limited (low) back extensor endurance (Biering-Sorensen,1984a). Unfortunately, this was the only study using this variable, but since it is consistent with the results of the retrospective studies it would seem that back extensor endurance needs to be given more attention. Recurrent back pain has been successfully predicted in about half of the studies of trunk and back extensor strength/endurance with, as expected, low scores preceding the reoccurrence of back pain (Plowman, 1992).

One prospective study found lumbar flexibility to be predictive of first time LBP (Biering-Sorensen, 1984b). In it, increased (not decreased as might be expected) lumbar mobility was found to be predictive of first-time back pain in males but not females. It is anatomically possible that extreme lumbosacral flexion stresses the discs at that site (Sharpe, Liehmon, and Snodgrass, 1988). Recurrent back pain has been found to be predictable from both low lumbar extension range of motion and low hamstring flexibility.

No specific level of strength, endurance and/or flexibility has emerged as critical in any of these studies. Hopefully, further research to clarify these issues will be forthcoming.

References

Battié, M.C., Bigos, S.J., Fisher, L.D>, Hansson, T.H., Nachemson, A.L., Spengler, D.M., Wortley, M.D., & Zeh, J. (1989). A prospective study of the role of cardiovascular risk factors and fitness in industrial back pain complaints. *Spine*, 12: 141-147.

Biering-Sorensen, F. (1984a). A one-year prospective study of low back trouble in a general population. *Danish Medical Bulletin*, 31: 362-375.

Biering-Sorensen, F. (1984b). Physical measurements as risk indicators for low-back trouble over a one-year period. *Spine*, 9: 106-119.

Cady, L.D., Thomas, P.C., & Karwasky, R.J. (1985). Program for increasing health and physical fitness for fire fighters. *Journal of Occupational Medicine*, 27:110-114.

Cailliet, R. (1988). *Low Back Pain Syndrome*, 4th edition. Philadelphia, PA: F.A. Davis.

DeVries, H.A. (1968). EMG fatigue curves in postural muscles. A possible etiology for idiopathic low back pain. *American Journal of Physical Medicine*, 47: 175-181.

Gracovetsky, S. Kary, M., Levy, S., Ben Said, R., Pitchen, I., & Helie, J. (1990). Analysis of spinal and muscular activity during flexion/extension and free lifts. *Spine*, 15: 1333-1339.

Kraus, H., & Raab, W. (1961). *Hypokinetic Disease*. Springfield, IL: Charles C. Thomas.

Plowman, S.A. (1992). Physical activity, physical fitness, and low back pain. In: Holloszy, J.O. (ed.), *Exercise and Sport Sciences Review*, 20: 221-242.

Porter, R.W., Adams, M.A., & Hutton, W.C. (1989). Physical activity and the strength of the lumbar spine. *Spine*, 14: 201-203.

Public Health Service. (1990). *Healthy People 2000*. Washington, D.C.: U.S. Government Printing Office.

Roy, S.H., DeLuca, C.J., Casavant, D.A. (1989). Lumbar muscle fatigue and chronic lower back pain. *Spine*, 14: 992-1001.

Roy, S.H., DeLuca, C.J., Snyder-Mackler, L., Emley, M.S., Crenshaw, R.L., & Lyons, J.P. (1990). Fatigue, recovery, and low back pain in varsity rowers. *Medicine and Science in Sports and Exercise*, 22: 463-469.

Sharpe, G.L., Liehman, W.P., & Snodgrass, L.B. (1988). Exercise prescription and the low back—kinesiological factors. *Journal of Health, Physical Education, Recreation and Dance*, 59(8): 74-78.

Chapter 36

Heredity and
Health-Related Fitness

Note from the Editors

In the February issue of the *Physical Activity and Fitness Research Digest* (see Chapter 33) we noted the importance of heredity as a factor affecting the development of health-related physical fitness. We cited the research of Claude Bouchard and colleagues and indicated that a forthcoming issue of the Digest would deal with the influences of heredity on physical fitness in greater detail.

In this issue of the *Digest* readers have the opportunity to read a synthesis paper on "Heredity and Health-Related Fitness" written by the most prominent scholar in the area. While we have known for some time that heredity was a factor affecting fitness performances, it was not until Dr. Bouchard and his colleagues began their in-depth studies in the area that we began to really know the extent of hereditary influences.

Dr. Bouchard has studied families, especially families with twins, to learn how heredity affects fitness. Heredity (genotypes) affects different fitness components (phenotypes) in different ways. For example two people of the same age and sex with similar lifestyles could vary in health-related fitness just because of the genes they inherited. As noted later in this paper, the heritability for body fatness is 25%+, muscle fitness 20-40%, and CV fitness 10 to 25%.

Physical Activity And Fitness Research Digest, Series 1, No. 4, November 1993.

But heritability only accounts for differences that heredity might make when comparing two people who have not trained. Bouchard and colleagues have been the pioneers who have demonstrated that not only do people differ in fitness based on heredity, but people of different genetic backgrounds respond differently to training. In other words, two people of different genetic background could do the exact same exercise program and get quite different benefits (see Figure 1). Some people get as much as 10 times as much benefit from activity as others who do the same program.

Though quite technical in some places, the following paper has many practical implications for teachers and professionals in physical activity and fitness. Some of these are listed below:

- Recognizing individual differences is critical in helping students, clients, and patients with fitness achievement. People do not enter our programs with similar backgrounds, nor do they respond similarly to training.

- Assumptions about a person's fitness cannot always be indicative of their current activity levels. The conclusion that the lower fitness of one person compared to another is a result of inactivity is a dangerous one. Those who do not adapt quickly to physical activity need encouragement to keep them involved, not discouragement associated with conclusions about their level of activity and effort.

- Different people (genotypes) respond differently to each part of fitness (phenotype). A person who has less hereditary predisposition to one type of fitness may respond well to another. For this reason we should be careful not to expect people to perform well on all health-related fitness tests just because they score well on one test.

Even those with little technical background can benefit from the paper that follows. Read on!

Introduction

Health is the culmination of many interacting factors, including the genetic constitution. Humans are genetically quite diverse. Current estimates are that each human being has about one variable DNA base for every 300 bases out of a total of about 3 billion base pairs. Variations in DNA sequence constitute the molecular basis of genetic individuality. Given genetic individuality, an equal state of health and of physical and mental well-being is unlikely to be achieved for all individuals even under similar environmental and lifestyle conditions. Some will thrive better than others and will remain free from disabilities for a longer period of time. Allowing for such individuality, it should thus come as no surprise that there is a minority of adults who remain relatively fit in spite of a sedentary lifestyle.

Genetic differences do not operate in a vacuum. They constantly interact with existing cellular and tissue conditions to provide a biological response commensurate with environmental demands. Genes are constantly interacting with everything in the physical environment as well as with lifestyle characteristics of the individual that translate into signals capable of affecting the cells of the body. For instance, overfeeding, a high fat diet, smoking, and regular endurance exercise are all powerful stimuli that may elicit strong biological responses. However, because of inherited differences at specific genes, the amplitude of adaptive responses varies from one individual to another. Inheritance is one of the important reasons why we are not equally prone to become diabetic or hypertensive or to die from a heart attack. It is also one major explanation for individual differences in the response to dietary intervention or regular physical activity.

Health-Related Fitness

There is no universally agreed upon definition of fitness and of its components. In the present context, we are particularly interested in what is now referred to as health-related fitness, i.e. in the physical and physiological components of fitness that impact more directly on health status. Health-related fitness refers to the state of physical and physiological characteristics that define the risk levels for the premature development of diseases or morbid conditions presenting a relationship with a sedentary mode of life (Bouchard and Shephard, 1993). Important determinants of health-related fitness include such factors as body mass for height, body composition, subcutaneous fat distribution, abdominal visceral fat, bone density, strength and endurance of the abdominal and dorso-lumbar musculature, heart and lung functions, blood pressure, maximal aerobic power and tolerance to submaximal exercise, glucose and insulin metabolism, blood lipid and lipoprotein profile, and the ratio of lipid to carbohydrate oxidized in a variety of situations. A favorable profile for these various factors presents a clear advantage in terms of health outcomes as assessed by morbidity and mortality statistics. The components of health-related fitness are numerous and are determined by several variables, including the individual's pattern and level of habitual activity, diet and heredity.

The Genetic Perspective

In general, genetic issues can be considered from two different perspectives. The first is from the genetic epidemiology perspective. Here the evidence is derived from samples of human subjects, particularly families, large pedigrees, relatives by adoption or twins. The data can be epidemiological in nature or be enriched by molecular studies. The second perspective is frankly molecular and pertains to transcription, translation, and regulatory mechanisms and how the genes adapt or come into play in response to various forms of acute exercise and of training. In this case, the tissue (generally heart muscle or skeletal muscle) is perturbed by an acute or a chronic stress and the changes are monitored. The emphasis is therefore on the molecular mechanisms involved in the adaptation.

Both approaches are very useful in delineating how important genes are for a given phenotype. However, they differ considerably in the type of information they can provide. The first approach is asking whether individual differences for a given phenotype are caused by DNA sequence variation, gene-environment interactions and gene-gene interactions seen among human beings and, ultimately, what are the genes involved and the specific DNA variants accounting for human heterogeneity. The second approach relies heavily on animal models with a focus on the role of various DNA sequences on regulatory mechanisms with no particular interest for the differences that may exist among members of the species.

The genetic epidemiology approach is of particular interest to us here because it deals with individual differences caused by inherited DNA sequence differences. Results available from the genetic epidemiology perspective will therefore constitute the essential of this review.

Heredity and Health-Related Fitness

Although the literature presents evidence for a role of genetic factors in most of the health-related fitness phenotypes, the quality of the evidence varies according to the phenotype considered. Four major components of health-related fitness will be considered here.

Morphological Component

Obesity (body fat content) and regional fat distribution are the phenotypes of morphological fitness that have been studied most by geneticists. Table 1 summarizes the trends emerging from several reviews regarding the contribution of genetic factors to obesity, regional subcutaneous fat distribution, abdominal visceral fat and bone density. The body mass index (BMI), subcutaneous fat (sum of skinfold thicknesses) and percent body fat derived from underwater weighing are among the most commonly used phenotypes in genetic studies of obesity. They are characterized by heritability levels reaching about 25% and at times higher. Results from a few studies suggest that BMI and percent body fat may be influenced by variation at a single or a few genes, although there are conflicting results. The phenotypes associated with regional fat distribution are generally characterized by slightly higher heritability levels with values reaching about 30% to 50% of the phenotypic variance. The trunk to extremity skinfolds ratio as a marker of regional subcutaneous fat distribution has been found to be influenced by major effects, possibly associated with variation at a single gene, suggesting that the pattern of fat deposition between the trunk and the limbs is significantly conditioned by genetic factors.

Muscular Component

This fitness component is probably the one for which the evidence for a contribution of genetic factors is the least abundant. Two studies used family data to study familial transmission of muscular fitness. In one study (Pérusse et al, 1988), muscular endurance and muscular strength measurements were obtained in 13,804 subjects who participated in the 1981 Canada Fitness Survey. The results showed that about 40% of the phenotypic variance in muscular endurance and muscular strength could be accounted for by factors transmitted from parents to offspring. In the Quebec Family Study (Pérusse et al, 1987), we found a genetic effect of 21% for muscular endurance and 30% for muscular strength. These results suggest that the heritability of muscular fitness is significant and ranges from low to moderate.

487

Table 1. *An overview of trends in heritability data for selected factors of morphological fitness*

Phenotype	Heritability[a]	Familial environment[b]
Body fat content	– 25%	Weak
Distribution of subcutaneous fat	30-50%	Weak
Visceral fat	30-60%	Unknown
Bone density	30-60%	Weak

a) Approximate proportion of the variation in the phenotype compatible with a genetic transmission after removing the effects of age and sex.
b) Conditions shared by individuals living together.

Cardiorespiratory Component

Cardiorespiratory fitness is a major component of health-related fitness and depends on a large number of phenotypes associated primarily with cardiac, vascular and respiratory functions. Measurements of submaximal exercise capacity and maximal aerobic power are generally performed to assess cardiorespiratory fitness. The contribution of genetic factors to these two phenotypes has been recently reviewed (Bouchard et al, 1992) and estimates of heritability were found to be lower for submaximal exercise capacity (about 10%) than for maximal aerobic power (about 25%). These inherited differences in cardiorespiratory fitness may be partly explained by interindividual differences in heart structures and functions, but relatively little is known about the role of heredity on these determinants despite evidence for significant familial aggregation.

Because of the high prevalence of hypertension in most developed countries and its association with an increased risk of death from myocardial infarction or stroke, the genetic and non-genetic determinants of blood pressure have been extensively studied in various populations. Overall, it is clearly established that blood pressure aggregates in families and heritability estimates reported from various populations are remarkably similar, accounting for about 30% of the interindividual differences. More recently, several specific genes have been implicated in the determination of the susceptibility to hypertension.

Metabolic component

There is increasing evidence that the metabolic component of health-related fitness should be considered as an important element of the relationship between physical activity and health. The metabolic component refers to normal blood and tissue carbohydrate and lipid metabolisms and adequate hormonal actions, particularly insulin. A large number of studies have been reported on the genetics of blood lipids and lipoproteins, because of their predominant role in the etiology of cardiovascular disease. Briefly, genetic factors contribute to interindividual differences in blood lipids and lipoproteins with heritability estimates generally accounting for about 25% to as much as 98% of the phenotypic variance, depending on the trait considered with an average value of 50%. Major gene effects have been reported for most of the phenotypes including total cholesterol, LDL-cholesterol, HDL-cholesterol, various apolipoprotein concentrations and Lpa. Highly significant genetic effects have also been reported for fasting glucose and insulin values as well as for plasma fibrinogen, a protein involved in blood clotting. The glucose and insulin responses to a carbohydrate meal appear to be characterized by lower heritability estimates ($< 25\%$) than for fasting values.

The contribution of heredity to the various health-related fitness components thus ranges from low to moderate and, except for some phenotypes pertaining to muscular fitness and metabolic fitness, it rarely exceeds 50% of the phenotypic variance and is often below 25%. These low to moderate heritabilities should not be interpreted as an indication that genes are not important in the determination of these phenotypes. These highly complex phenotypes are undoubtedly influenced by a variety of interactions. There is increasing evidence to the effect that interactions between genes and environmental factors or between various genes are common and contribute to interindividual differences in health-related fitness phenotypes and, consequently, cannot be any longer ignored in the field of physical activity, fitness and health.

Heredity and Response to Exercise

Research has amply demonstrated that aerobic performance, stroke volume, skeletal muscle oxidative capacity and lipid oxidation rates are phenotypes that can adapt to training. For instance, the VO_2max of sedentary persons increases, on the average, by about 20 to 25 percent after a few months of training. The skeletal muscle oxidative potential can easily increase by 50 percent with training and, at times, it may even double. However, if one is to consider a role for the genotype in such responses to training, there must be evidence of individual differences in trainability. There is now considerable support for this concept (Bouchard, 1986; Lortie et al, 1984). Some indications about the extent of individual differences in the response of maximal oxygen uptake to training are shown in Figure 1. Following exposure to training programs lasting from 15 to 20 weeks in 47 young men, some exhibited almost no change in VO_2max, while others gained as much as one liter of O_2 uptake. Such differences in trainability could not be accounted for by age (all subjects were young adults, 17 to 29 years of age) or gender (all young men). The initial (pre-training) level accounted for about 25 percent of the variance in the response of VO_2max; the lower the initial level the greater the increase with training. Thus about 75% of the heterogeneity in response to regular exercise was not explained.

Similar individual differences were observed for other relevant phenotypes such as indicators of endurance, markers of skeletal muscle oxidative metabolism, markers of adipose tissue metabolism, relative ratio of lipid and carbohydrate oxidized, fasting glucose and insulin levels as well as in their response to a glucose challenge, and fasting plasma lipids and lipoproteins (Bouchard et al, 1992). All these phenotypes respond to regular exercise in the young adults of both sexes. However, there are considerable individual differences in the response of these biological markers to exercise-training, some exhibiting a high responder pattern, while others are almost non-responders and with a whole range of response phenotypes between these two extremes.

What is the main cause of the individuality in the response to training? We believe that it has to do with as yet unidentified genetic characteristics (Bouchard, 1986). To test this hypothesis, we have now performed several different training studies with pairs of identical (MZ) twins, the rationale being that the response pattern can be observed for individuals having the same genotype (within pairs) and for subjects with differing genetic characteristics (between pairs). We have concluded from these studies that the individuality in trainability of cardiovascular fitness phenotypes and in response to exercise-training of cardiovascular risk factors is highly familial and most likely genetically determined. The data are expressed in terms of the ratio of the variance between genotypes to that within geno-

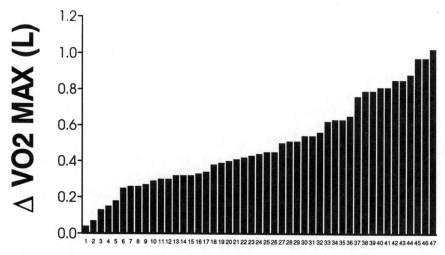

Figure 1. *Individual differences in the response of 47 young men to training programs lasting from 15 to 20 weeks. Results are expressed as gains of VO₂max in liters of O₂ per min.*

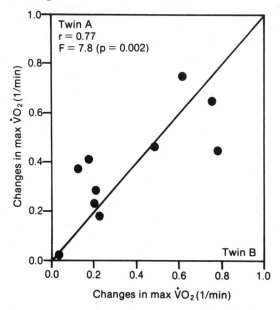

Figure 2. *Intrapair resemblance in 10 pairs of monozygotic twins for training changes in VO₂max (liters of O₂ per min) after 20 weeks of endurance training. Adapted from Prud'homme et al, Medicine and Science in Sports and Exercise, 1984.*

types in the response to standardized training conditions. The similarity of the training response among members of the same MZ pair is illustrated in Figure 1 for the VO_2max phenotype based on the result of our first study on this issue (Prud'homme et al, 1984). In this case, 10 pairs of MZ twins were subjected to a fully standardized and laboratory controlled-training program for 20 weeks and gains of absolute VO_2max showed almost 8 times more variance between pairs than within pairs.

Over a period of several years, 26 pairs of MZ twins were trained in our laboratory with standardized endurance and high intensity cycle exercise programs for periods of 15 or 20 weeks (Bouchard et al, 1992). After 10 weeks of training, the twins were exercising 5 times per week, 45 min. per session at the same relative intensity in each program. These training programs caused significant increases in VO_2max and other indicators of aerobic performance. They were also associated with a decrease in the intensity of the cardiovascular and metabolic responses at a given submaximal power output. For instance, when exercising in relative steady state at 50 watts, there were decreases in heart rate, oxygen uptake, pulmonary ventilation, ventilatory equivalent of oxygen and with an increase in the oxygen pulse. These various metabolic improvements were, however, all characterized by a significant within-pair resemblance (Bouchard et al, 1992). We have made the same observation for the alterations seen in skeletal muscle metabolism following training studies performed on skeletal muscle biopsies obtained before and after the training program in a good number of MZ twin pairs (Simoneau et al, 1986).

Nonpharmacological interventions designed to improve the cardiovascular risk profile center around the cessation of smoking, weight loss by means of dietary restriction and at times regular physical activity, dietary modifications aimed at fat, sodium and fiber intake, and regular exercise in order to improve health-related fitness. Among the expected changes associated with a regular exercise regimen, one finds in a group of sedentary and unfit adults a decrease in resting heart rate and blood pressure, a reduction in fasting plasma insulin level and in its response to a glucose load, a decrease in plasma triglycerides and, occasionally, in LDL-cholesterol and total cholesterol, and an increase in plasma HDL-cholesterol. Little is known about the individual differences in the response of these important clinical markers to regular exercise and about the role of genetic variation. We have used the MZ twin design to explore these issues in two studies. In one experiment, 6 pairs of young adult male MZ twins exercised on the cycle ergometer 2 hours per day for 22 consecutive days (Poehlman et al, 1986). The mean intensity of training reached 58 percent of VO_2max and the program was designed to induce an energy deficit of about 1,000 kcal per day. Baseline energy intake was assessed and prescribed for the 22 days of the training program. The diet prescription was fully enforced for each subject in the metabolic ward where they lived for the duration of the experiment. The second study was performed on 7 pairs of MZ twins who followed the same regimen for 100 days. The results of both studies are quite concordant. The program induced a significant increase in VO_2max and a significant decrease in body fat content. Significant changes were observed in fasting plasma insulin and in the insulin response to an oral glucose tolerance test. Plasma triglycerides, total cholesterol, LDL-cholesterol and apo B as well as the HDL-cholesterol to total cholesterol ratio were also modified. However, again, significant within MZ pair resemblance was observed for the response of fasting plasma insulin, and LDL-cholesterol, HDL-cholesterol, the HDL-cholesterol to total cholesterol ratio and for the improvement in body fat content and in fat topography. Thus being genetically different translates into heterogeneity in the adaptation to exercise programs.

Conclusions

Genetic individuality is important because it has an impact on the physical activity, fitness and health paradigm. The results summarized here reveal that there is highly suggestive evidence that genetic variation accounts for most of the individual differences in the response to regular exercise of health-related fitness components and of various risk factors for cardiovascular disease and diabetes. Not only is it important to recognize that there are individual differences in the response to regular physical activity but research also indicates that there are nonresponders in the population. Typically, there is a 3 to 10 fold difference between low responders and high responders, depending upon the phenotype considered, as a result of exposure to the same standardized physical activity regimen for a period of 15 to 20 weeks.

An appreciation of the critical role of DNA sequence variation in human responses to a variety of challenges and environmental conditions has become essential to those interested in the physical activity, fitness and health paradigm. It can only augment our understanding of human individuality and make us more cautious when defining fitness and health benefits that may be anticipated from a physically active lifestyle. Incorporating biological individuality into or thinking will increase the relevance of our observations to the true human situation.

References

Bouchard, C. (1986). Genetics of aerobic power and capacity. In R.M Malina, & C. Bouchard (Eds.), *Sport and human genetics* (pp. 59-88). Champaign, IL: Human Kinetics Publishers.

Bouchard, C., & Shepard, R.J. (1993). Physical activity, fitness and health: The model and key concepts. In C. Bouchard, R.J. Shepard, & T. Stephens (Eds.), *Physical activity, fitness, and health: Consensus Statement* (pp. 11-20). Champagne, IL: Human Kinetics Publishers.

Bouchard, C., Dionne, F.T., Simoneau, J.A., & Boulay, M.R. (1992). genetic of aerobic and anaerobic performances. *Exercise and sport Sciences Reviews*, 20, 27-58.

Lortie, G., Simoneau, J.A., Hamel, P., Boulay, M.R., Landry, F., & Bouchard, C. (1984). Responses of maximal aerobic power and capacity to aerobic training. *International Journal of Sports Medicine*, 5, 232-236.

Pérusse, L., Leblanc, C., & Bouchard, C. (1988). Inter-generation transmission of physical fitness in the Canadian population. *Canadian Journal of Sport Sciences*, 13, 8-14.

Pérusse, L., Lortie, G., Leblanc, C., Tremblay, A., Thériault, G., & Bouchard, C. (1978). Genetic and environmental sources of variation in physical fitness. *Annals of Human Biology*, 14, 425-434.

Poehlman, E.T., Tremblay, A., Nadeau, A., Dussault, J., Thériault, G., Bouchard, C. (1986). Heredity and changes in hormones and metabolic rates with short-term training. *American Journal of Physiology: Endocrinology and Metabolism*, 250, E711-E717.

Prud'homme, D., Bouchard, C., Leblanc, C., Landry, F., & Fontaine, E. (1984). Sensitivity of maximal aerobic power to training is genotype-dependent. *Medicine and Science in Sports & Exercise*. 16, 489-493.

Simoneau, J.A., Lortie, G., Boulay, M.R., Marcotte, M., Thibault, M.C., & Bouchard, C. (1986). Inheritance of human skeletal muscle and anaerobic capacity adaptation to high-intensity intermittent training. *International Journal of Sports Medicine*, 7, 167-171.

Chapter 37

Readiness for Physical Activity

Current practice in physical education and sports medicine emphasizes the twin goals of reducing the risk of illness and increasing quality-adjusted life expectancy through the development of health-related fitness (Bouchard et al., 1990). The average city-dweller currently takes insufficient habitual physical activity to realize these goals, but involvement in a regular, well-designed program of aerobic training, supplemented by moderate resisted muscle exercises could satisfy both objectives (American College of Sports Medicine (ACSM), 1991; ACSM, 1993). What are the risks of engaging in such activity, and how can a person determine if they are ready to undertake such a program?

Risks of Exercise

Excessive physical activity can provoke a variety of musculo-skeletal injuries, but the big fear, highlighted by such events as the sudden death of Jim Fixx and other high-profile exercisers, is that the program will provoke a fatal heart attack. Studies from our own laboratory and elsewhere (Cobb & Weaver, 1986; Northcote & Ballantyne, 1984; Sadaniantz & Thompson, 1990; Shephard, 1974, 1981; Vuori et al., 1982) show that (at least in symptom-free men) the risk of fatal and nonfatal heart attacks during physical activity is from 4 to 56

Physical Activity And Fitness Research Digest, Series 1, No. 5, February 1994.

times higher than it is while sitting at home reading a book. Maron et al. (1986) suggested that the main causes of sudden death in exercisers under 35 years of age were hypertrophic cardiomyopathy (48%: particularly a thickening of the septum between left and right ventricles) and unexplained enlargement of the left ventricle (18%). In those over the age of 35 years, 80% of exercise-related deaths were attributed to disease of the coronary arteries. The overall risk that vigorous physical activity will provoke a cardiac emergency is quite low, about one death per 400,000 hours of jogging (Thompson et al., 1982), and furthermore the risk seems even lower in regular than in occasional exercisers (Siscovick et al., 1984).

Implications for Pre-exercise Screening

Ideally, regular physical activity should be conceived as a simple, safe, and natural part of healthy living, a lifestyle to which the human body has adapted over many centuries of evolutionary struggle as a hunter and primitive agriculturalist (Shephard, 1993), rather than as a dangerous medical intervention that requires extensive, high-technology pre-exercise evaluation.

For a long period, physicians in the United States adopted a somewhat restrictive approach to exercise prescription, suggesting that a stress electrocardiogram was needed in all men over the age of 35 years who wanted to increase their habitual physical activity (Cooper, 1970). Their starting point was the now largely discredited assumption (Shephard, 1984; Siscovick et al., 1991) that a medically-supervised exercise stress ECG could predict and thus avert the occasional exercise-induced cardiac arrest. Northcote and Ballantyne (1984) have pointed out that it would cost $13 billion to screen even current athletes over the age of 35 years; moreover, it would be necessary to screen 10,000 potential exercisers to find one who might die, and four other individuals who had been cleared by exercise stress testing would die unexpectedly while exercising (Epstein & Maron, 1986). Finally, the stress test itself has a significant morbidity and mortality (Van Camp, 1988), and a heavy emotional, financial and medical burden is generated by the high proportion of false positive test results.

The need for extensive preliminary screening is particularly questionable, given that moderate exercise decreases rather than increases a person's overall risk of cardiac death (Siscovick et al., 1984). The Swedish physiologist P.O. Astrand has often suggested in his lectures that it would be more logical to focus detailed medical attention on sedentary people than on those who are about to enter a conditioning program. Nevertheless, potential exercisers can be offered some practical advice that will reduce the likelihood of an exercise catastrophe. A review of such incidents (Johnson, 1992; Shephard, 1974, 1981) suggests that risks are increased if:

1. There is a history of fainting or chest pain during exercise.

2. There is a family history of sudden death at a young age.

3. The intensity and duration of activity are much greater than the subject has recently experienced.

4. Competition, publicity or pride encourages persistence with exercise in the face of warning symptoms.

5. The individual exercises while under pressure of time, or when oppressed by business or social problems.

6. The activity involves heavy lifting or prolonged isometric effort.

7. The weather is unduly hot or cold.

8. The participant has a viral infection, senses chest discomfort or cardiac irregularity, or feels "unwell."

The corresponding precautions are all matters of common sense, readily understood by the general public, but rarely discussed in the course of the usual clinical examination. There has thus been increasing acceptance of the Canadian viewpoint (Shephard, 1976, 1988), that (in symptom-free people from adolescence through to early old age) simple advice and self-administered questionnaires provide the most appropriate method of determining readiness for a modest increase of physical activity.

Current U.S. Screening Recommendations

The current U.S. recommendation for pre-exercise screening has moved much closer to the Canadian position (Table 1). It looks at the age of the subject (males > 40 and females > 50 years, American College of Sports Medicine, 1991, p.37), the proposed intensity of effort, and associated symptoms or major cardiac risk factors.

If the subject is planning no more than a moderate increase of habitual activity (an intensity of less than 60% of peak aerobic effort, which the person can sustain comfortably for an hour or longer), is symptom-free and has no more than one major coronary risk factor, then a preliminary medical examination is no longer recommended. Indications for medical advice are (1) the presence of disease, (2) the intent to undertake vigorous exercise above the specified age limit, and (3) two or more major risk factors, or symptoms suggestive of cardiopulmonary or metabolic disease.

Simple Approaches to Screening

Although the expense and anxiety associated with a formal medical examination is unwarranted for the great majority of people who plan to begin a simple exercise program, there remains merit in simple screening procedures, either self-administered or carried out by staff of a fitness center.

Bailey et al. (1976) first suggested such an approach when screening candidates for the Canadian Home Fitness Test. In the following year, Chisholm and associates (1975, 1978) surveyed 1253 apparently healthy adults who were attending an exhibition. They evaluated a potential list of some 19 self-administered screening questions against a medical examination that included a physical examination, the measurement of resting blood pressure, and recordings of resting and exercise electrocardiograms. As a result of this research, a brief self-administered questionnaire (the Physical Activity Readiness Questionnaire, or PAR-Q) was developed. This incorporated the 7 questions they judged had been the most effective in identifying individuals who needed a medical examination prior to exercise testing or conditioning.

The original version of the PAR-Q was quickly endorsed by the Canadian federal government fitness agency (Fitness Canada), and it has since been widely used, both in Canada and abroad (Shephard, 1986). Indeed, the American College of Sports Medicine recently recommended adoption of the PAR-Q procedure for healthy adults (men > 40, women > 50 years) who wish to increase their habitual physical activity (American College of Sports Medicine, 1991). Nearly two decades of experience has shown that the original PAR-Q procedure is remarkably safe (Shephard 1988, 1991). Given the low inherent risk of exercise for the healthy adult, and the fact that even clinical examination and an exercise stress ECG provide a rather dubious "gold standard" of exercise readiness, it is difficult to assess the sensitivity (the percentage of subjects unready for exercise who are detected) and the specificity (the percentage of individuals who are screened needlessly) of the PAR-Q procedure. Sensitivity seems adequate, since the PAR-Q has been used to screen as many as half a million people, without any reported adverse events in subsequent exercise testing or programs. On the other hand, about 20% of would-be exercisers "fail the test" by responding positively to one or more questions (Shephard et al., 1981), and in those aged 60-69 years, as many as 55% are "screened out" (Fitness Canada, 1983; Shephard, 1986). Moreover, subsequent examination of the medical records, blood pressure readings and electrocardiograms on positive responders suggests that at all ages from adolescence onward, many of the PAR-Q exclusions are unnecessary (Shephard et al., 1981).

Accordingly, the detailed wording of individual PAR-Q questions has recently been reviewed and revised by an expert committee of Fitness Canada (Figure 1). Given the absence of any clear gold standard of exercise readiness, the rewording was agreed through the Delphic process of circulating repeated drafts of the questionnaire for critical comment. The principal objective was to increase specificity without an undue sacrifice of sensitivity. The revised wording of the questionnaire reduced the overall number of individuals who were "screened out" from 17% to 12%. In all, 7.3% who had originally made positive responses were cleared by the rPAR-Q, but 2.3% of new candidates were cautioned about exercising.

The trend was for the revised format to allow exercise in a higher proportion of elderly subjects. The largest change of response patterns occurred on the question relating to blood pressure, which had been a major cause of erroneous exercise exclusions when using the original PAR-Q (Shephard et al., 1981).

Current Evaluation of Screening Questionnaires

The specificity of any screening test can only be improved at the price of some loss of sensitivity. A further decade of usage will be needed to decide whether the shift in this balance has been gauged correctly in the rPAR-Q, although preliminary data are encouraging in this regard. Unfortunately, there are major obstacles to an objective comparison of the two questionnaire wordings. Cost is a significant barrier, given the required sample size, but the cost/effectiveness of a validation against clinical examination is also questionable, given the lack of agreement between doctors on appropriate criteria for exclusion from conditioning programs, and the high proportion of false positive stress ECGs in symptom-free adults (Shephard, 1981). Physician-exclusion rates can range from 1% to 15% in comparable samples of the general adult population (Shephard, 1988). Moreover, high physician exclusion rates apparently lack validity, since they do not reduce the number of electrocardiographic abnormalities and other minor complications that are encountered during exercise testing.

When developing the original PAR-Q, Chisholm et al. (1975,1978) did attempt to validate their list of 19 potential questions against physician records, blood pressures and electrocardiographic tracings. The final, reduced list of seven questions did not receive any formal clinical validation. Nevertheless, less direct validation has been possible, coupling the International Classification of Diseases (ICD) codings reported in a national health survey (Health a Welfare, Canada, 1982) with PAR-Q responses. Trial of this approach has shown remarkable success (Arraiz et al., 1992). Over a seven year follow up, 1644 of 31,668 subjects died (Table 3). PAR-Q responses were divided into 3 categories: pass (no positive responses), conditional pass (positive response about hypertension, not under treatment or supervision for elevated blood pressure), and failure (other positive response). In those failing the test (Table 2), the crude overall mortality risk ratio was 2.2 (or 2.1, after adjustment for age, sex, body mass index and smoking behavior). Moreover, the relative risk of cardiovascular death was 9.1 (or 7.8 after adjusting for age, sex, body mass index and smoking behavior). Interestingly, the relative risk was moderately greater than that associated with a poor performance on the Canadian Home Fitness Test, and was much greater than would have been obtained by use of an exercise stress ECG. Siscovick et al. (1991) found a relative risk of only 2.6 when asymptomatic hypercholesterolemic men with exercise-induced ST segmental depression were followed for a seven year period. The PAR-Q responses remained of prognostic value when cases with known heart disease, stroke and high blood pressure were deleted (Table 2).

When the Canadian governmental committee revised the PAR-Q, changes from the original format were deliberately held to minor clarifications of wording, and the number of questions was unchanged. It already seems a very useful screening tool. However, the questionnaire may pass through several further revisions and refinements of wording before all of its potential has been realized. Issues that remain to be addressed include the need for age-specific questionnaires for children and for the very old, the level of certification needed by paramedical professionals who are now urged to discuss client responses to questions 5 and 6, the need to caution those cleared by the

Table 1.

Indications for preliminary medical screening among those who wish to increase their habitual physical activity (based on the recommendations of the American College of Sports Medicine, 1991; see original article for details).

Variable	Indication for Medical Screening
Known disease	Yes, if cardiac, pulmonary, or metabolic
Symptoms or signs suggesting disease[a]	Yes, if cardiac, pulmonary, or metabolic
Major cardiac risk factors[b]	Yes, if two or more
Vigorous exercise[c]	Yes, if man > 40 yr or woman > 50 yr

[a]Pain or discomfort in chest, shortness of breath with mild exertion, dizziness or sudden loss of consciousness, shortness of breath while sleeping, swelling of the ankles, palpitations or racing heart beat, pain in the calves on walking, or known heart murmur.

[b]Blood pressure higher than 160 mm Hg systolic or 90 mm Hg diastolic on two occasions, or use of medication to reduce blood pressure; serum cholesterol higher than 6.2 mmol/L (240 mg/dL); cigarette smoking; diabetes mellitus; family history of coronary or atherosclerotic disease in parents or siblings before the age of 55 years.

[c]Exercise that represents a substantial challenge; usually higher than 60% of maximal oxygen intake, and causing fatigue within 20 minutes or less.

rPAR-Q against large and sudden increases in habitual activity, the value of additional questions, and the potential to add information about lifestyle and conditioning techniques to the back of the questionnaire.

Summary

The risk that exercise will induce a cardiac catastrophe is low, and a medically-supervised exercise ECG is not a cost-effective approach to the pre-exercise screening of symptom-free adults. However, a questionnaire (whether self-administered, or completed by fitness center staff) is a useful safety precaution. The Canadian Physical Activity Readiness Questionnaire (PAR-Q) has proven a very safe screening tool, and comparison of responses with findings from the Canada

Table 2.

Validation of the original PAR-Q test against a 7-year prospective study of data from the Canada Health Survey (data abstracted from the paper of Arraiz et al., 1992).

Source of Risk	Relative risk if failed PAR-Q	
Crude	**Adjusted**	
All-causes	2.2	2.1
Cardiovascular disease	9.1	7.8
CVD (omitting if history of CVD)	5.4	
CVD (omitting if history of CVD, stroke, HBP)	2.9	
Cancer	2.1	1.6
Other causes	2.4	2.1

Health Survey has shown remarkable success in detecting potential contraindications to exercise. Nevertheless, the PAR-Q also "screens out" an excessive proportion of apparently healthy older adults. To reduce unnecessary exclusions, the questionnaire wording has now been revised (rPAR-Q). The balance of sensitivity to specificity is apparently improved in the revised questionnaire, particularly in regard to the question about an elevation of blood pressure. The rPAR-Q is thus the currently recommended method of determining exercise readiness in symptom-free adults with no more than one major cardiac risk factor.

References

Adams, R. (1991). *Report of Expert Committee on Revision of the Physical Activity Readiness Questionnaire*. Ottawa: Fitness and Amateur Sport.

American College of Sports Medicine. (1991). *Guidelines for Graded Exercise Testing and Prescription*. 4th Ed. Philadelphia: Lea & Febiger.

American College of Sports Medicine. (1993). Summary Statement: Workshop on Physical Activity and Public Health, *Sports Medicine Bulletin*, October - November, page 7.

Arraiz, G.A., Wigle, D.T. & Mao, Y. (1992). Risk assessment of physical activity and physical fitness in the Canada Health Survey mortality follow up. *Journal of Clinical Epidemiology* 45: 419-428.

Bailey, D.A., Shephard, R.J., Mirwald, R.L. and McBride, G.A. (1974). A current view of Canadian cardio-respiratory fitness. *Canadian Medial Association Journal* 111: 25-30.

Bailey, D.A., Shephard, R.J. and Mirwald, R.L. (1976). Validation of a self-administered home test for cardio-respiratory fitness. *Canadian Journal Of Applied Sport Sciences* 1: 67-78

Bouchard, C., Shephard, R.J. Stephens, T., Sutton, J. & Mcpherson, B. (1990). *Exercise, Fitness and Health*. Champaign, IL.: Human Kinetics Publishers.

Chisholm, D.M., Collis, M.L., Kulak, L.L., Davenport, W. and Gruber, N. (1975). Physical activity readiness. *British Columbia Medical Journal* 17: 375-378.

Chisholm, D.M., Collis, M.L., Kulak, L.L., Davenport, W., Gruber N. and Stewart, G. (1978). *PAR-Q Validation Report: The Evaluation of a Self-administered Pre-exercise screening Questionnaire for Adults*. Vancouver: B.C. Ministry of Health.

Cobb, L.A., & Weaver, W.D. (1986). Exercise a risk for sudden death in patients with coronary heart disease. *Journal of the American College of Cardiology* 7: 215-219.

Cooper, K.H. (1970). Guidelines in the management of the exercising patient. *Journal of the American Medical Association* 211: 1163-1167.

Epstein, S.E. & Maron, B.J. (1986). Sudden death and the competitive athlete: perspectives on preparticipation screening studies. *Journal of the American College of Cardiology* 7: 220-230.

Fitness Canada (1983). *Fitness and Lifestyle in Canada*. Ottawa: Fitness and Lifestyle Research Institute.

Health & Welfare Canada (1982). *Canada Health Survey*. Ottawa: Health & Welfare Canada.

Maron, B.J., Epstein, S.E. & Roberts, W.C. (1986). Causes of sudden death in competitive athletes. *Journal of the American College of Cardiology* 7: 204-214.

Northcote, R.J. & Ballantyne, D. (1984). Sudden death and sport. *Sports Medicine* 1: 181-186.

Sadaniantz, A. & Thompson, P.D. (1990). The problem of sudden death in athletes as illustrated by case studies. *Sports Medicine* 9: 199-204.

Shephard, D.A.E. (1976). Home fitness testing of Canadians. *Canadian Medical Association Journal* 114: 662-663.

Shephard, R.J. (1974). Sudden death—A significant hazard of exercise? *British Journal of Sports Medicine* 8: 101-110.

Shephard, R.J. (1984). Can we identify those for whom exercise is hazardous? *Sports Medicine* 1: 75-86.

Shephard, R.J. (1981). *Ischemic Heart Disease and Exercise.* London: Croom Helm.

Shephard, R.J. (1986). *Fitness of a Nation: Lessons from the Canada Fitness Survey.* Basel: Karger Publications.

Shephard, R.J. (1988). PAR-Q, Canadian Home Fitness Test and exercise screening alternatives. *Sports Med.* 5: 185-195.

Shephard, R.J. (1991). Safety of exercise testing—the role of the paramedical specialist. *Clin. J. Sports Med.* 1: 8-11.

Shephard, R.J. (1993). *Physical Activity and Health-Related Fitness.* Champaign, IL.: Human Kinetics Publishers.

Shephard, R.J., Cox, M. and Simper, K. (1981). An analysis of PAR-Q responses in an office population. *Canadian Journal of Public Health* 72: 37-40.

Shephard, R.J., Thomas, S. and Weller, I. (1991). The Canadian Home Fitness Test: 1991 Update. *Sports Medicine* 11: 358-366.

Siscovick, D.S., Weiss, N.S., Fletcher, R.H. & Lasky, T. (1984). The incidence of primary cardiac arrest during vigorous exercise. *New England Journal of Medicine* 311: 874-877.

Siscovick, D.S., Ekelund, L.G., Johnson, J.L., Truong, Y. & Adler, A. (1991). Sensitivity of exercise electrocardiography for acute cardiac events during moderate and strenuous physical activity. *Archives of Internal Medicine* 151: 325-330.

Thompson, P.D., Funk, E.J., Carleton, R.A. et al. (1982). Incidence of death during jogging in Rhode Island from 1975 through 1980. *Journal of the American Medical Association* 247: 2535-2538.

Van Camp, S.P. (1988). Exercise-related sudden death: risks and causes. *Physician and Sportsmedicine* 16 (5): 97-112.

Vuori, I., Suurnakki, L. & Suurnakki, T. (1982). Risk of sudden cardiovascular death (SCVD) in exercise. *Medicine and Science in Sports and Exercise* 14: 114-115.

Chapter 38

Influences on Physical Activity of Children, Adolescents, and Adults, Or: Determinants of Active Living

The U.S. Department of Health and Human Services has adopted a policy of increasing regular physical activity of children, adolescents and adults, because of the numerous health benefits that have been documented through research (Bouchard et al., 1994). The physical activity guidelines are published in *Healthy People 2000* (USDHHS, 1990), and even a casual inspection of the data accompanying the guidelines leads to the conclusion that most Americans are not physically active enough to optimize their health, and a sizable percent of adults are extremely sedentary.

Before launching large-scale programs to stimulate more physical activity, it is widely accepted that a better understanding of the various influences on physical activity habits is needed. If the most important influences can be identified, then they could be targeted for change in educational or other intervention programs. In this chapter, some of the theory and research on "determinants" of physical activity are summarized, and both the commonalities and differences between youth and adults are described. An attempt is made to apply these findings to the improvement of physical activity intervention programs.

Physical Activity And Fitness Research Digest, Series 1, No. 7, August 1994.

Explaining Human Behavior

Human behavior is complex enough to frustrate all attempts to explain it, but the attempts continue because of the importance of the task Efforts to explain individual differences in physical activity are further complicated by variations in frequency, intensity, duration, and type. The objectives in *Healthy People 2000* (USDHHS, 1990) call for decreases in sedentary behaviors and increases in light-to-moderate, vigorous, strength-building and flexibility-promoting activities. The influences may differ for each of these categories of physical activity. Most of the research work to date has focused on vigorous exercise in leisure time, but some studies are beginning to examine the influences on moderate intensity activities, like walking (Hovell et al., 1992), that are increasingly being recommended because of their health benefits. There are many studies of special populations, such as cardiac patients, but the present paper focuses on physical activity in the general population.

Theoretical models are the starting point for research on human behavior, because theories simplify the complex phenomena under study by suggesting which factors should be studied. Psychological models that emphasize the role of knowledge, beliefs, attitudes, motivations, and emotions have been dominant and have inspired studies that have shown many psychological factors influence physical activity patterns of adults and youth. These models include the theory of planned behavior (Godin & Shephard, 1990) and the intrinsic motivation model that was presented in a previous issue of this publication (Whitehead, 1993).

Other models take into consideration that beliefs and perceptions are not the only influences on physical activity. The behavior of others and factors in the external environment can also play a role in influencing physical activity. Social cognitive theory (Bandura, 1986) emphasizes multiple influences from within the person, the social environment, and the physical environment.

Over 300 studies of the influences on physical activity have produced a scientific literature rich with information, but the picture is not yet entirely clear The following sections summarize some of the major findings, and readers desiring more detailed information can consult recent reviews (Dishman & Sallis, 1994; King et al., 1992; Sallis, Simons-Morton, Stone et al., 1992; Sallis & Hovell, 1990).

Biological and Psychological Influences

Biologic factors are strongly associated with level of physical activity, even though it is not clear these factors actually "cause" physical activity to vary. Age is a potent predictor, and the level of physical activity is known to decrease throughout the entire age span, beginning at least with entry into school. During the school years, the activity level declines about 50% (Sallis, 1993), and the decline continues until the typical elderly person is almost entirely sedentary (Stephens & Caspersen, 1994). Females are less physically active than males at virtually all ages (Sallis, 1993; Stephens & Caspersen, 1994), but many people feel this difference is due to socialization rather than biology.

A biological reason why adults drop out of vigorous exercise programs is musculoskeletal injuries. In one study, injuries were the most common reason for dropping out (Sallis et al., 1990), and the history of injuries is a good predictor of future injuries. Though most people believe the obese are less active than the normal weight, it is difficult to find evidence to support this notion in either adults or youth. However, recent studies indicate that a substantial portion of physical activity may be explained by genetic factors (Perusse et al., 1989).

The personal characteristics of being well educated and affluent are consistently associated with higher levels of leisure time physical activity. African Americans and Latinos are usually found to be less active than Anglos, even in childhood (McKenzie et al., 1992). However, these ethnic differences are largely due to socioeconomic factors (Shea et al., 1991). It is surprising that health behaviors such as cigarette smoking, dietary habits, and alcohol consumption are not consistently related to physical activity habits, but it appears that people selectively choose their health behaviors. Recent physical activity predicts future activity in leisure time, but activity levels in childhood are not reliable predictors of exercise habits in adulthood. One explanation is that children may be taught activities, like team sports, that are difficult to carry over to adulthood.

A wide variety of psychological factors appear to influence participation in physical activity among adults. Much of our current understanding can be summarized by stating that beliefs and perceptions that are not personal in nature, such as knowledge about exercise, personality traits, and general attitudes, are weakly related to behavior. Personal beliefs about one's own physical activity are usually found to be significant influences on physical activity. One of the strongest predictors of future activity is perceptions of personal efficacy, or confidence regarding one's ability to be active on a regular basis. Simple ratings are useful in predicting activity levels among adolescents (Reynolds et al., 1990) and adults of all ages (Garcia & King, 1991; McAuley, 1992; Sallis, Hovell, Hofstetter et al., 1992). Program leaders could use such ratings to estimate which participants are likely to continue activity and which are at risk of dropping out.

There is a growing literature that supports the common belief that people must enjoy physical activity if they are to continue. Enjoyment appears to influence the activity levels of both children (Stucky-Ropp & DiLorenzo, 1993) and adults (Garcia & King, 1991). One of the main influences on enjoyment is the amount of exertion required by the activity. Children (Epstein et al., 1991) and adults (Garcia & King, 1991) prefer activities with lower levels of exertion, and dropout rates are higher from vigorous activity than from moderate intensity activity (Dishman & Sallis, 1994). One of the reasons behind the recent emphasis on encouraging people to engage in moderate activities (USDHHS, 1990) is that more people are expected to adhere.

Every sedentary person seems to have a reason for not being active, and knowing what those reasons are can provide clues about how to design an intervention. It is well known that the most common reason is "lack of time". In addition, the number and strength of perceived barriers to activity are consistently related to physical activity in both adults (Sallis, Hovell, Hofstetter et al., 1992) and adolescents (Tappe et al., 1989).

Psychological influences on children's physical activity have not been widely researched, in part because of the difficulties of assessing psychological states in children, and in part because parents and teachers select and control many of children's physical activities. Most children enjoy "playing", but our research group has encountered many children in elementary schools who complain, in the same way adults do, they do not have the time for physical activity.

Social and Physical Environment Influences

Significant others can make it more or less likely that a person is active on a regular basis. Social influences on physical activity are strong for people for all ages, but the nature of the support varies with developmental level. Social support for adults can come from friends, coworkers, or family members, and the main types of support are encouragement, participating in physical activities, and providing

512

assistance, such as child care (Dishman & Sallis, 1994). For adolescents, the influence of peers is paramount. If a given adolescent identifies with a peer group that values and participates in physical activity, the group creates a supportive environment for its members. If the main peer group devalues physical activity, this is an effective deterrent.

The younger the child, the more influential parents are. Studies of children aged 9 to 13 years have shown there are several ways that parents can support children's physical activity. Serving as active role models and providing encouragement may have limited influence, but two studies show that parents can have the most impact by directly helping children be active. Parents who participate in activities with their children (Stucky-Ropp & DiLorenzo, 1993), organize activities (Anderssen & Wold, 1992), or transport children to places where they can be active are the most effective supporters. For preschool children, prompts and encouragement to be active can be helpful (Sallis et al., 1993).

It seems self-evident that physical environmental factors such as climate and weather can have a major effect on physical activities, but few of many possible environmental factors have been documented in research. It is probable that changes in the environment have made it necessary to focus attention on increasing physical activity. Automobiles, television, computers, labor saving devices, and sedentary jobs have created an environment that makes possible a profoundly sedentary lifestyle for large numbers of people, maybe for the first time in history. Thus, it is critical to be aware of the effect of our artificial environments on physical activity levels.

A supportive environment for adults might consist of a safe and attractive space for outdoor activities, exercise equipment or supplies in or near the home, and convenient access to exercise facilities and programs. One study showed that adults were more likely to be active if they had a number of exercise facilities within a short distance from their homes (Sallis et al., 1990). For adolescents, it may be especially important to have organized activities in convenient locations, such as after-school intramural teams.

A supportive environment is essential for younger children. Because it is difficult for children to be active indoors, time spent outdoors is highly correlated with physical activity levels (Klesges et al., 1990; Sallis et al., 1993). Many parents are concerned about the safety of their neighborhoods and prohibit children from going outside to play. Unfortunately, the more parental rules that limit children's play, the less physically active young children are (Sallis et al., 1993). The more places the child can play that are within walking distance from home, the more active the child is (Sallis et al., 1993). Balancing safety concerns with the need to let children play outdoors is a serious challenge.

Television is a ubiquitous part of the environment of children, adolescents, and adults that encourages sedentary behavior. However, there is little indication that children or adults who watch the most television are the least active. There is reason to limit the hours per week children watch television, because of associations between amount of television viewing and obesity (Robinson et al., 1993).

Applying the Research to the Improvement of Programs

The research on influences on physical activity provides information that may be useful in more effectively promoting physical activity in individuals or groups of adults and youth.

Table 1 is a checklist that can be used to assess some of the key influences. Steps can then be taken to modify these influences so that physical activity is facilitated.

The biological and demographic influences are not easily changeable, but they provide some index of risk. A person or group with a low score on this section may need additional assistance in developing regular physical activity habits.

The higher the scores on the Psychological, Social, and Physical Environment sections, the more likely the person or group is to be physically active. Ideally, there are some checks in all of the sections. If there are few checks in a section, consider how to make changes in some of the influences listed. This checklist provides a rough assessment of existing resources and strengths as well as an indication of areas that need improvement. The reader is challenged to use this assessment to guide appropriate changes in personal or other physical activity programs.

Summary

Many health benefits of physical activity are documented, but large numbers of Americans are not engaging in the recommended levels of physical activity. Understanding the many factors that influence physical activity may help improve the effectiveness of physical activity intervention programs. Research suggests that the effectiveness of programs should be maximized when participants' confidence about

Table 1. Assessing Influences on Physical Activity.

Check those that apply. Each check represents an influence that supports physical activity.

Biological and Demographic Influences

____ Age. One check if less than 50; two checks if less than 18 years.
____ Male sex.
____ No (or minor) history of activity-related injuries.
____ Genetics. Both parents led active lifestyles.
____ Graduated college (for children, one parent graduated college).
____ White collar occupation (for children, parents have white collar occupation).

Psychological Influences

____ Self-efficacy. High level of confidence in ability to do regular physical activity.
____ Enjoys physical activity.
____ Belief that time for physical activity can be found.
____ Perceives few barriers to doing regular physical activity.
____ Strong intentions to be physically active.
____ Belief that personal benefits of physical activity outweigh the costs.

Social Influences

____ Friends or family are active role models
____ Friends or family encourage physical activity.
____ Friends or family participate in physical activity with you.
____ Friends or family directly help you be physically active.

Physical Environment

____ Weather or climate is favorable for preferred activities.
____ Feel safe being active outdoors near home.
____ Attractive outdoor space is convenient.
____ Exercise facilities or programs are convenient and affordable.
____ Exercise equipment or supplies in home.

their ability to continue physical activities is nurtured, they enjoy the activities they have chosen, receive encouragement and assistance from other people in their lives, and reside in a supportive environment that provides convenient, attractive, and safe places for physical activity.

References

Anderssen, N., & Wold, B. (1992). Parental and peer influences on leisure-time physical activity in young adolescents. *Research Quarterly for Exercise and Sport*, 63, 341 348.

Bandura, A. (1986). *Social Foundations of Though and Action*. Englewood Cliffs, NJ: Prentice-Hall.

Bouchard, C., Shephard, R.J., & Stephens, T. (Eds.) (1994). *Physical Activity, Fitness, and Health: International Proceedings and Consensus Statement*. Champaign, IL: Human Kinetics.

Dishman, R.K., & Sallis, J.F. (1994). Determinants and interventions for physical activity and exercise. pp. 214-238. In C. Bouchard, R.J. Shephard, & T. Stephens (Eds.), *Physical Activity, Fitness, and Health: International Proceedings and Consensus Statement*. Champaign, IL: Human Kinetics.

Epstein, L.H., Smith, J.A., Vara, L.S., & Rodefer, J.S. (1991). Behavioral economic analysis of activity choice in obese children. *Health Psychology*, 10, 311-316.

Garcia, A.W., & King, A.C. (1991). Predicting long-term adherence to aerobic exercise: A comparison of two models. *Journal of Sport and Exercise Psychology*, 13, 394-410.

Godin, G., & Shephard, R.J. (1990). Use of attitude-behaviour models in exercise promotion. *Sports Medicine* 10, 103-121.

Hovell, M.F., Hofstetter, C.R., Sallis, J.F., Rauh, M.J.D., & Barrington, E. (1992). Correlates of change in walking for exercise: An exploratory analysis. *Research Quarterly for Exercise and Sport*, 63, 425-434.

King, A.C., Blair, S.N., Bild, D.E., Dishman, R.K., Dubbert, P.M., Marcus, B.H.,

Klesges, R.C., Eck, L.H., Hanson, C.L., Haddock, C.K., & Klesges, L.M. (1990). Effects of obesity, social interactions, and physical environment on physical activity in preschoolers. *Health Psychology* 9, 435-449.

McAuley, E. (1992). The role of efficacy cognitions in the prediction of exercise behavior in middle-aged adults. *Journal of Behavioral Medicine*, 15, 65-88.

McKenzie, T.L., Sallis, J.F., Nader, P.R., Broyles, S.L., & Nelson, J.A. (1992). Anglo- and Mexican-American preschoolers at home and at recess: Activity patterns and environmental influences. *Journal of Developmental and Behavioral Pediatrics*, 13, 173-180.

Oldridge, N.B., Paffenbarger, R.S., Powell, K.E., & Yeager, K.K. (1992). Determinants of physical activity and interventions in adults. *Medicine and Science in Sports and Exercise*, 24, S221-S236.

Perusse, L., Tremblay, A., Leblanc, C., & Bouchard, C. (1989). Genetic and environmental influences on level of habitual physical activity and exercise participation. *American Journal of Epidemiology*, 129, 1012-1022.

Reynolds, K.D., Killen, J.D., Bryson, S.W., Maron, D.J., Taylor, C.B., Maccoby, N., & Farquhar, J.W. (1990). *Preventive Medicine*, 19, 541-551.

Robinson, T.N., Hammer, L.D., Killen, J.D., Kraemer, H.C., Wilson, D.M., Hayward, C., & Taylor, C.B. (1993). Does television viewing increase obesity and reduce physical activity? Cross-sectional and longitudinal analyses among adolescent girls. *Pediatrics*, 91, 273-280.

Sallis J.F., & Hovell, M.F. (1990). Determinants of exercise behavior. *Exercise and Sports Sciences Reviews*, vol. 18 Baltimore: Williams & Wilkins, 307-330.

Sallis J.F., Hovell, M.F., Hofstetter, C.R., Elder, J.P., Caspersen, C.J., Hackley, M., & Powell, K.E. (1990). Distance between homes and exercise facilities related to the frequency of exercise among San Diego residents. *Public Health Reports*, 105, 179-185.

Sallis, J.F. (1993). Epidemiology of physical activity and fitness in children and adolescents. *Critical Reviews in Food Science and Nutrition*, 33, 403-408.

Sallis, J.F., Alcaraz, J.E., McKenzie, T.L., Hovell, M.F., Kolody, B., & Nader, P.R. (1992). Parent behavior in relation to physical activity and fitness in 9-year-olds. *American Journal of Diseases of Children*, 146, 1383-1388.

Sallis, J.F., Hovell, M.F., Hofstetter, C.R., & Barrington, E. (1992). Explanation of vigorous physical activity during two years using social learning variables. *Social Science and Medicine*, 34, 25-32.

Sallis, J.F., Hovell, M.F., Hofstetter, C.R., Elder, J.P., Faucher, P., Spry, V.M., Barrington, E., & Hackley, M. (1990). Lifetime history of relapse from exercise. *Addictive Behaviors,* 15, 573-579.

Sallis, J.F., Nader, P.R., Broyles, S.L., Berry, C.C., Elder, J.P., McKenzie, T.L., & Nelson, J.A. (1993). Correlates of physical activity at home in Mexican-American and Anglo-American preschool children. *Health Psychology,* 12, 390-398.

Sallis, J.F., Simons-Morton, B.G., Stone, E.J., Corbin, C.B., Epstein, L.H., Faucette, N., Iannotti, R.J., Killen, J.D., Klesges, R.C., Petray, C.K., Rowland, T.W., & Taylor, W. (1992). Determinants of physical activity and interventions in youth. *Medicine and Science in Sports and Exercise,* 24, S248-S257.

Shea, S., Stein, A.D., Basch, C.E., Lantigua, R., Maylahn, C., Strogatz, D.S., Novick, L. (1991). Independent associations of educational attainment and ethnicity with behavioral risk factors for cardiovascular disease. *American Journal of Epidemiology,* 134, 567-582.

Stephens, T., & Caspersen, C.J. (1994). The demography of physical activity. pp. 204-213. In C. Bouchard, R.J. Shephard, & T. Stephens (Eds.), *Physical Activity, Fitness, and Health: International Proceedings and Consensus Statement.* Champaign, IL: Human Kinetics.

Stucky-Ropp, R.C., & DiLorenzo, T.M. (1993). Determinants of exercise in children. *Preventive Medicine,* 22, 880-889.

Tappe, M.K., Duda, J.L., & Ehrnwald, P.M. (1989). Perceived barriers to exercise among adolescents. *Journal of School Health,* 59, 153-155.

U.S. Department of Health and Human Services. (1990). *Healthy people 2000.* Washington, D.C.: U.S. Government Printing Office.

Whitehead, J.R. (1993). Physical activity and intrinsic motivation. *Physical Activity and Fitness Research Digest,* 1 (2), 1 -6.

Chapter 39

Toward an Understanding of Appropriate Physical Activity Levels for Youth

Summary

In the not so distant past, children were protected from vigorous physical activity. Even leading educators felt that children were incapable of exercise that caused high heart rates. In the last half century science has found that children can safely perform high intensity exercise. However, many of the guidelines for physical activity for children formulated in the last thirty years have been based on what is often called the Exercise Prescription Model (EPM), an approach developed primarily for adults. Since 1985, there has been a shift from the EPM to a Lifetime Physical Activity Model (LPAM) as the basis for establishing activity guidelines for adults. This model suggests that moderate daily lifetime exercise such as walking results in an energy expenditure of 3 to 4 kcal/kg/day (1000 to 2000 calories per week) which is sufficient to produce health benefits. Because high intensity activity is a deterrent to some, this model is offered as a "new strategy" for health risk reduction through physical activity.

Just as the LPAM is more appropriate for many adults than the EPM, the LPAM is better suited for children than the EPM. Like many adults, children often do not respond well to high intensity physical activity. The LPAM standards for minimal activity requirements necessary to gain the health benefits of physical activity (3 to 4 cal/kg/

Physical Activity And Fitness Research Digest, Series 1, No. 8 November 1994.

day) provide the basis for a child specific physical activity model called the Children's Lifetime Physical Activity Model (C-LPAM). This model suggests that children should, as a minimum, expend the same number of kcal/kg/day as adults. However, it also suggests that optimally, children should be encouraged to do additional physical activity (6 to 8 kcal/kg/day) because children have different needs than adults and it is during childhood that lifetime activity patterns are developed.

Physical Activity and Children

In 1879 a German physician named Behnke warned of the danger of vigorous physical activity among children (Karpovich, 1937). He cautioned adults to restrict activity among children because of the "natural disharmony" between the development of the size of the heart muscle and the size of the large vessels. He suggested that the blood vessels develop at a relatively slower rate than the heart muscle making the vessels unable to accommodate the faster growing heart. He concluded that there would be "grave danger" for the exercising child because of high blood pressure and accompanying circulatory problems.

Physical and health educators (Van Hagen, Dexter, and Williams, 1951; Young, 1923) perpetuated this myth as did "experts" in child growth and development (Hurlock, 1967). A widely used textbook in elementary school physical education warned that "...the heart increases greatly in size during this growth period (11-14 years), with veins and arteries developing much more slowly. The heart, therefore, should not be overtaxed with heavy and too continuous activity (Van Hagen et al., 1951, p. 52)." As late as 1967 Hurlock's text on adolescent development indicated that until late adolescence when the size of the blood vessels catches up with the size of the heart, "...too strenuous exercise may cause an enlargement of the heart and result in valvular disease (Hurlock, 1967, p. 47)." Apparently these experts had cited other experts each of whom had relied on Behnke or other uninformed sources.

The myth of children being unable to perform vigorous exercise persisted in the literature well into the 1960s even though published data had been presented in 1937 debunking the ideas of Behnke. Karpovich (1937) reexamined Behnke's data and showed that a simple mathematical error had been made. Though the circumference of the artery of children is proportionally small compared to the size of the heart, the bloodcarrying capacity of the artery is proportional to increases in heart size. Behnke assumed that the blood carrying capacity of the artery could be measured using the circumference of the artery when in fact it is the cross-sectional area of the interior of the artery that is critical. Karpovich was not the only one to debunk the "child's heart" myth. Another researcher, Boas (1931) conducted studies with exercising children that led him to conclude that during vigorous exercise the muscles will "flag" so that the child will "collapse before the heart is called for its last ounce of effort."

Even though research discredited the notion that children were incapable of vigorous exercise, many educators were skeptical about prescribing strenuous activity for children well into the 1960s. Texts for elementary school physical educators began to include sections documenting the cardiovascular capabilities of children (Corbin, 1969) and repudiating earlier incorrect statements. Still, not all physical educators were convinced of the capabilities of children as evidenced by the fact that the 600 yard run/walk (introduced in 1958) continued as the measure of cardiovascular fitness for children in the 1965 and 1975 national youth fitness battery (AAHPERD, 1980). Many physical educators continued to believe that children were not physically able to run long distances or to per form endurance activities and thought it was dangerous for them to do so.

Further evidence about the concern for exercising children was the resistance researchers experienced from human subject's committees that were just being organized in the 1960s and early 1970s. An example was an initial rejection by a human subjects committee for a study of the heart rates of children using telemetry during various distance runs (Corbin, 1972). The committee felt that children should be stopped from running if heart rates exceeded 170 bpm and if distances exceeded 600 yards. It was necessary to educate the committee members including medical doctors. The study was ultimately approved even though heart rates often exceeded 200 bpm and distances were as long as 800 yards.

It was not until 1978 that an American Academy on Pediatrics position paper (cited in AAP, 1991) noted that many children who had previously been screened out of physical education were capable of "full and active" participation. In 1980 longer runs became part of national physical fitness test batteries for children (AAHPERD, 1980).

The Exercise Prescription Model

The health fitness movement for adults began to gain momentum in the 1960s. Paul Dudley White, physician for President Eisenhower during the 1950s, emphasized the health value of physical activity (Pomroy and White, 1958) and his national visibility brought attention to the health benefits of activity. The classic study of Morris, Hady, Raffle, Roberts, and Parks (1953) on London transportation workers was published providing good evidence for the health value of physical activity. By the early 1960s, Taylor and colleagues (1962) had added to the body of literature supporting the value of physical activity for health. Rehabilitation programs for cardiac patients using physical activity were gaining credibility due to the work of pioneers such as Hellerstein and Wolffe. The exercise prescription model (EPM) was developed and served as the basis for most cardiovascular exercise for the next two decades.

During the late 1950s and 1960s, considerable work was conducted regarding the EPM in an attempt to define the intensity and frequency of short duration exercise required to promote gains in cardiovascular fitness as measured by VO_2max. Karvonen's classic research (1959) identified the threshold of training and provided a basis for the EPM. By 1966, widely used exercise physiology texts cited Karvonen's formula for fitness development. DeVries (1966), for example, cited the work of Karvonen and noted that exercise must be performed at 60% of heart rate reserve. This guideline was similar to "rules of thumb advocated for performance improvement by swimming and track coaches of the era. Whatever the original reasons for research concerning the EPM and the related concepts of threshold of training and target zone heart rates, the major emphasis in exercise prescription was on physiological VO_2max and performance improvement.

By the 1970s, the EPM and its focus on higher intensity and shorter duration activity (using percentage of maximum heart rate or O_2 consumption as the criterion for intensity) was firmly established for adults. In 1972, the American Heart Association published an exercise testing and training handbook (AHA, 1972) and by 1978 the emerging American College of Sports Medicine (ACSM, 1978) published its first position statement outlining the frequency, intensity, duration and mode of exercise prescription necessary to produce cardiovascular fitness gains for the adult population. This statement was updated in 1990 (ACSM, 1990).

The EPM and the exercise guidelines developed based on this model have been useful and effective. For young adults of Western cultures, exercise programs based on the EPM are useful because cardiovascular fitness can be achieved without a major time commitment. Improved fitness can be accomplished by performing continuous exercise in as few as three days per week. This allows busy people to fit moderate to high intensity exercise into their otherwise sedentary lifestyles. In addition, the EPM is particularly effective for athletes and those interested in optimal physical performance.

Ironically, the model for prescribing adult physical activity that gained the greatest attention (EPM) was quite different than the type of activity that seemed effective for public health promotion. Although the epidemiological literature suggested exercise of longer duration and relatively low intensity reduced heart disease risk (Morris, et al, 1953; Taylor, et al, 1962), the type of exercise prescription gaining notoriety was shorter in duration and of higher intensity.

Because improvement in cardiovascular fitness (rather than the reduction of health risk) was central to the EPM measures of cardiovascular fitness were of particular importance. The twelve minute run developed by Cooper to test the cardiovascular fitness of military personnel was popularized for the general public in the book *Aerobics* (Cooper, 1968). Shorter runs were developed for children and in 1980, the health related physical fitness test which included a mile run was adopted by AAHPERD (1980). By 1985, all of the major national fitness tests included a distance run of at least a mile in length. The capability of children to perform vigorous physical activity was acknowledged. In the absence of specific research to guide recommendations, the EPM was used to design exercise programs for children. Professionals had come full circle. Instead of fearing for the health of children who participated in vigorous exercise, guidelines for physical activity were similar to those designed for adults.

A Lifestyle Physical Activity Model: The New Strategy[2]

In July of 1992 the American College of Sports Medicine and the Centers for Disease Control and Prevention (CDC), in cooperation with the President's Council on Physical Fitness and Sports, issued a statement acknowledging the importance of lifestyle physical activity as a means of reducing disease risk. The new recommendation is to accumulate throughout the day a minimum of 30 minutes of moderate intensity physical activity over the course of most days of the week. Examples of such activities are "...walking up stairs (instead of taking the elevator), gardening, raking leaves, dancing, and walk-

---

[2] For comprehensive coverage of the scientific basis for the LPAM, readers are referred to articles by Blair (1993), Blair et al. (1992),and Haskell (1994). See references.

ing all or part of the way to work. Activity can also come from planned exercise or recreation such as jogging, playing tennis, swimming, and cycling (CDC & ACSM, 1994, p. 7)." Another example of lifestyle exercise that can be used to meet CDC/ACSM guidelines is a two mile walk daily.

Blair and colleagues have called this "new strategy" the Lifestyle Exercise Model (Blair, Kohl, and Gordon, 1992). Haskell (1994), in his recent Wolffe lecture to the American College of Sports Medicine also advocated the adoption of a lifestyle exercise model he calls the Physical Activity Health Paradigm. In this article, this model is referred to as the Lifetime Physical Activity Model (LPAM). Strong scientific evidence exists to support the LPAM (Haskell, 1994). The work of Paffenbarger and colleagues (Paffenbarger, Hyde, Wing, and Hsueh, 1986; Paffenbarger, Hyde, Wing, and Steenmetz, 1984; Paffenbarger, Wing, and Hyde, 1978) showed that the expenditure of 2000 kcals per week resulted in a significant reduction in morbidity and mortality among Harvard alumni. Those who expended 2000 to 3500 kcal per week attained the optimal value from their exercise. The studies of Harvard men showed that lifestyle activities such as climbing stairs, walking, doing physically active household activities and participating in active sports helped reduce disease risk not only for heart disease but for cancer and other types of hypokinetic conditions. Leon and colleagues (1987), studying a different group of adults, found that a 1500 kcal per week expenditure through moderate intensity physical activity produced similar health benefits to those found for the Harvard alums. Haskell (1985), based on a literature review, suggested 150 kcal per day (1050 kcal per week) as the minimum threshold for lifestyle exercise. These studies have demonstrated that health benefits accrue from lower intensity, longer duration exercise.

Blair et al. (1992), based on research at the Cooper Institute for Aerobics Research, have proposed that adults expend 3 kilocalories per kilogram of body weight per day (kcal/kg/day) in physical activity to achieve the benefits of regular physical activity. This standard is similar to the one used by previous researchers to classify people as "very active" (Montoye, 1987) and amounts to approximately 200 kcal per day for a 150 pound person or 1400 kcal per week. The kcal/kg/day standard allows individuals to calculate the caloric expenditure (based on their body weight) required to obtain health benefits. The physical activity necessary to expend 1000 to 2000 calories per week or 3 kcal/kg/day is the basis on which the CDC/ACSM guidelines for lifestyle physical activity were developed.

The LPAM differs from the EPM in several ways. First, the LPAM focuses on the amount of physical activity necessary to produce health benefits as associated with reduced morbidity and mortality rather than fitness and performance benefits. While the LPAM promotes fitness as it relates to good health, it does not focus on fitness performance as does the EPM. Moderate to high intensity exercise of shorter duration as outlined by the EPM was designed to promote changes on fitness tests such as VO$_2$*max*. Second, the LPAM recognizes the value of a wide range of physical activities that expend calories throughout the day rather than requiring the need for continuous moderate to vigorous physical activity done in one exercise bout. Finally, the LPAM acknowledges that some activity is better than none at all, and that up to a point, progressively increasing amounts of physical activity provide added health benefits.

The shift to the LPAM from the EPM does not mean, however, that the EPM is no longer a useful model. For young adults with limited amounts of time, moderate to vigorous physical activity is still an effective approach to achieving health benefits. For those who are interested in enhancing fitness for relatively high level performance such as sport involvement or active careers (law enforcement, military, etc.), the EPM is also an effective model. However, the type of exercise prescribed in the EPM is not necessarily the best approach for the general population that wants to receive substantial health benefits.

Children and the EPM

Just as most physical activity recommendations for adults have been based on the EPM for the past 20 to 30 years, recommendations for children have been based principally on guidelines evolving from the EPM. Rowland (1985) concluded that children need to follow the same exercise prescription as adults to achieve cardiovascular fitness. Using Karvonen's heart rate reserve method for calculating target heart rates, Sady (1986) estimated a heart rate of 159 as the threshold for aerobic exercise for most children. These results and the findings of other studies have served as the basis for recommendations suggesting that children need to perform 20 to 30 minutes of continuous moderate to vigorous physical activity (MVPA) at least three times a week. Typically heart rate standards are used as the indicator of MVPA. Recommendations vary but, in general, heart rates advocated are 140 bpm and higher.

Using heart rate standards as indicators has caused several researchers to conclude that many, if not most, children are inactive. Some examples illustrate the point. Using heart rates above 140 for 20 minutes of continuous exercise as the criterion of MVPA, Armstrong and Bray (1990) studied children and found 77% of boys and 88% of girls to be inactive by this measure. In a subsequent study of younger children, Armstrong, Balding, Gentle, and Kirby (1991) found 61 % of boys and 66% of girls to be inactive. Using observation techniques to assess 20 minutes of MVPA as the standard, Sleap and Warburton (1992) found 86% of children to be inactive and Baranowski, Hooks, Tsong, Cieslik, and Nader (1987) found 89.6% of children to be inactive. In another study involving 177 trials of day long monitoring of children averaging 703 minutes a day, Welk (1994) found 17% of children to have heart rates above 140 bpm for 20 consecutive minutes. If EPM were used to evaluate activity, it would be easy to conclude that most children are inactive.

Using data from the same studies but applying standards that are more consistent with the LPAM a different conclusion is reached. When minutes of physical activity during the day are determined for these same studies, the data of Armstrong and Bray (1990) show that on the average boys were active 45 minutes and girls 31 minutes of each day (above 140 but not consecutive minutes). In a second study (Armstrong & Bray, 1991) found younger boys were active 68 minutes and girls 59 minutes each day. Similarly, children studied by Baranowski, Hooks, Tsong, Cieslik, and Nader (1987) performed 60 to 70 minutes of activity per day even though 89% would be classified as inactive by the EPM standard. Eighty six percent of the children Sleap and Warburton (1992) studied were inactive in terms of EPM exercise yet, on average, they participated in 88 minutes of activity. Data from Welk's study (1994) using activity and heart rate monitors at the same time showed that 99% of boys and 98% of girls exceeded an energy expenditure of 4 kcal/kg/day, a standard that is slightly higher than the 3 kcal/kg/day, advocated by proponents of the LPAM.

It is apparent that the same children who fail to meet activity standards based on the EPM generally meet standards established for the LPAM. Rather than judge children as inactive based on MVPA data, it seems more reasonable to suggest the EPM is an inappropriate model for judging activity levels of most children. Children are sporadic exercisers who alternate between vigorous activity and rest. They are high volume exercisers who generally do not engage in continuous high intensity exercise. See Table 1 for a listing of concepts and implications concerning physical activity and children.

Table 1. Physical Activity and Children: Basic Concepts

Concept	Implication
Young animals, including humans, are inherently active.	Children will be active if given encouragementand opportunity.
Children are concrete rather than abstract thinkers.	Children are often unwilling to persist in activity if they see no concrete reason to do so.
The relationship between activity and fitness is weak among children.	Children may receive little feed back for their efforts in some activities.
Childhood activity is often intermittent and sporadic in nature.	Children will not likely do prolonged exercise without rest periods.
Total volume is a good indicator of childhood activity.	Given the opportunity, many children will perform relatively large volumes of intermittent physical activity.
Physical activity patterns vary with children of different developmental and ability levels.	Young children are not attracted to high intensity exercise but highly skilled older children may see its value for enhancing performance in sports.

The Children's Lifetime Physical Activity Model (CLPAM)

Evidence suggests that among adults 3 to 4 kcal/kg/day is a good minimum standard for producing the health benefits of physical activity. A similar minimum standard for children (3 to 4 kcal/kg/day) seems appropriate in light of recent evidence that show active children have a more beneficial coronary risk profile than their sedentary counterparts (Raitakara, Porkka, Taimela, Telama, Rasanen, & Viikari, 1994) and that many children already meet this standard (Blair, Clarke, Cureton, & Powell, 1989; Welk, 1994). Also, it is a standard that inactive children, those who need activity the most, can achieve with a modest commitment to childhood games and activities or lifestyle activities appropriate for children such as walking or riding a bicycle to school and performing physical tasks around the home.

It is not unreasonable, however, to establish a goal for children of expending 6 to 8 kcal/kg/day. Unlike adults, children have the time and energy for activity above the minimum standards if they see a reason to be active. There are at least five reasons why this goal of higher energy expenditure is appropriate.

1. During childhood children learn basic motor skills that provide the basis for lifetime activity. Proper skill development requires substantial practice time and energy expenditure. If motor skills are not learned early in life such skills may never be developed and the opportunities for lifetime activity will be limited.

2. Lifetime physical activities learned early in life (such as walking, riding bicycles, and doing active physical tasks around home) contribute to active lifestyles and help obese children maintain healthy body fat levels later in life (Epstein, Wing, Koeske, Ossip, & Beck, 1982).

3. Children need activity for the development of all parts of health related physical fitness including aerobic fitness, muscle strength and endurance, flexibility, and desirable level of body fatness as well as activity to promote a high peak bone density. To promote fitness development and to learn appropriate activities for development of these fitness parts, physical activity is essential.

4. Given the opportunity and encouragement, most children will choose to be active. This is especially true if time is provided for activity.

5. People who do no physical activity are at increased risk of disease and death compared to those who are physically active. The largest decrease in risk is associated with the expenditure of approximately 3 to 4 kcal/kg/day. Additional risk reduction is associated with increased amounts of physical activity (6 to 8 kcal/kg/day). To a point, activity be-

yond 6 to 8 kcal/kg/day produces additional benefits, but the relative benefits decrease as more activity is performed. The 6 to 8 kcal/kg/day standard seems a reasonable one for children. Evidence suggests that people become less active as they grow older (Rowland, 1990) and that people who are active when they are young are more likely to be active in later life (Raitakara, et al., 1994). This being the case, meeting a higher caloric expenditure as a child may interpret into greater activity as an adult.

High Performance Standards

As children grow older the EPM may become more important, especially if students make personal choices to perform high intensity physical activity designed to achieve optimal levels of fitness. For example, adolescents may wish to do EPM exercise to increase their chances of success in school or community sports. As noted earlier, children can participate in high intensity activity safely. However, the effort/benefit ratio (Fox and Biddle, 1988) for children is not good. To assure persistence in physical activity, children must believe the benefits of the activity are equal to or greater than the amount of effort expended. Because children are concrete thinkers they often see little benefit to high intensity training which makes their perception of effort high. Thus EPM exercise often produces a poor effort/benefit ratio.

Some children express a personal interest in EPM training. If their interest is strong and they perceive the benefits as great enough, they may successfully use the EPM exercise formula. However, because response to training is less in childhood compared to adolescence, there is some danger that children may lose interest in high intensity exercise. This is because of the lack of feedback from performance improvements. Learning skills through physical practice is often more rewarding and likely to enhance effort/benefit ratios for children. Generally, EPM physical activity designed to enhance high level performance in fitness is more appropriate and successful for adolescents and young adults than for children. Interestingly, evidence exists to suggest that the relationship between physical activity and aerobic fitness is not strong among children (Pate, Dowda, & Ross, 1990) or adolescents (Morrow & Freedson, in press).

529

Implications

Determining Activity Levels of Children

The best evidence suggests that children are among the most active segment of the population. Yet, using adults EPM standards, some have concluded that large numbers of children are inactive. This occurs in spite of the fact that the same children usually meet adult health standards for activity based on the scientifically documented LPAM. The C-LPAM is proposed as a more suitable model for judging the activity of children. National studies of the activity levels of children are needed, especially in attempt to determine if children are meeting appropriate standards.

Activity Recommendations for Children

As is inevitably the case, guidelines that gain national acceptance provide the basis for recommendations to be used in schools and other programs. In the case of physical activity, EPM guidelines have provided the basis for recommendations for children in schools as well as in community sports programs. Following the lead of scholars who have applied EPM guidelines to children, some professionals have advocated implementing programs that elevate heart rates of children to 140 or higher for 20 or more consecutive minutes. In some cases, heart rate monitors have been recommended to assure that exercise intensity levels are achieved among children (Strand and Reeder, 1993a; Strand and Reeder, 1994b).

Although programs using continuous high intensity (high heart rate) activity are not physiologically harmful to children, they are not the most appropriate for children. It is possible, given what we know about effort/benefit ratios and developmental needs of children that such activity can decrease rather than increase motivation for future activity. A more reasonable recommendation is that children perform C-LPAM activity as outlined here. In physical education programs, youth sports programs, or any other program designed to encourage current and lifetime activity for children, there are five guidelines that seem important:

1. Activity for children should focus on high volume and moderate intensity which includes sporadic activities such as active play performed in several activity sessions daily.

2. Lifestyle activity such as walking or riding bikes to and from school or performing active physical tasks at home (e.g., yard work) should be encouraged.

3. Opportunities to learn basic motor skills and develop all parts of health related physical fitness through appropriate moderate intensity activity should be included in the activity program.

4. Children should be afforded opportunities to begin developing behavioral skills that lead to lifetime activity.

5. EPM guidelines can be applied to individuals who are especially interested in high level physical performance, but only when it is developmentally appropriate.

References

American Academy of Pediatrics. (1991). *Sports Medicine: Health Care for Young Athletes*. (2nd ed.) Elk Grove Village, IL: American Academy of Pediatrics.

American Alliance of Heath, Physical Education, Recreation, and Dance. (1980). *Health Related Physical Fitness Test Manual*. Reston VA: American Alliance of Health, Physical Education, Recreation, and Dance.

American Association of Health, Physical Education, and Recreation. (1958) *Youth Fitness Testing Manual*. Washington, DC: American Association o Health, Physical Education, and Recreation.

American College of Sports Medicine. (1978). The recommended quantity and quality of exercise for developing and maintaining cardiorespiratory and muscular fitness of healthy adults. *Medicine and Science in Sports and Exercise*, 10, viix.

American College of Sports Medicine. (1990) The recommended quantity and quality of exercise for developing and maintaining fitness of healthy adults. *Medicine and Science in Sports and Exercise*, 22, 265-274.

American Heart Association. (1992). Medical/scientific statement on exercise: Benefits and recommendations for physical activity programs for all Americans. *Circulation*, 86(1), 2726-2730.

American Heart Association. (1972). *Exercise Testing And Training Of Apparently Healthy Individuals: A Handbook For Physicians.* Dallas: American Heart Association.

Armstrong, N., Balding, J., Gentle, P., Kirby, B. (1990) Patterns of physical activity among 11-16 year old British Children. *British Medical Journal,* 301, 203-205.

Armstrong, N. & Bray, S. (1991). Physical activity patterns defined by continuous heart rate monitoring. *Archives of Disease in Children,* 66, 245-247.

Baranowski, T., Hooks, P., Tsong, Y., Cieslik, C. & Nader, P.R. (1987) Aerobic physical activity among third to sixth grade children. *Developmental and Behavioral Pediatrics,* 8(4), 203-206.

Blair, S.N. (1993) C.H. McCloy Research Lecture: Physical activity, physical fitness, and health. *Research Quarterly for Exercise and Sport,* 64(4), 365-376.

Blair, S.N., Clarke, D.G., Cureton, K.J., & Powell, K E. (1989) Exercise and fitness in childhood: Implications for a lifetime of health. In C.V. Gisolfi and Lamb, D.V. (Eds.), *Perspectives in Exercise Science and Sports Medicine: Volume 2 Youth Exercise and Sport* (pp. 401-430). Indianapolis: Benchmark Press.

Blair, S.N., Kohl, H.A.W. III, Paffenbarger, R.S., Clark, D.B., Cooper, K.H., & Gibbons, L.W. (1969) Physical fitness and allcause mortality. *The Journal of the American Medical Association,* 262, 2395-2401.

Blair, S.N., Kohl, H.W., & Gordon, N.F. (1992). Physical activity and health: A lifestyle approach. *Medicine, Exercise, Nutrition, and Health,* 1, 54-57.

Boas, E.P. (1931) The heart rate of boys during and after exhausting exercise. *Journal of Clinical Investigation,* 10, 145-147.

Cooper, K.H. (1968). *Aerobics.* New York: M. Evans.

Corbin, C.B. (1989) *Becoming Physically Educated In The Elementary School.* Philadelphia: Lea & Febiger.

Corbin, C.B. (1972). Relationships between PWC and running performance of young boys. *Research Quarterly,* 43, 235-238.

DeVries, H.A. (1986). *Physiology Of Exercise Or Physical Education And Athletics.* Dubuque, IA: W. C. Brown.

Epstein, L.H., Wing, R.R., Koeshe, R., Ossip, D., & Bech, S. (1982). A comparison of lifestyle change and programmed aerobic exercise on weight loss in obese children. *Behavior Therapy,* 13, 651-665.

Fox, K. & Biddle, S. (1966). Children's participation motives. *British Journal of Physical Education,* 19, 34-38.

Haskell, W.L. (1985) Physical activity and health: Need to define the required stimulus. *American Journal of Cardiology,* 5, 4D-9D.

Haskell, W.L. (1994) Heath consequences of physical activity: Understanding and challenges regarding dose response. *Medicine and Science in Sport and Exercise,* 26(6), 649-660.

Hurlock, E.B. (1987) *Adolescent Development.* New York: McGraw Hill.

Karpovich, P.V. (1937). Textbook fallacies regarding the development of the child's heart. *Research Quarterly,* 6, 33.

Karvonen, M.J. (1969).The effects of vigorous exercise on the heart, In Rosenbaum, F.F. & Belknap, E.L. (Ed.), *Work and the Heart.* New York: P.B. Hoebner.

Leon, A.S., Connett, J., Jocobs, D.R., & Rauramaa, R. (1987). Leisuretime physical activity levels and risk of coronary heart disease and death. *Journal of the American Medical Association,* 266, 2388-2395.

Montoye, H.J. (1987). How active are modern populations? *The Academy Papers,* 21, 34-45.

Morris, J.N., Hady, J.A., Raffle, P.A., Roberts, C.B, & Parks, J.W. (1953). Coronary heart disease and physical activity of work. *Lancet,* 2,1053-1057, 1111-1120.

Morrow, J.R. & Freedson, P.S. (in press). Relationship between habitual physical activity and aerobic fitness in adolescents. *Pediatric Exercise Science.*

Paffenbarger, R.S., Hyde, R.T., Wing, A.L., & Hsueh, R.T. (1986). Physical activity, all-cause mortality, and longevity of college alumni. *New England Journal of Medicine,* 314, 605-613.

Paffenbarger, R.S., Hyde, R.T., Wing, A.L., & Steenmetz, C.H. (1984). A natural history of athleticism and cardiovascular health. *Journal of the American Medical Association,* 252, 491-495.

Paffenbarger, R.S., Wing, A.L. & Hyde, R.T. (1976). Physical activity as an index of heart attach risk in college alumni. *American Journal of Epidemiology,* 108,161-176.

Pate, R.R., Dowda, M., & Ross, J.G. (1990) Associations between physical activity and physical fitness in American children. *American Journal of Diseases in Children,* 144,1123-1129.

Pomroy, W.C. & White, P.D. (1956). Coronary heart disease in former football players. *The Journal of the American Medical Association,* 167, 711-714.

Raitakari, O.T., Porkka, K., V., K, Taimela, S, Telama, R., Rasanen, L., & Viikari, J.S.A. (1994) Effects of persistent physical activity and inactivity on coronary risk factors in children and young adults. *American Journal of Epidemiology,* 140(3), 195-205.

Rowland, T.W. (1986). Aerobic response to endurance training in prepubescent children: A critical analysis. *Medicine and Science in Sports and Exercise,* 17.493-497.

Rowland, T.W. (1990). *Exercise And Children's Health.* Champaign, IL: Human Kinetics.

Sady, S.P. (1986). Cardiorespiratory exercise training in children. *Clinics in Sports Medicine.* 493-514.

Sleap, M., & Warburton, P. (1992) Physical activity levels of 5 11 year old children in England as determined by continuous observation. *Research Quarterly for Exercise and Sport.* 63(3), 238-245.

Strand, B. & Reeder, S. (1993a). Analysis of heart rate levels during middle school physical education activities. *Journal of Physical Education, Recreation, and Dance,* 64(3), 65-91.

Strand, B. & Reeder, S. (1993b). Physical education with a heartbeat. *Journal of Physical Education, Recreation, and Dance,* 64(3), 61-64.

Taylor, H.L., et al. (1982). Death rates among physically active and sedentary employees of the railway industry. *American Journal of Public Health,* 52,1697-1707.

U.S. Centers for Disease Control & Prevention and American College of Sports Medicine (1994) Summary statement: Workshop on physical activity and public health. *Sports Medicine Bulletin*, 26(4), 7.

Van Hagen, W.V., Dexter, G, & Williams, J.F. (1961). *Physical Education In The Elementary School*. Sacramento, CA: California State Department of Education.

Welk, G.J. (1994). A comparison of methods for the assessment of physical activity in children. Unpublished doctoral dissertation, Arizona State University. Tempe AZ.

Young, E. (1923) *Hygiene in the Schools*. Philadelphia: W.B. Saunders.

Chapter 40

Physical Activity in the Prevention and Management of Coronary Heart Disease

Introduction

The concept that a sedentary lifestyle leads to an increase in the clinical manifestations of coronary heart disease (CHD), especially myocardial infarction and sudden death, has become generally accepted by the public and many health professionals. Most often, the idea has been expressed that regular exercise, in conjunction with other risk-reducing behaviors, will help protect against an initial cardiac episode (primary prevention); will aid in the recovery of patients following myocardial infarction, coronary artery bypass surgery, or coronary angioplasty (cardiac rehabilitation); and will reduce the risk of recurrent cardiac events (secondary prevention).

Evidence relating level of habitual exercise to risk of CHD has been derived from a variety of sources including animal studies, clinical impressions, observational surveys of the general population or special groups, and experimental studies in which the exercise of subjects assigned to "treatment" was increased in relation to sedentary control subjects. No one of these studies provides irrefutable evidence of a casual relationship between exercise status and CHD pathology, even though many sources of information do generally support such a contention. This situation is not unique to our understanding of the preventive role of exercise as it relates to CHD since a similar situation exists for all other "lifestyle" risk factors.

Physical Activity And Fitness Research Digest, Series 2, No. 1, March, 1995.

The presentation of information in this edition of the *Digest* is designed to provide the scientific basis for making decisions regarding the potential value of exercise in the primary and secondary prevention of CHD. Data on the relationship of exercise to CHD are reviewed, the possible biologic mechanisms by which beneficial effects may occur are summarized, the risks of developing cardiac complications during exercise are briefly discussed, and physical activity guidelines for promoting cardiovascular health are provided.

Physical Activity and the Primary Prevention of Coronary Heart Disease

During the past half century more than 50 studies have been published reporting on the association between habitual level of physical activity and the prevalence or incidence of initial clinical manifestations of CHD, especially myocardial infarction and sudden cardiac death (Berlin & Colditz, 1990; Powell et al., 1987). These studies have included the determination of on-the-job or leisure-time activity in free-living populations of many men and relatively few women with activity classifications based on job category, self-report questionnaires, or interviewer determinations. Manifestations of CHD were established by examination of death certificates, hospital or physician records, questionnaires completed by the subjects or physicians, and medical evaluations conducted by the investigators. Reported activity levels range from daily caloric expenditures exceeding 6,000 kilocalories (kcal) per day in Finnish lumberjacks at one extreme to very sedentary civil servant mangers and postal clerks at the other. Studies have been conducted in major industrial environments as well as rural and primate living areas.

As a result of the diverse protocols used in the various studies, including sample-selection procedures, physical activity classification methods, clinical event determination criteria, and statistical treatment of the data, it is not possible to collate the results into a single summary statement or interpretation. However, certain findings, although not universally obtained, occur sufficiently frequently to warrant the formulation of preliminary conclusions to use as a basis for program recommendations and planning future research.

More Active Persons Appear to be at Lower Risk

The general impression obtained as the result of a comprehensive review of the scientific reports containing data on the primary preventive effect of physical activity is that more active people develop less CHD than their inactive counterparts, and when they do develop CHD, it occurs at a later age and tends to be less severe (Berlin & Colditz, 1990: Powell et al, 1987). The results of the numerous reports are quite variable, with some studies demonstrating a highly significant beneficial effect of exercise (Lakka et al, 1994; Morris et al, 1980; Paffenbarger, Wing and Hyde, 1978; Shapiro et al, 1969; Shaper & Wannamethee, 1991), others showing a favorable but nonsignificant trend in favor of the more active (Costas et al, 1978; Salonen, Puska and Tuomilehto, 1982), and a few early studies showing no difference in CHD rates (Chapman and Massey, 1964; Paul, 1969). Of major importance is the consistent finding that being physically active does not increase an individual's overall risk of CHD.

No specific study characteristics can be identified that explain the differences in results among the various studies, but in some cases the physical activity measure is not very accurate or reliable and the activity gradient among the population is quite small (Shapiro et al, 1969). Also, with populations in whom CHD mortality is exceptionally high and in whom major risk factors such as hypercholesterolemia, hypertension, and cigarette smoking are prevalent, even very high levels or physical activity do not appear to exert a major protective effect. Finnish lumberjacks are an example of very physically active individuals in whom CHD risk remains high (Karvonen et al, 1961). It appears that in observational studies that are well designed, the inverse association between activity and CHD mortality is stronger than reported in scientifically less rigorous studies (Powell et al, 1987).

Moderate Amounts of Exercise May Be Protective

A striking feature of many studies demonstrating a reduced CHD risk for more active individuals is that the greatest difference in risk is achieved between those people who do almost nothing and those who perform a moderate amount of exercise on a regular basis. Much smaller differentials in risk are observed when moderately active individuals are compared with the most active persons (Leon et al, 1987; Lakka et al, 1994; Paffenbarger et al, 1993).

The amount of activity, in both intensity and duration, that is associated with a decrease in CHD clinical manifestations varies substantially among the different reports. Several studies have observed significant differences in CHD indicators with quite small differences in habitual activity level at a relatively low intensity (Leon et al, 1987; Kahn, 1963; Shapiro et al, 1969), whereas other authors interpret their data to indicate that a 'threshold' of higher intensity or amount of activity is needed in order to obtain a benefit (Cassel et al, 1971; Morris et al, 1980; Paffenbarger, Wing, and Hyde, 1978). The types of activity performed by the more active groups include brisk walking on level or hilly ground, climbing stairs, lifting and carrying light objects, lifting heavy objects, operating machinery or appliances, light and heavy gardening, performing home maintenance or repairs, and participating in active games and sports. The results of several studies, however, indicate that an intensity threshold of approximately 7 kcal/min (e.g. brisk walking, heavy gardening) may exist, with exercise more vigorous than this providing greater protection than a similar amount of less vigorous activity (Cassel et al, 1971; Morris, et al, 1990). Of greatest benefit seems to be large muscle dynamic or "aerobic" activity that substantially increases cardiac output with rather small increases in mean arterial blood pressure. Such activity is in contrast to heavy resistance or isometric exercise that substantially increases arterial blood pressure with a relatively small increase in cardiac output. Participation in "physical fitness" or "athletic conditioning" programs contributes little to the more active classification in most observational studies so far reported.

On-The-Job Activity

Most of the initial observations establishing an association between physical activity status and CHD manifestations used on-the-job activity. It is much easier (but likely less accurate) to classify individuals as inactive or active according to their job title or description that it is to obtain self-assessments by interview, questionnaire, or direct observation of job-related or leisure-time activity. The early studies that obtained a difference in CHD rates between inactive and active classifications, such as the reports by Morris on London busmen (Morris et al, 1953), Kahn's observation on Washington, D.C., postal workers (Kahn, 1963) or Taylor's studies on U.S. railroad workers (Taylor et al, 1970) included job situations in which the major exercise of the more active groups was walking on flat ground, up stairs, or up and down hills. If the more physically active status is responsible for the lower CHD rates in these populations, the intensity threshold for an activity-related benefit is not high. Other on-the-job studies, however, have not found any protective association with activity level until a classification of "heavy work" was obtained (Cassel et al, 1971; Morris et al, 1953; Morris et al, 1990).

The estimated net energy expenditure (above the energy expenditure of the inactive group) associated with a decrease in CHD mortality in the various occupational studies ranges from 300 to 800 kcal/day. The intensity of the activity contributing to this increased energy expenditure includes walking, lifting and carrying objects, farming, and laboring-type jobs. In most cases, the higher-intensity activities (i.e., heavy lifting or carrying) are performed in relatively short bursts throughout the workday with the lower intensities (i.e., walking) being carried out for longer durations.

Leisure-Time Activity

Accurate quantitative assessments of leisure time or non-job activity status are difficult to obtain on samples of the size needed to evaluate the relationship of habitual activity status and CHD clinical events. Various diary and recall techniques have been used, and they all present significant administration and scoring difficulties. However, in the studies that have attempted to quantitate various aspect of non-job activities, several have identified an inverse association between activity status and CHD similar to the relationship reported in the earlier occupational-based studies.

Evidence of some protection possibly being provided by nonjob, low-intensity activity on a regular basis was first reported by Rose (1969). He observed that the prevalence of "ischemic-type" resting electrocardiographic (ECG) abnormalities was inversely associated with duration of walking to work among 8,948 executive grade civil service workers in London. Those employees who walked 20 or more minutes to work on a regular basis had one third fewer ECG abnormalities than their counterparts who rode to work. This association could not be accounted for as a result of differences in age, grade of employment, smoking habits, serum cholesterol, or glucose tolerance. Those who walked regularly, however, tended to be a little less overweight.

The relationship of leisure-time activity to CHD mortality among middle-aged male civil servant workers in Britain has been studied using a two-day activity recall procedure (Morris et al, 1980; Morris et al, 1990). Morris and co-workers reported that nonjob activity, as assessed by a self administered 48-hour recall questionnaire completed on a Monday for the preceding Friday and Saturday, was significantly associated with CHD mortality only when activities requiring a peak energy expenditure of 7.5 kcal/min for 30 minutes or longer each day were performed ("vigorous activity"). Lesser amounts of activity appeared to carry no protective benefit. This apparent protective action of "vigorous activity" was not related to plasma total cholesterol, blood pressure, cigarette smoking, or adiposity, and it occurred at all ages from 40 to 69 years.

Paffenbarger and colleagues (Paffenbarger et al, 1986, 1993) have continued to evaluate the relationship between past and recent physical activity habits and cardiovascular health in Harvard University alumni. Analyses of 572 first heart attacks among 16,936 men between 1962 and 1972 and 1,413 total deaths between 1962 and 1978 showed that it was habitual post-college exercise, not student sports play, that predicted low coronary heart disease risk. They have shown that sedentary alumni who were ex-varsity athletes had high risk while sedentary students who became active in later life seem to acquire a low risk. These results are similar to several reports of job-related activity and heart disease risk where more physically active jobs early in a career followed by years of sedentary work resulted in higher risk than when the active job was continued throughout a person's career.

The relationship of self-selected leisure-time physical activity (LTPA) to first major CHD events and overall mortality was studied in 12,138 middle-aged men participating in the Multiple Risk Factor Intervention Trial (Leon et al, 1987). Total LTPA over the preceding year was quantitated in mean minutes per day at baseline by questionnaire, with subjects classified into tertiles (low, moderate, and high) based on LTPA distribution. During seven years of follow-up, moderate LTPA was associated with 64% as many fatal CHD events and sudden deaths, and 73% as many total deaths as low LTPA (P <.01). Mortality rates with high LTPA were similar to those in moderate LTPA; however, combined fatal and nonfatal major CHD events were 20% lower with high as compared with low LTPA (P <.05). These risk differentials persisted after statistical adjustments for possible confounding variables, including other baseline risk factors.

Physical activity at work and in leisure time was studied by questionnaire in a random sample residents living in Eastern Finland (Salonen, Puska and Tuomilehto, 1982). The study population consisted of 3,978 men aged 30-59 years and 3,688 women aged 35-59 years. During a seven-year follow-up, low physical activity at work was associated with an increased risk of myocardial infarction, cerebral stroke and death due to any disease in both men and women, even after controlling for age, cholesterol, diastolic blood pressure, weight and smoking status using a multiple logistic model. The relative risk for myocardial infarction was 1.5 (95% confidence interval = 1.2-2.0) for men and 2.4 (95% confidence interval = 1.5-3.7) for women. Men and women at highest risk were those that reported no vigorous exercise during either work or leisure time while those at lowest risk reported vigorous exercise during both times.

Recently Lakka and colleagues (1994) reported the results of following 1,453 men aged 42 to 60 years for about 5 years. In the more active third of the men (>2.2 hours per week of activity) the relative risk of a myocardial infarction was 0.31 (95% confidence interval = 0.12 to 0.85; p = 0.02) compared to the least active third. Similar results were obtained when aerobic capacity as determined by maximal oxygen uptake was related to risk of myocardial infarction.

A major criticism of the observational studies which demonstrate a protective effect of exercise is that the differences in CHD rates between active and inactive individuals may be due to less healthy people selecting a less active lifestyle, not that increased activity prevents disease. Such self-selection may account for some of the differences reported; but in several reports, the investigators considered this problem in their data analyses and still found that being physically active was of significant benefit (Kahn, 1963; Paffenbarger, Wing and Hyde, 1978). Also, Paffenbarger and colleagues (1993) recently reported that an increase in activity from one examination to the next was associated with a lower CHD mortality rate. These results strengthen the argument that it is an increase in activity that causes the reduction in mortality.

Physical Fitness and Primary Prevention

Only in the past decade have studies been published that have adequately measured cardiovascular functional capacity or physical fitness on a sample of sufficient size and then followed their clinical status long enough to be able to effectively evaluate the relationship of physical fitness to future CHD or total mortality. If a higher level of habitual activity causes a reduction in cardiovascular morbidity and mortality, then a similar association should be observed with an accurate and reliable measure of fitness.

This issue was examined in a study of 4,276 men, 30 to 69 years of age who were screened as part of the Lipid Research Clinic's prevalence survey and followed for an average of 8.5 years (Ekelund et al, 1988). Examination at baseline included assessment of conventional coronary risk factors and treadmill exercise testing. The heart rate during submaximal exercise (stage 2 of the Bruce exercise test) and the duration of exercise were used as measures of physical fitness. After adjustment for age and cardiovascular risk factors, a lower level of physical fitness was associated with a higher risk of death from CVD and CHD. The relative risk for death due to CVD for the least fit healthy men versus the most fit healthy men was 3.6 (95% confidence interval = 1.6 to 5.6; p = 0.0004) and for death due to CHD it was 2.8 (95% confidence interval = 1.3 to 6.1; p = 0.007). Highly significant associations were also seen for men that had CVD at their initial evaluation and for all-cause mortality. Thus, a low level of physical fitness is associated with a higher risk of death, especially from CVD and CHD, in men independent of conventional risk factors.

The relationship of physical fitness, as measured by maximal treadmill performance, to all-cause and cause-specific mortality was evaluated in 10,224 men and 3,120 women who had completed comprehensive medical examinations at the Cooper Clinic (Blair et al, 1989). Average follow-up was slightly more than 8 years, for a total of 110,482 person-years of observation. There were 240 deaths in men and 43 deaths in women. Age adjusted all-cause mortality rates declined across physical fitness quintiles from 64.0 per 10,000 person-years in the least-fit men to 18.6 per 10,000 person-years in the most-fit men. Corresponding values for women were 39.5 per 10,000 person-years to 8.5 per 10,000 person-years. These trends remained after statistical adjustments for age, smoking habit, cholesterol level, systolic blood pressure, fasting blood glucose level, parental history of coronary heart disease, and follow-up interval. Higher levels of physical fitness appeared to delay all-cause mortality primarily due to lowered rates of cardiovascular disease and cancer.

The relationship of maximal oxygen uptake measured during a maximal test on a cycle ergometer to CVD mortality during a 16-year follow-up was reported for 2,014 Norwegian men initially aged 40 to 59 years (Sandvick et al, 1993). The relative risk of death from any cause in fitness quartile 4 (highest) as compared with quartile 1 (lowest) was 0.54 after adjustment for age, smoking status, serum lipids, blood pressure, resting heart rate, vital capacity, body mass index, level of physical activity and glucose tolerance. The adjusted relative risk of death from CVD in fitness quartile 4 as compared with quartile 1 was 0.41 (p = 0.013). The corresponding relative risks for quartile 3 and 2 (as compared to quartile 1) were 0.45 (p = 0.026) and 0.59 (p = 0.15), respectively.

The results of these three physical fitness studies and the data reported by Sobolski, Kornitzer, and De Backer (1987) and Lakka and colleagues (1994) are highly consistent with the observational data on physical activity and cardiovascular mortality: the least fit and active have the highest rate of disease with only moderate increases in fitness and activity associated with a significant reduction in risk. There is a continued dose-response relationship at higher levels of fitness, but the magnitude of the benefit tends to decline as fitness levels increase, with the most fit generally having the lowest CHD mortality rate.

Secondary Prevention of Coronary Heart Disease

As with primary prevention, there is no definitive study demonstrating a significant reduction in new cardiac events as a result of exercise training in patients with established CHD. But in addition to studies that have simply compared morbidity or mortality rates in active with inactive cardiac patients, controlled experimental trials have been conducted in which myocardial infarction patients have been randomly assigned to exercise and control groups.

Here again, the trend in mortality favors the more physically active patients, with benefits apparently derived from an increase in caloric expenditure of no more than 300 to 400 kcal per session three to four times per week at a moderate intensity (60 to 75% of maximal erertion or aerobic capacity). All of the studies published, which show either no differences or lower mortality rates in the active population, have either design or implementation flaws that prohibit definitive conclusions regarding the hypothesis, "Does an increase in exercise reduce the future likelihood of recurrent myocardial infarction, cardiac arrest, or sudden cardiac death?"

Randomized clinical trials of cardiac rehabilitation following hospitalization for myocardial infarction usually have demonstrated a tendency for lower mortality in treated patients, but a statistically significant reduction occurred in only one trial (Wilhelmsen et al, 1975; Rechnitzer et al, 1983; Shaw, 1981). To overcome the problem of inadequate power of any one study to detect small but clinically important benefits on cardiovascular morbidity and mortality in randomized trials of rehabilitation, a meta-analysis was performed on the combined results of ten clinical trials (Oldridge et al, 1988). All of the trials had to have good documentation of myocardial infarction, randomization of patients, a rehabilitation program lasting at least six weeks, follow up for 24 months or longer and comprehensive documentation of outcome. Data on a total of 4,347 patients were analyzed. The pooled odds ratio of 0.76 (95% confidence interval, 0.63 to 0.92) for all-cause deaths and of 0.75 (95% confidence intervals, 0.62 to 0.93) for cardiovascular death were significantly lower for the rehabilitation group than the control group, with no significant difference for recurrent myocardial infarction. A similar review, but evaluating a total of 22 randomized trials of rehabilitation after myocardial infarction reached a very similar conclusion (O'Conner, 1989).

Biologic Mechanisms Protecting Against Coronary Heart Disease

A variety of biologic changes or mechanisms have been proposed to explain how physical activity might decrease the development of CHD clinical manifestations or improve the clinical status of patients with CHD (Table 1). Most of these changes either decrease myocardial oxygen demand or increase myocardial oxygen supply and thus decrease the likelihood of myocardial ischemia at rest or during exercise. These mechanisms can be classified as either those that contribute to the maintenance or increase of oxygen supply to the myocardium or those that contribute to a decrease in myocardial work and oxygen demands. Also, it is possible that exercise training enhances the intrinsic mechanical or metabolic functioning of the myocardium or increases its electrical stability. It is these very same mechanisms through which all preventive and therapeutic measures for reducing clinical manifestations of CHD work. The specific data supporting the possible existence of these mechanisms have been extensively reviewed recently (Bouchard, Shephard and Stephens, 1994).

Cardiovascular Risks During Exercise

When someone dies suddenly due to a "heart attack" during vigorous recreational or sporting activities the event receives much more publicity than if the same individual had died while at home or work. Because of this publicity, the percentage of all sudden cardiac deaths

(SCD) that occur during sporting activities in the general population probably is lower than it would seem based on casual observation. However, if an individual has underlying cardiac disease that significantly reduces myocardial perfusion, the increased myocardial oxygen demand imposed by either vigorous static or dynamic exercise can precipitate sudden cardiac arrest or sudden death (Thompson and Mitchell, 1984).

Adults in the general population who participate in vigorous activities such as jogging, long-distance running, cross-country skiing, cycling, or vigorous sports may be at greater risk of SCD during exercise than when not exercising (Siscovick et al, 1984; Thompson et al, 1982; Vuori, Makarainen, and Jaaselainen, 1978). For example, in a study of 133 men who died suddenly of cardiac arrest without known prior heart disease, Siscovick et al. (1984) reported that while the overall risk of cardiac arrest was lower in men performing habitual physical activity, the risk of primary cardiac arrest was transiently increased during vigorous exercise compared to that at other times. Among men who performed vigorous activity very infrequently the risk of cardiac arrest during that activity was 56 times greater (95% confidence limits = 23 to 131) than at other times, but this risk decreased to a factor of S (95% confidence limits = 2 to 14) among men at the highest level of vigorous activity. Based on the circumstances surrounding 2,606 sudden deaths in Finland during one year, Vuori and colleagues (1978) concluded that SCD in connection with sporting activities in the general population are quite rare; instantaneous deaths were even rarer (<1% of all incidences of SCD) and occurred only with coexisting activity. Of the deaths associated with exercise, 73% were caused by acute or chronic ischemic heart disease and most of the subjects had serious cardiovascular risk factors that were known in advance or could have been identified easily.

In adults who have had a recent medical evaluation, the risk for SCD during exercise is extremely small. Gibbons and colleagues (1980) documented only two nonfatal cardiac arrests and no deaths in 374,798 person-hours of vigorous exercise. In a very large experience obtained by Vander and associates (Vander, et al, 1982) from 40 exercise facilities over five years, the fatality rate associated with exercise in the general population was quite low. In 33,726,000 participant-hours of exercise, only 38 fatal cardiovascular complications occurred for a fatality rate of one death every 887,526 hours of participation. This means one could expect one death per year if 3,400 adults were exercising five hours per week each. Also, the mortality

Table 1.

Biological mechanisms by which exercise may contribute to the primary or secondary prevention of coronary heart disease*

Maintain or increase myocardial oxygen supply
Delay progression of coronary atherosclerosis (possible)
Improve lipoprotein profile (increase HDL-C/LDL-C ratio) (probable)
Improve carbohydrate metabolism (increase insulin sensitivity) (probable)
Decrease platelet aggregation and increase fibrinolysis (probable)
Decrease adiposity (usually)
Increase coronary collateral vascularization (unlikely)
Increase epicardial artery diameter by dilitation or remodeling (possible)
Increase coronary blood flow (myocardial perfusion) or distribution (possible)

Decrease myocardial work and oxygen demand
Decrease heart rate at rest and during and submaximal exercise (usually)
Decrease systolic and mean arterial pressure during submaximal exercise (usually) and at rest (possible)
Decrease cardiac output during submaximal exercise (possible)
Decrease circulating plasma catecholamine levels (decrease sympathetic tone) at rest (probable) and at submaximal exercise (usually)

Increase myocardial function
Increase stroke volume at rest and in submaximal and maximal exercise (likely)
Increase ejection fraction at rest and during exercise (likely)
Increase intrinsic myocardial contractility (possible)
Increase myocardial function resulting from decreased "afterload" (probable)
Increase myocardial hypertrophy (probable); but this may not reduce CHD risk

Increase electrical stability of myocardium
Decrease regional ischemia at rest or at submaximal exercise (possible)
Decrease catecholamines in myocardium at rest (possible) and at submaximal exercise (probable)

Increase ventricular fibrillation threshold due to reduction of cyclic AMP (possible)

*Expression of likelihood that effect will occur for an individual participating in endurance type training program for 16 weeks or longer at 65% to 80% of functional capacity for 25 minutes or longer per session (300 kilocalories) for three or more sessions per week ranges from unlikely, possible, likely, probable, to usually.

Abbreviations: **HDL-C** = high density lipoprotein cholesterol **LDL-C** = low-density lipoprotein cholesterol: **CHD** = coronary heart disease; **AMP** = adenosine monophosphate.

---

rate while exercising in this group is about one percent per year, nearly the same as the annual CHD mortality rate for middle-aged men in the United States.

Physical Activity to Promote Cardiovascular Health

Recently a consensus was reached by an expert panel working under the auspices of the Centers for Disease Control and Prevention and the American College of Sports Medicine on a "public health recommendation" for promoting physical activity (Pate et al, 1995). While these recommendations were made on the basis that improvement in overall health of the person was the primary goal, much of the data supporting these recommendations was derived from the favorable relationship between physical activity and improved CHD risk factor status and lower CHD mortality. Thus, these guidelines provide a useful framework for recommending a program of physical activity to promote cardiovascular health. The essence of these recommendations is that all adults will benefit by performing at least 30 minutes of physical activity at a moderate intensity or higher on most days. For maximum cardiovascular benefits, this exercise should be of the endurance or aerobic type using the larger muscles of the legs or trunk including brisk walking, jogging, hiking, cycling, swimming, rowing, aerobic and active social dancing, selected calisthenics, and a variety of active games or sports.

A new twist in these recommendations as compared to those issued previously by various organizations is that the 30 minutes of activity can be achieved by performing short bouts of moderate intensity activity throughout the day in addition to performing a single bout of activity for 30 minutes or longer. These recommendations are not precise on the issue of how long these short bouts of activity need to be to warrant credit as time exercising. My suggestion, until more scientific data are available, is to assign credit to only those bouts of activity that last for five minutes or longer. The activity during these bouts need to be of at least moderate intensity (defined as activity equivalent in intensity to that of brisk walking). These guidelines emphasize that prior guidelines by the President's Council on Physical Fitness and Sports, the American College of Sports Medicine, and the American Heart Association are still valid and that these new recommendations are an attempt to expand the opportunity for adults to exercise for health benefits. These guidelines do not change either the recommended intensity or amount of activity to be performed. Similar guidelines for children and youth were recently published (Sallis, et al, 1994).

Existing scientific data strongly support the value of frequently performed activity of moderate intensity as part of a comprehensive program of heart disease prevention and cardiac rehabilitation. Physical activity and endurance fitness make contributions to decreased risk independent of other established heart disease risk factors and can provide substantial health benefits beyond cardiovascular health (Bouchard, Shephard and Stephens, 1994). Along with stopping smoking, maintaining a physically active lifestyle is one of the least expensive and most productive health behaviors available to the public.

References

Berlin, J.A., Colditz, G.A. (1990). A meta-analysis of physical activity in the prevention of coronary heart disease. *American Journal of Epidemiology*, 132, 612-628.

Blair, S.N., Kohl, H.W., Paffenbarger, R.S., Clark, D.G., Cooper, K.H., Gibbons, L.W (1989). Physical fitness and all-cause mortality: A prospective study in healthy men and women. *Journal of the American Medical Association*, 262, 2395-2399.

Bouchard, C., Shephard, R.J., Stephens, T (Eds.) (1994). *Physical Activity, Fitness and Health. International Proceedings and Consensus Statement.* Champaign, IL: Human Kinetics.

Cassel, J., Heyden, S., Bartel, A.G., et al. (1971). Occupation and physical activity and coronary heart disease. *Archives of Internal Medicine*, 128, 920-926.

Chapman, J.M., Massey, F.J. (1964). The interrelationship of serum cholesterol, hypertension, body weight and risk of coronary disease. *Journal of Chronic Diseases*, 17, 933-941.

Costas, R., Garcia-Palmieri, M.R., Nazario, E., and Sorlie, P. (1978). Relation of lipids, weight and physical activity to incidence of coronary heart disease. *The Puerto Rico Heart Study American Journal of Cardiology*, 42, 653-660.

Ekelund, L.G., Haskell, W.L., Johnson, J.L, Wholey, F.S., Criqui, M.H., Sheps, D.S. (1988) Physical fitness as a prevention of cardiovascular mortality in asymptomatic North American men. *New England Journal of Medicine*, 319, 1379-1384.

Gibbons, L.W., Cooper, K.H., Myer, B., Ellison, C. (1980) The acute cardiac risk of strenuous exercise. *Journal of the American Medical Association*, 244, 1799-1804.

Kahn, H.A. (1963). The relationship of reported coronary heart disease mortality to physical activity of work. *American Journal of Public Health*, 53, 1058-1063.

Karvonen, M.J., Rautaharju, P.M., Orma, E., et al. (1961). Heart disease and employment: Cardiovascular studies on lumberjacks. *Journal of Occupational Medicine*, 3, 49-57.

Lakka, T.A., Venalainen J.M., Rauramaa, R., et al. (1994). Relation of leisure-time activity and cardiorespiratory fitness to the risk of acute myocardial infarction in men. *New England Journal of Medicine*, 330, 1549-1554.

Leon, A.S., Cornett, J., Jacobs, D.R., Rauramaa, R. (1987). Leisure-time physical activity levels and risk of coronary heart disease and death: The multiple risk factor intervention trial. *Journal of the American Medical Association*, 258, 2388-2395.

Morris, J.N., Heady, J.A., Raffle, R.A.B., et al. (1953). Coronary heart disease and physical activity of work. *Lancet*, 1053, 1111-1120.

Morris, J.N., Polland, R., Everitt, M.G., and Chave, S.P.W. (1980). Vigorous exercise in leisure time: Protection against coronary heart disease. *Lancet*, 8206, 1207-1210.

Morris, J.N., Clayton, D.G., Everitt, M.G., Semmence, A.M., Burgess, E.H (1990). Exercise in leisure time: Coronary attack and death rates. *British Heart Journal*, 63, 325- 334.

O'Conner, G.T., Boving, J.E., Yusuf, S. et al. (1989). An overview of randomized trials of rehabilitation with exercise after myocardial infarction. *Circulation,* 80, 234-244.

Oldridge, N.B., Guyatt, G.H., Fisher, M.E., Rimm, A.A. (1988). Cardiac rehabilitation after myocardial infarction: Combined exercise of randomized clinical trials. *Journal of the American Medical Association,* 260, 945-950.

Paffenbarger, R.S., Wing, A.L., Hyde, R.T. (1978). Physical activity as an index of heart attack in college alumni. *American Journal of Epidemiology,* 108, 161-167.

Paffenbarger, R.S., Hyde, R.T., Wing, A.L., Hsieh, C. (1986). Physical activity, all-cause mortality, and longevity of college alumni. *New England Journal of Medicine,* 314, 605-613.

Paffenbarger, R.S., Hyde, R.T, Wing, A.L., Lee, I.M., Jung, D.L., Kampert, J.B. (1993). The association of changes in physical activity level and other lifestyle characteristics with mortality among men. *New England Journal of Medicine,* 328, 538-545.

Pate, R.R., Pratt, M., Blair, S.N., Haskell W.L., et al. (1995). Physical activity and public health: A recommendation from the Centers for Disease Control and Prevention and the American College of Sports Medicine. *Journal of the American Medical Association,* (in press).

Paul, O. (1969). Physical activity and coronary heart disease, Part II. *American Journal of Cardiology.* 23, 303-318.

Powell, K.E., Thompson, P.D., Caspersen, C.J., Kendrech, J.S. (1987). Physical activity and incidence of coronary heart disease. *Annual Review of Public Health,* 8, 253-287.

Rechnitzer, P.A., Cunningham, D.A., Andre, G.M., et al. (1983). Relation of exercise to the recurrence rate of myocardial infarction in men. *American Journal of Cardiology,* 51:65-69.

Rose, G. (1969). Physical activity and coronary heart disease. *Proceedings of the Royal Society of Medicine.* 62, 1183-1187.

Sallis, J.F. (Editor) (1994). Physical activity guidelines for adolescents. *Pediatric Exercise Science,* 6, 299-465.

Salonen, J.T., Puska, P., and Tuomilehto, J. (1982). Physical activity and risk of myocardial infarction, cerebral stroke and death: A longitudinal study in Eastern Finland. *American Journal of Epidemiology,* 115, 526-537.

Sandvick, L., Erikssen, J., Thaulow, E., et al. (1993). Physical fitness as a predictor of mortality among healthy middle-aged Norwegian men. *New England Journal of Medicine,* 328, 533-537.

Shaper, A.G., Wannamethee, G. (1991). Physical activity and ischemic heart disease in middle-aged British men. *British Heart Journal,* 66, 384-394.

Shapiro, S., Weinblatt, E., Frank, C.W., and Sager, R.V. (1969). Incidence of coronary heart disease in a population insured for medical care (HIP). *American Journal of Public Health* (Suppl.), 59, 1-101.

Shaw, L. (1981). Effects of a prescribed supervised exercise program on mortality and cardiovascular morbidity in patients after myocardial infarction. *American Journal of Cardiology,* 48, 39-48.

Siscovick, D.S., Weiss, N.S., Fletcher, R.H., Lasky, T. (1984). The incidence of primary cardiac arrest during vigorous exercise. *New England Journal of Medicine,* 311, 874-877.

Sobolski, J., Kornitzer, M., De Backer, G. (1987). Protection against ischemic heart disease in the Belgian Physical Fitness Study: Physical fitness rather than physical activity. *American Journal of Epidemiology,* 125, 601-610.

Taylor, H.L., Blackburn, H., Keys, A., Parlin, R.W., Vasquez, C., Pucher, T. (1970). Five-year follow-up of employees of selected U.S. railroad companies. *Circulation,* 41 (Suppl. 1), 20-39.

Thompson, P., Funk, E., Carleton, R., and Sturner, W. (1982). Incidence of death during jogging in Rhode Island from 1975 through 1980. *Journal of the American Medical Association,* 247, 2535-2538.

Thompson, P.D., Mitchell, J.H. (1984). Exercise and sudden cardiac death. Protection or provocation? *New England Journal of Medicine,* 311, 914-915.

Vander, L., Franklin, B., and Rubenfire, M. (1982). Cardiovascular complications of recreational physical activity. *The Physician and Sports Medicine*, 10, 89-95.

Vuori, I., Makarainen, M., and Jaaselainen, A. (1978). Sudden death and physical activity. *Cardiology*, 63, 287-304.

Wilhelmsen, L., Sanne, H., Elmfeldt, D., et al. (1975). A controlled trial of physical training after myocardial infarction: Effects on risk factors, nonfatal reinfarction and death. *Preventive Medicine*, 4, 491-508.

Chapter 41

Physical Activity and Cancer

Introduction

Cancer is the second leading cause of death, after heart disease, in the United States today (Boring et al., 1994). In 1994, the American Cancer Society estimated that 540,000 Americans died from cancer, while 1,210,000 new cases of this disease occurred that same year (Boring et al., 1994).

Two of the important avoidable causes of cancer are cigarette smoking and alcohol consumption. If we totally eliminated these two factors, perhaps one-third of all cancers might be avoided (Doll & Peto, 1981). In the search for other modifiable aspects of human behavior that potentially may reduce risk of developing cancer, physical activity emerges as a promising candidate. Higher levels of exercise have been shown to be associated with numerous health benefits, including decreased incidence of coronary heart disease (Berlin & Colditz, 1990), hypertension (Hagberg, 1990), non-insulin-dependent diabetes mellitus (Helmrich et al., 1991) and increased longevity (Paffenbarger et al., 1993). Is there also an association between physical activity and reduced rates of cancer occurrence? This hypothesis—that exercise can reduce cancer risk—is not new; in fact, in the early twentieth century, Cherry (1922) observed that men involved in physically active occupations experienced lower cancer mortality rates than their fellow men engaged in less strenuous jobs.

Physical Activity and Fitness Research Digest, Series 2, No. 2, June, 1995.

In this review, we first will discuss potential biologic mechanisms whereby exercise might be expected to reduce cancer risk, then proceed to explore the epidemiologic data on the relation between physical activity and cancer of various sites.

Potential Biologic Mechanisms Underlying an Exercise-Cancer Association

Among the many complex functions of the human immune system is the regulation of susceptibility to cancer. Thus, if exercise can enhance the immune system, it is plausible for physical activity to reduce cancer risk.

As far back as 1902, investigators observed that vigorous exercise (i.e., running a marathon) could influence certain components of the immune system (Larrabee, 1902). Today, investigators have attempted to study the effects of exercise on the immune system in several ways. Markers of immune function examined have included susceptibility to upper respiratory infections and the function of cells (e.g., cells of the monocyte-macrophage system and natural killer or NK cells) that serve as the body's first line of defense against the development and spread of cancer (Mackinnon, 1989; Roitt et al., 1989; Shephard, 1991). Upper respiratory infections have been studied because the human immune system also is responsible for regulating susceptibility to infection.

Available evidence suggests that increasing levels of physical activity, up to a certain point, enhance the immune function; beyond this, immune system function appears instead to decrease (Nieman, 1994; Pedersen & Ullum, 1994; Woods & Davis, 1994). What this cut-point is remains unclear. Moderate amounts of physical activity (e.g., brisk walking) have been shown to reduce risk of upper respiratory infection (Nieman, 1994), as well as enhance the function of cells of the monocyte-macrophage system (Woods & Davis, 1994) and NK cells (Pedersen & Ullum, 1994). At more intense levels of exercise, however, immune suppression appears to occur instead. For example, following marathon type races, runners appear to have increased rates of upper respiratory tract infections for a one to two week period (Nieman, 1994). Also, elite athletes (e.g., cyclists) have increased NK cell activity at rest, but depressed function following intense activity (Pedersen & Ullum, 1994).

To summarize, then, it appears plausible for exercise—at least, in moderate amounts—to reduce cancer risk by enhancing the function of the human immune system.

Physical Activity and Reduced Cancer Risk: Potential Biologic Mechanisms

Cancer Type	Potential Mechanisms
• Most cancer types	• Enhanced immune system
• Colon cancer	• Shortened intestinal transit time • Decreased body fat
• Breast cancer	• Hormone level changes • Decreased body fat
• Prostate cancer	• Hormone level changes

For site-specific cancers, other mechanisms may operate. With colon cancer, it has long been postulated that a shortened intestinal transit time may reduce cancer incidence by decreasing the amount of contact between potential carcinogens, co-carcinogens or promoters in the fecal stream and colonic mucosa (Burkitt et al., 1971; 1972). Thus, if exercise can reduce transit time within the colon, risk of this cancer may be decreased. However, whether exercise does or does not reduce transit time within the intestine is unclear. Several investigators have shown that exercise does indeed decrease transit time (Holdstock et al., 1970; Cordain et al., 1986; Oettlé, 1991); others have not (Bingham & Cummings, 1989; Lampe et al., 1991; Coenen et al., 1992). Apart from the methodologic limitations of these studies, it is possible that the inconsistent findings resulted because exercise may shorten transit time within certain segments of the gut without affecting total (i.e., oral-anal) transit time (Lupton & Meacher, 1988).

Turning to cancers of the reproductive system, various hormones are necessary for their development. Thus, if exercise can alter the levels of these hormones, this represents another plausible mechanism for physical activity to decrease cancer risk. In females, estrogen, as well as the combination of estrogen and progesterone, stimulate cell proliferation in the breast and so have been implicated in the development of breast cancer (Henderson et al, 1993). Studies of female athletes have shown that training can lower estrogen and progesterone levels (Shangold 1984). Further, in young girls, strenuous training also can delay the onset of menarche (Warren, 1980), thus, reducing a woman's total lifetime exposure to these hormones. In males, testosterone appears to be important in the development of prostate cancer (Gittes, 1991). Strenuous exercise may lower basal testosterone levels, potentially reducing risk of this cancer (Lee et al., 1992).

Finally, exercise may influence cancer risk via its effect on decreasing body weight and reducing body fat. For certain cancers such as colon cancer (Lew & Garfinkel, 1979) and breast cancer (Kelsey & Gammon, 1991), obesity is associated with increased risk.

Physical Activity and Colon Cancer

Of the various site-specific cancers, colon cancer has been the most commonly studied cancer. The first detailed epidemiologic study was conducted by Garabrant et al. (1984). They examined the occupation of men, aged 20-64 years, who had developed colon cancer. Based on the estimated amount of physical activity required on the job, men were classified as sedentary, moderately active or highly active. Investigators also examined occupational data among similarly aged men with cancers other than colon cancer. Using this comparison, investigators reported that sedentary men had a 1.6 times the risk of developing colon cancer. when compared with highly active men.

It could be argued that the increased risk observed by Garabrant et al. may have been due to higher consumption of fat in the diet among sedentary men, since dietary fat is associated with increased colon cancer risk (Willett et al., 1990). However, another study by Slattery et al., conducted in Utah, did take into account differences in dietary patterns, as well as differences in body weight (1988). When investigators compared the occupational and leisure-time activities of men and women with colon cancer against the activity patterns of a random sample of the population without this disease, they also found sedentary individuals to be at increased risk. The magnitude of this increased risk was approximately two-fold.

In their study of over 17,000 men, followed for up to 26 years, Lee et al. observed that physical activity, assessed at one point in time, did not predict risk of subsequent colon cancer (1991). However, men who were sedentary (expending < 1,000 kcal/week) at two time points, separated by 11 to 15 years, had twice the risk of those active (expending >2,500 kcal/week) at both times. This led investigators to postulate that for physical activity to protect against colon cancer, it may be necessary for the activity to be sustained over time. Investigators also put forward an alternate hypothesis: In this study, men were asked, on questionnaires, how much walking and stair climbing they did, the kinds of leisure-time sports and recreational activities they engaged in and the frequency and time spent on these activities. Investigators then calculating the energy expenditure for each subject, based on these data. Thus, two assessments of physical activity may have increased the precision of activity measurement, and allowed investigators to better distinguish between the sedentary and the active men.

To date, 33 publications on the relation between physical activity and colon cancer have resulted (reviewed in Lee, 1994; Markowitz et al., 1992; Vetter et al., 1992; Arbman et al., 1993; Chow et al., 1993; Dosemeci et al., 1993; Fraser & Pearce, 1993; Vineis et al., 1993). The majority—25 publications—have shown that individuals who exercise have a lower incidence of colon cancer than their sedentary counterparts. This relation has been described in the United States, Europe, the Far East and Australia. The magnitude of increased risk experienced by sedentary persons has been reported to be 1.2 to 3.6 times, with most studies describing the magnitude of increased risk to be between one-and-a-half to two-fold. From currently available data, it is unclear whether a gradient relation, i.e., increasing protection with increasing activity, exists (Lee, 1994).

Physical Activity and Rectal Cancer

Many of the studies of colon cancer above also examined rectal cancer (reviewed in Lee, 1994). In contrast to colon cancer, most studies in which rectal cancer was studied separately (as opposed to those that grouped colorectal cancers into a single category) found no significant relation between increased physical activity and risk of this cancer. Where colorectal cancer was studied as a single entity, investigators tended to report a protective effect of physical activity, perhaps reflecting the relation with colon cancer instead.

Physical Activity and Breast Cancer

While it is attractive to postulate that exercise can decrease risk of breast cancer as few modifiable risk factors for this cancer exist, available data do not consistently support this hypothesis. Frisch, et al. first described an inverse relation between physical activity and breast cancer in 1985. They contacted 5,398 surviving alumnae of the classes of 1925-1981 from 10 colleges or universities by questionnaire and asked them to report whether they had developed breast cancer. These women represented 2,622 former athletes from the institutions and a random sample of non-athletes. A total of 69 breast cancers had developed among these surviving alumnae. When investigators compared the prevalence of breast cancer among athletes with non-athletes, they found that the latter had 1.9 times the risk of the former, after taking into account differences in reproductive characteristics between the two groups.

Subsequent studies did not consistently reproduce this findings (reviewed in Lee, 1994; Pukkala et al., 1993; Zheng et al., 1993; Bernstein et al., 1994; Dorgan et al., 1994). Of eight other publications, three described an inverse relation between physical activity and breast cancer risk, four, no relation and one, a suggestion of a direct association, i.e. risk increased with increasing physical activity.

This last publication used data from the Framingham Heart Study, a study ongoing since 1948 (Dorgan et al., 1994). Subjects in this study are brought in every two years to be examined. In this analysis of physical activity and breast cancer, 2,307 women reported their physical activity to physicians in 1954-1956. They then were followed for the development of breast cancer until 1984. A total of 117 women were diagnosed with breast cancer during follow-up. Investigators divided women into quartiles, based on their level of physical activity. They found that women in the highest quartile of physical activity had 1.6 times the breast cancer risk of those in the least active quartile, and this finding was of borderline statistical significance.

Most recently, Bernstein et al. (1994) hypothesized that the timing of physical activity is pertinent with respect to risk for breast cancer. They studied 545 women, aged 40 years or younger, with breast cancer, and compared their physical activity patterns to those of 545 women without breast cancer, who were from the same neighborhood and of the same age, race and parity. Investigators divided subjects into five categories, depending on the number of hours per week that a woman spent in physical activity, after she had reached menarche. Women who did not spend any time in physical activity had 2.4 times the breast cancer risk of their colleagues who exercised for 23.8 hours per week. There was a strong gradient of increasing risk with decreasing hours of physical activity. Investigators did take into account differences in reproductive history, use of oral contraceptives, a family history of breast cancer and obesity in their analysis. The protective effect of physical activity during young adulthood appeared stronger for women having borne children than for women never having borne children.

Physical Activity and Prostate Cancer

As with breast cancer, the epidemiologic data do not consistently support an association between physical activity and risk of this cancer, even though a plausible hypothesis has been put forward to explain the biologic basis for an inverse association (Lee et al., 1992). Of 10 epidemiologic studies on this topic, five observed inverse relations between physical activity and risk of this cancer (reviewed in Lee, 1994). For example, Lee et al. (1992) followed 17,719 men, initially aged 30-79 years, for up to 26 years for the development of prostate cancer. For men aged >70 years, those who expended <1,000 kcal/week in walking, climbing stairs and leisure-time sports and recreational activities had 1.9 times the risk of their more active colleagues who expended >4,000 kcal/week. For younger men, there was no significant association between level of exercise and risk of this cancer.

Another three studies found significant direct associations between level of physical activity and prostate cancer risk. That is, these studies observed risk of this cancer to increase with increasing levels of physical activity. For example, Le Marchand et al. (1991) examined the lifetime occupational physical activity of 452 Hawaiian men with prostate cancer and compared this with the lifetime occupational activity of 899 men without such cancer. Men were classified into five categories of activity, depending on the proportion of their life that they had spent in sedentary jobs or jobs involving only light work. Among men aged 270 years, the most sedentary fifth of men had only half the risk of prostate cancer of the least sedentary fifth of men. There also was a gradient relation, with risk decreasing as sedentariness increased. For men aged younger than 70 years old, no clear pattern emerged.

Two other indices of lifetime occupational activity also were created: the proportion of life spent in moderately active jobs and the proportion of life spent in heavy or very heavy work. Neither of these two indices were significantly related to prostate cancer risk. The remaining two studies reported no significant relation between the amount of exercise in men and risk of prostate cancer.

Physical Activity and Other Site-Specific Cancers

Because of the potential for physical activity to influence levels of reproductive hormones, investigators have postulated that active individuals may experience lower risks of other reproductive cancers, in addition to breast and prostate cancers. In their study of college alumnae, Frisch et al. (1985) also examined the relation between college athleticism and all reproductive cancers (i.e., cancers of the breast, uterus, cervix, vagina and ovary). Women who had been non-athletes had 2.5 times the risk of these cancers, compared with women who had been college athletes. In another study conducted in Italy and Switzerland, the most sedentary women, based on self-reported physical activity, had 2.4 to 8.6 times the risk (for physical activity at different ages) of endometrial cancer, compared with the most active women (Levi et al., 1993). However, a study from China did not find risk of cancers of the corpus uteri or ovary to differ between women who were inactive or active on the job (Zheng et al., 1993).

Meanwhile, among men, investigators from the United Kingdom have reported that physical activity is inversely related to risk of testicular cancer in those aged 15-49 years. Men who did not exercise experienced a doubling of risk of this cancer, compared with those who spent 215 hours a week in exercise (United Kingdom Testicular Cancer Study Group, 1994). Using a different measure of physical activity, men who spent 210 hours a day sitting had 1.7 times the risk of testicular cancer of those who spent only 0-2 hours sitting.

Other site-specific cancers that have been studied in relation to physical activity include lung and pancreatic cancers (reviewed in Lee, 1994). Currently, the data are insufficient to conclude whether any association exists. For the remaining site-specific cancers, the data have been even more sparse (reviewed in Lee, 1994).

Physical Activity and Patients with Cancer

There is little information on whether patients who already have developed cancer do or do not benefit from physical activity. In animal experiments, investigators found that among tumor-bearing rats which were allowed to feed freely, those rats allowed to exercise spontaneously experienced delayed onset of appetite loss when compared with non-exercised rats (Daneryd et al., 1990). In addition, exercised animals were found to have reduced tumor weights. In humans, exercise has a mood elevating affect and, thus, may improve the quality of life of cancer patients. In a study of 24 women with breast cancer, investigators developed a moderate exercise program for each patient and followed women for six months (Peters et al., 1994). After five weeks, but not at six months, satisfaction with life was significantly enhanced when compared with baseline attitude. Investigators postulated that this may have been due to decreased adherence to the exercise protocol between five weeks and six months. Further, at the end of the six months, these women were found to have increased NK cell activity at rest compared with baseline NK cell activity, indicating enhancement of this aspect of the immune system.

Summary

Exercise has been shown to be inversely related to risk of developing a whole host of chronic diseases in humans, including coronary heart disease, hypertension and non-insulin-dependent diabetes mellitus. Over the last decade, there has been accumulating epidemiologic data suggesting that exercise also may decrease risk of cancer, in particular, colon cancer. However, exercise appears to be unrelated to rectal cancer risk. With regard to other cancers, because physical activity can alter levels of reproductive hormones, investigators have hypothesized that active individuals should experience decreased incidence of breast or prostate cancer. However, the epidemiologic data do not consistently support this hypothesis. Data on other site-specific cancers have been sparse. Finally, preliminary data suggest that exercise also may be beneficial for cancer patients by improving the quality of life and enhancing immune function; while promising, this needs more careful research.

References

Arbman, G., Axelson, O., Fredriksson, M, Nilsson, E., Sjîdahl, R. (1993). Do occupational factors influence the risk of colon and rectal cancer in different ways? *Cancer,* 72: 2543-2549.

Berlin, J.A., Colditz, G.A. (1990). A meta-analysis of physical activity in the prevention of coronary heart disease. *American Journal of Epidemiology,* 132: 612-28.

Bernstein, L., Henderson, B.E., Hanisch, R., Sullivan-Halley, J., Ross, R.K. (1994). Physical exercise and reduced risk of breast cancer in young women. *Journal of the National Cancer Institute,* 86: 1403-1408.

Bingham, S.A., Cummings, J.H. (1989). Effect of exercise and physical fitness on large intestinal function. *Gastroenterology,* 97: 1389-1399.

Blot, W.J. (1993). Physical activity and occupational risk of colon cancer in Shanghai, China. *International Journal of Epidemiology,* 22: 23-29.

Boring, C.C., Squires, T.S., Tong, T., Montgomery, S. (1994). Cancer statistics 1994. *CA,* 44: 7-26.

Burkitt, D.P. (1971). Epidemiology of cancer of the colon and rectum. *Cancer,* 28: 3-13.

Burkitt, D.P., Walker, A.R.P., Palmer, N.S. (1972). Effect of dietary fibre on stools and transit-times, and the role in the causation of disease. *Lancet,* ii: 1408-1411.

Cherry, T. (1922). A theory of cancer. *Medical Journal of Australia,* 1: 425-438.

Chow, W-H., Dosemeci, M. Aheng, W., Vetter, R., McLaughlin, J.K., Gao, Y-T.

Coenen, C., Wegener, M., Wedmann, B., Schmidt, G., Hoffmann, S. (1992). Does physical exercise influence bowel transit time in healthy young men? *American Journal of Gastroenterology,* 87: 292-295.

Cordain, L., Latin, R.W., Behnke, J.J. (1986). The effects of an aerobic running program on bowel transit time. *Journal of Sports Medicine,* 26: 101-104.

Daneryd, P.L.E., Hafstrim, L.R., Karlber, I.H (1990). Effects of spontaneous physical exercise on experimental cancer anorexia and cachexia. *European Journal of Cancer,* 10: 1083-1088.

Doll, R., Peto, R. (1981). *The Causes of Cancer: A Quantitative Estimates of the Avoidable Risks of Cancer in the United States Today* (pp. 1220-1256). New York: Oxford University Press.

Dorgan, J.F., Brown, C., Barrett, M., Splansky, G.L., Kreger, B.E., D'Agostino, R.B., Albanes, D., Schatzkin, A. (1994). Physical activity and risk of breast cancer in the Framingham Heart Study. *American Journal of Epidemiology,* 139: 662-669.

Dosemeci, M., Hayes, R.B., Vetter, R., Hoover, R.N., Tucker, M., Engin, K., Unsal, M., Blair, A. (1993). Occupational physical activity, socioeconomic status, and risks of 15 cancer sites in Turkey. *Cancer Causes and Control,* 4: 313-321.

Fraser, G., Pearce, N. (1993). Occupational physical activity and risk of cancer of the colon and rectum in new Zealand males. *Cancer Causes and Control,* 4: 45-50.

Frisch, R.E., Wyshak, G., Albright, N.L., Albright, T.E., Schiff, I., Jones, K.P., Witschi, J., Shiang, E., Koff, E., Marguglio, M. (1985). Lower prevalence of breast cancer and cancers of the reproductive system among former college athletes compared to non-athletes. *British Journal of Cancer,* 52: 885-891.

Garabrant, D.H., Peter, J.M., Mack, T.M., Bernstein, L. (1984). Job activity and colon cancer risk. *American Journal of Epidemiology,* 119: 1105-1014.

Gittes, R.F. (1991). Carcinoma of the prostate. *New England Journal of Medicine,* 324: 236-24.

Hagberg, J.M. (1990). Exercise, fitness, and hypertension. In: Bouchard, C., Shephard, R.J., Stephens, t., Sutton, J.R., McPherson, B.D., (eds.). *Exercise, Fitness, and Health: A consensus of Current Knowledge* (pp. 455-466). Champaign, Ill.: Human Kinetics Publishers.

Helmrich, S.P., Ragland, D.R., Leung, R.W., Paffenbarger, R.S., Jr. (1991). Physical activity and reduced occurrences of non-insulin-dependent diabetes mellitus. *New England Journal of Medicine,* 147-152.

Henderson, B.E., Ross, R.K., Pike, M.C. (1993). Hormonal chemoprevention of cancer in women. *Science,* 259: 633-638.

Holdstock, D.J., Misiewicz, J.J., Smith, T., Rowlands, E.N. (1970). Propulsion (mass movements) in the human colon and its relationship to meals and somatic activity. *Gut,* 11: 91-99.

Kelsey, J.L., Gammon, M.D. (1991). The epidemiology of breast cancer. *CA,* 41: 146-165.

Lampe, J.W., Slavin, J.L., Apple, F.S. (1991). Iron status of active women and the effect of running a marathon on bowel function and gastrointestinal blood loss. *International Journal of Sports Medicine,* 12: 173-179.

Larrabee. R.C. (1902). Leukocytosis after violent exercise. *Journal of Medical Research,* 7: 76-82.

Lee, I-M. (1994). Physical activity, fitness and cancer (pp. 814-831). In: Bouchard, C., Shephard, R.J., Stephens, T. (eds.). *Physical Activity, Fitness, and Health: International Proceedings and Consensus Statement.* Champaign, Ill.: Human Kinetics, Publishers.

Lee, I-M., Paffenbarger, R.S. Jr., Hsieh, C-c (1992). Physical activity and risk of prostate cancer among college alumni. *American Journal of Epidemiology,* 135: 169-179.

Lee, I-M., Paffenbarger, R.S. Jr., Hsieh, C-c. (1991). Physical activity and risk of developing colorectal cancer among college alumni. *Journal of the National Cancer Institute,* 83: 1324-1329.

Levi, F., La Vecchia, C., Negri, E., Franceschi, S. (1993). Selected physical activities and risk of endometrial cancer, *British Journal of Cancer,* 67: 846-851.

Lew, E.A., Garfinkel, L. (1979). Variations in mortality by weight among 750,000 men and women. *Journal of Chronic Disease,* 32: 563-576.

Lupton, J.R., Meacher, M.M. (1988). Radiographic analysis of the effect of dietary fibres on rat colonic transit time. *American Journal of Physiology,* 255: G633-639.

Mackinnon, L.T. (1989). Exercise and natural killer cells: What is the relationship? *Sports Medicine,* 7: 141-149.

Markowitz, S., Morabia, A., Garibaldi, K., Wynder, E. (1992). Effect of occupational and recreational activity on the risk of colorectal cancer among males: A case-control study. *International Journal of Epidemiology,* 21: 1057-1062.

Nieman, D.C. (1994). Exercise , upper respiratory infection, and the immune system. *Medicine & Science in Sport & Exercise.* 26: 140-146.

Oettlé, G.J. (1991). Effect of moderate exercise on bowel habit. *Gut,* 32: 941-944.

Paffenbarger, R.S. Jr., Hyde, R.T., Wing, A.L., Lee, I-M., Jung, S.L., Kamper, J.B., (1993), The association of changes in physical activity level and other lifestyle characteristics with mortality among men. *New England Journal of Medicine,* 538-545.

Pedersen, B.K., Ullum, H. (1994). NK cell response to physical activity: Possible mechanisms of action. *Medicine & Science in Sports & Exercise,* 26: 140-146.

Peters, C., Litzerich, H., Niemeier, B., SchÅle, K., Uhienbruck, G. (1994). Influence of moderate exercise on natural killer cytotoxicity and personality traits in cancer patients. *Anticancer Research,* 14: 1033-1036.

Pukkala, E., Poskiparta, M., Apter, D., Vihko, V. (1993). Life-long physical activity and cancer risk among Finnish female teachers. *European Journal of Cancer Preview,* 2: 369-376.

Roitt, I.M., Broskoff, J., Male, D.K. (1989). *Immunology,* 2nd. ed. (pp. 18.1-18.17). London: Gower Medical Publishers.

Shangold, M.M. (1984). Exercise and the adult female: Hormonal and endocrine effects. *Exercise and Sport Science Review,* 12: 53-79.

Shephard, R.J. (1991). Physical activity and the immune system. *Canadian Journal of Sports Science,* 16: 169-185.

Slattery, M.L., Schumacher, M.C., Smith, K.R., West, D.W., Abd-Elghany N. (1988). Physical activity, diet and risk of colon cancer in Utah. *American Journal of Epidemiology,* 128: 989-999.

United Kingdom Testicular Cancer Study Group (1994). Aetiology of testicular cancer: Association with congenital abnormalities, age at puberty, infertility, and exercise. *British Medical Journal,* 308: 1393-1399.

Vetter, R., Dosemeci, M., Blair, A., Wacholder, S., Unsal, M., Engin, K., Fraumeni, J.F. Jr. (1992). Occupational physical activity and colon cancer risk in Turkey. *European Journal of Epidemiology,* 8: 845-850.

Vineis, P., Ciccone, G., Magnino, A. (1993). Asbestos exposure, physical activity and colon cancer: A case-control study. *Tumori,* 79: 301-303.

Warren, M.P. (1980). The effects of exercise on pubertal progression and reproductive function in girls. *Journal of Clinical Endocrinology Metabolism,* 51: 1150-1157.

Willett, W.C., Shampfer, M.J., Colditz, G.A., Rosner, B.A., Speizer, F.E. (1991). Relation of meat, fat, and fiber intake to the risk of colon cancer in a prospective study among women. *New England Journal of Medicine,* 323: 1664-1672.

Woods, J.A., Davis, J.M. (1994). Exercise, monocyte/macrophage function, and cancer. *Medicine & Science in Sports & Exercise,* 26: 147-156.

Zheng, W., Shu, X.O., McLaughlin, J.K., Chow, W.H., Gao, Y.T., Blot, W.J. (1993). Occupational physical activity and the incidence of cancer of the breast, corpus uteri and ovary in Shanghai. *Cancer,* 71: 3620-3624.

Chapter 42

Osteoporosis and Physical Activity

Introduction

The National Osteoporosis Foundation (NOF) has defined osteoporosis as a disease characterized by low bone mass and microarchitectural deterioration of bone tissue leading to enhanced bone fragility and a consequent increase in fracture risk. In other words, osteoporosis is the loss of bone tissue that makes bones weaker. It has been projected that over 5 million fractures of the hip, spine, and wrist will occur in women over the age of 45 which will account for more than 45 billion dollars in direct health care costs over the next ten years (Chrischilles, Shireman, & Wallace, 1994). This is a conservative estimate of the future public health impact of osteoporosis, since the projections are based on only three fracture sites and limited to females. No doubt the estimate would be greater if it included men who also are at risk of osteoporosis as they grow older.

In addition to the financial burden attributed to this disease, osteoporosis has a profound effect on the quality of life of older individuals. Those afflicted typically experience reduced mobility, pain, loss of independence, and psychological distress associated with postural disfigurement and the fear of additional fractures. Hip fractures are the most severe fractures since they carry the highest incidence

Physical Activity And Fitness Research Digest, Series 2, No. 3, September, 1995.

of morbidity and mortality. The postural abnormality associated with vertebral fractures results in reduced cardiovascular capacity and affects other internal organs due to compression of the chest and abdominal regions. In order to define effective preventive strategies, it is important to determine the lifestyle factors which influence fracture risk. The two primary determinants of fracture risk are low bone mass and falls.

Physical activity has been proposed as one strategy to reduce fractures by increasing bone mass and by preventing falls through improved functional ability. Although the mechanism by which exercise increases bone mass is not clear, it likely influences bone directly through mechanical forces (loading) transferred to bone. Bone responds to changes in mechanical loading and the regulation of bone strength is a function of the loads to which the skeleton is exposed. The most striking examples of this adaptation are the reports which demonstrate marked bone loss in the absence of weight bearing activity, such as occurs in space travel and prolonged bedrest (Mack, et al., 1967; Nishimura, et al., 1994). Conversely, many reports have shown that bone mass among physically active individuals and athletes is significantly higher compared to their non-active and non-athletic counterparts. Some studies which have imposed significant mechanical forces via exercise intervention report positive effects on bone mass, although the magnitude of effect is much less impressive than would be predicted from studies on athletes and active individuals. Therefore, the ideal exercise program that maximizes bone response remains elusive. Evidence is accumulating to suggest, however, that exercise which increases muscle strength, mass, and power, may provide the best osteogenic stimulus. Activities of this type provide additional skeletal protection in the older adult by preventing falls, which are highly related to the incidence of fractures, particularly at the hip.

This review will serve to present the most recent literature in the field and provide recommendations for exercise design which may aid in fracture prevention. In this review, the terms "bone mass" and "bone mineral density (BMD)" will be used as synonyms.

Physical Activity and Bone Mass

Physical activity transmits loads to the skeleton in two ways: by muscle pull and by gravitational forces from weight bearing activity. It is generally assumed that a high level of activity corresponds to a high level of mechanical loading. However, despite the intensity of muscular activity associated with competitive swimming, studies comparing athletic groups have demonstrated that swimmers generally have BMD values lower than those of non-athletic controls (Taaffe, et al., 1995). Therefore, activities that require full support of body weight (i.e., those that are performed on the feet) are recommended if skeletal response is a desired outcome of exercise participation. Sports with unilateral activity, such as tennis, continue to provide the best representation of the positive effects of exercise on bone in humans (Huddleston, et al., 1980; Kannus, et al., 1994). These studies have demonstrated greater BMD in the dominant playing arm vs the nondominant arm across different age groups. However, most forms of activity are not as easily characterized by such specific, localized loading patterns.

Other indicators that physical activity exerts a positive influence on the skeleton is the finding that certain measures of physical fitness are correlated with BMD. Specifically, body composition and muscular strength exhibit positive associations with bone mass. Investigations of BMD and body composition have arisen out of the common finding that body weight is associated with bone density. Research has attempted to specify which aspect of body composition, lean (muscle) or fat mass, is the best predictor of bone mass. Muscle directly attaches to bone and may influence the skeletal system via this mechanism, while fat mass contributes to body weight in a nonspecific manner. It has been proposed that fat mass has the potential to increase circulating levels of estrogen, although this explanation for its beneficial influence on bone has yet to be established. Associations between both fat and lean mass and BMD have been demonstrated (Reid, Plank, & Evans, 1992; Sowers, et al., 1992). Although fat mass has been associated with bone and can provide cushioning in the fall-prone elderly, there are known health problems associated with excess body fat (e.g., cardiovascular disease, type II diabetes). On the other hand, adequate muscle mass is necessary for optimal function throughout the lifespan and muscular atrophy that accompanies the aging process is associated with falling and fracture. Therefore it is prudent to recommend that a fracture prevention program include activities that encourage muscle mass development.

Mechanical forces are directly applied to bone by muscular attachments and individuals with high muscle strength are able to generate large forces during contraction. Thus, muscle strength is a measure of physical fitness which has been studied with respect to skeletal health. Research has shown that the relationship between muscle strength and bone demonstrates site-specificity. Strength of the hip muscles has been related to hip BMD, and grip strength has been associated with forearm BMD (Snow-Harter, et al., 1993; Snow-Harter, et al., 1990). The contribution of muscle strength to BMD in various cross-sectional studies has ranged from 9 to 38% in nonathletic adults. Since approximately 60-80% of bone mass is estimated to be genetically determined, the relationship between muscle strength and bone is not trivial and again points to the importance of the muscular system with respect to bone health.

Research has demonstrated that male and female athletes who participate in sports that require muscular strength and power (e.g., weight lifting, gymnastics, wrestling) exhibit higher bone mass than those whose sports involve primarily muscular endurance (e.g., distance running, triathlon) (Robinson, et al., 1995). Information on the loading characteristics of various activities suggests that walking and slow running provide loads equal to or slightly higher than body weight alone at the spine. In comparison, forces at the spine have been estimated to be 5 to 6 times body weight while weight lifting (Granhad, Jonson, & Hansson, 1987). Jumping associated with gymnastics training may elicit forces as high as 10 to 12 times body weight.

The research on athletes and the size of the load for a specific sport suggests that the skeleton's response to mechanical loading depends on the magnitude of the force. In practical terms, the skeleton must encounter forces that are greater than those it experiences on a day-to-day basis Even though walking is a weight-bearing activity, its ability to evoke a skeletal response is limited to the older adult who was previously bedridden and unable to ambulate for a period of time. On the other hand, one who performs activities of daily living without assistance will be in a weight bearing posture much of the day. For this person, walking as an exercise will not exceed the loading threshold of daily activities and therefore will not improve bone mass.

Exercise intervention studies have attempted to introduce various exercise programs in humans to determine the best exercise prescription for bone health. The results of these studies are equivocal. While some reports indicate that BMD increases slightly with exercise, some report no change or slight decreases. In order to detect changes in bone mass, an intervention must be several months in duration, depending on the age group and type of program (6 months minimum). Relative to other exercise interventions, these are long time intervals (e.g., muscular strength increases can be observed in 8 weeks). Over the life span, however, these time intervals are relatively short. This may be one reason why remarkable changes have not been observed within the time frame of training studies. In addition, the expected magnitude of skeletal response is much less than that observed in the muscular system. To illustrate, muscular strength improvements on the order of 50-100% during the course of a resistance training program are not unusual, especially if initial values were low. A 1.5% increase in bone mass over a period of 9 months is meaningful, since average rates of loss are approximately 0.5-1% per year. To date, most exercise studies have not designed their exercise training programs according to the principles of training. This may be the main reason why many studies have observed minimal or no training effects on the skeleton (Drinkwater, 1994). The application of these principles to bone loading is outlined in Table 1.

Table 1. Principles of Training

Specificity
The impact of the training should be at the bone site of interest since loading seems to have a localized effect.

Overload
The training stimulus must include forces much greater than that afforded by habitual activity.

Reversibility
In the absence of the training stimulus, the positive effect on bone will be lost.

Initial Values
Indiviuals with low BMD will have the greatest potential to gain from increased mechanical loading.

Diminishing Returns
Each individual's biological ceiling determines the extent of adaptation to the training.

Prevention Strategies Throughout the Lifespan

Bone is a dynamic tissue that is constantly undergoing remodeling activity, a function of bone cells, during which old bone is removed and new bone is formed. The factors which determine the level of bone cell activity are mechanical loading, calcium intake, and reproductive hormones. Strategies to decrease risk for osteoporotic fracture should take these factors into consideration throughout the lifespan since bone mass in the older adult is a product of the amount of bone acquired during growth and subsequent rates of loss during adulthood.

Physical activity has been shown to be an important contributor to bone mass in children prior to adolescence (Slemenda, et al., 1991). In addition, this group should have adequate calcium intake so that the necessary blocks for building bone mineral are present during growth. It has been proposed that young bone may be more responsive to mechanical loading than old bone (Forwood & Burr, 1993). Given that approximately 60% of the final skeleton is acquired during adolescence, one preventive strategy is to maximize skeletal loading during this rapid phase of growth. It is also important to consider reproductive endocrine status at this time of life. The negative effects of abnormally low estrogen on BMD in amenorrheic women with a high volume of physical training and very low body weight (primarily distance running and ballet dancing) are well documented (Drinkwater, et al., 1984). These effects are even more dramatic in amenorrheic women with anorexia nervosa. Although there is little if any documentation in men, abnormally low testosterone levels are theoretically detrimental for bone.

Preventive strategies in adults are generally aimed at maintaining bone mass or reducing the rate of loss. However, recent studies on young adult women indicate that physical activity may play an important role with respect to the capacity to increase bone mass after growth has stopped (Recker, et al., 1992; Bassey & Ramsdale, 1994). Recker and colleagues observed increases in spine BMD over a period of 5 years in a large group of women in their twenties. The increases were related to self-selected physical activity patterns. Bassey and Ramsdale (1994) administered high and low impact exercise programs to young women for 6 months and observed BMD increases at the hip in the high impact group only. The authors note that small improvements in bone mass in young to middle adulthood may result in quite significant reductions in risk for osteoporotic fracture in later years. It is important to note that BMD increases with physical activity are likely to be most dramatic in young adulthood when bone appears to be more responsive to mechanical loading. In addition, loading characteristics must be substantial, as demonstrated by the high impact activity administered by Bassey and Ramsdale (1994) which included jumping. Adequate calcium intake and maintenance of normal circulating levels of reproductive hormones are still important factors for optimal bone health in adulthood. However, since growth has ceased, recommendations for calcium intake are slightly lower than in adolescence.

Older adults face multiple challenges with advancing age. Age-related reductions in bone mass, muscle strength and power, and postural stability make this group at highest risk for fracture. Impaired musculoskeletal function and dynamic balance associated with aging and disuse ultimately result in decreased mobility. In addition, these declines in musculoskeletal function have been associated with an increase in falls and incidence of hip fracture. Vandervoort, et al. (1990) report that once function has declined to the point where mobility is significantly reduced, older individuals may refuse to ambulate due to a fear of falling, which is the beginning of a downward spiral which ultimately results in loss of independence. This situation, in which very few physical attempts are made, leads to marked reductions in strength and power of the lower extremities which have specifically been linked to fall risk. Although bone mass is a major risk factor for osteoporosis, falls and their severity are highly related to fractures in the elderly. In fact, 90% of all hip fractures occur with a fall (Melton, 1993).

Falls are caused by many different factors. Epidemiological research has consistently found that lower limb strength, reaction time, sensory impairment, and postural instability are important risk factors for falls. Greenspan, et al. (1994) have proposed that not all falls are potentially injurious and that fall severity in combination with bone mass at the hip are the two primary determinants of hip fracture in ambulatory elderly. Specifically, those who fall to the side and have no ability to alter fall direction or speed of impact and land directly on the hip, are more likely to fracture, particularly if BMD at that site is low (Hayes, et al., 1993). The link of muscular strength and power to fall risk is most logically in the stabilization and control required for voluntary movements as well as for the ability to recover from a stumble. One study determined that leg extensor (quadriceps) power in older men and women was the best predictor of functional performance (Bassey, et al., 1992).

Strategles to prevent fracture in older adults must target bone mass as well as factors associated with falls. Several studies have observed beneficial effects of weight training in older populations including increased bone mass, muscular strength, power, dynamic balance, and functional independence. Thus, this may be the best choice of exercise training at this stage in the lifespan. Most research has focused on machine-based training (e.g., Universal Gym, Nautilus), which requires a seated posture for lower body exercises. While this isolates muscle groups in the legs, it effectively reduces loads at the hip and does not require postural control and balance. To encourage optimal function in a standing posture, older adults should be encouraged to perform exercises such as stepping and rising from a chair. These exercises target muscle groups and actions which are important for everyday function. While it may seem dangerous for older adults to engage in this type of training, resistance training has proven successful in nursing home residents, even among quite old adults. The benefits of participation clearly outweigh the risks of immobility, decreased function and increased likelihood of falls and fracture.

Assessing Your Risk for Osteoporosis

For each of the following questions, check either yes or no.

		Yes	No
1.	Do you have a family history of osteoporosis? (Have any of your relatives broken a wrist or hip or had a dowager's hump?)	___	___
2.	Did you go through menopause or have your ovaries removed by surgery before age 50?	___	___
3.	Did your menstrual periods ever stop for more than a year for reasons other than pregnancy or nursing?	___	___
4.	Did your ancestors come from England, Ireland, Scotland, Northern Europe, or Asia, or do you have a small, thin body frame?	___	___
5.	Have you had surgery in which a part of your stomach or intestines was removed?	___	___
6.	Are you taking or have you taken drugs like cortisone, steroids, or anticonvulsants over a prolonged period?	___	___

7. Do you have a thyroid or parathyroid disorder (hyper-   ___ ___
    thyroidism or hyper parathyroidism)?

8. Are you allergic to milk products or are you lactose   ___ ___
    intolerant?

9. Do you smoke cigarettes?   ___ ___

10. Do you drink wine, beer, or other alcoholic beverages   ___ ___
    daily?

11. Do you do less than 1 hour of exercising such as aer-   ___ ___
    obics, walking, or jogging per week?

12. Have you ever exercised so strenuously that you had   ___ ___
    irregular periods or no periods at all?

13. Have you ever had an eating disorder (bulimia or ano-   ___ ___
    rexia nervosa)?

If you answered "yes" to many of these questions, you may be at an increased risk for osteoporosis.

From Donatelle, Snow-Harter, Wilcox. *Wellness: Choices for Health and Fitness*,
Brooks Cole Publishing Co., 1995. Published with permission.

Summary and Conclusions

Exercise may benefit the skeleton and reduce osteoporosis and fracture risk in the following ways: 1) increase bone mass up to and
through adolescence which will result in higher BMD levels across
the lifespan; 2) improve and maintain bone density during early adulthood; and, 3) reduce or slow the rate of age-related loss during middle
and older age. In order to have an effect on bone, exercise must be
different from daily activities, that is, an overload must be applied to
the skeleton. It is important to remember that physical activity has
not been shown to offset the transient increase in bone loss resulting
from estrogen deficiency that is observed in the first 5-7 years past
menopause. Although still uncertain, the gap is beginning to narrow
with respect to the types and amount of activities which confer the
best osteogenic stimulus. Participation in activities of high load and
low repetitions which increase muscle strength and power may ulti-

mately prove to be the most beneficial to bone mass. Research to quantify forces from activities that promote strength and power will substantiate these predictions and the models should be evaluated in populations at different stages of skeletal development.

The importance of building lower extremity strength and cardiovascular health cannot be overemphasized with respect to fall prevention and general health. Low bone mass is a primary risk factor for fractures, with 90% of hip fractures occurring as the result of a tall. Perhaps the most significant benefit of participation in exercise relates to improvements in neuromuscular function. Sound neuromuscular function is essential for both static and dynamic postural stability. The ability to avoid an obstacle, recover from a stumble or alter the direction of a fall may significantly reduce tall severity. (Greenspan, et al., 1994). Muscle mass. strength, and power decline with age, particularly in the lower extremities (Annianson, et al., 1984) and this has been attributed, in part, to a decrease in physical activity. As a result, it is more difficult for the elderly to perform activities of daily living, particularly ambulation Resistance training programs have demonstrated significant improvement in neuromuscular function in the elderly through the tenth decade, which translates to reduced risk of tall-related fractures.

References

Annianson, A.C., Zitterberg, C., Hedberg, C., et al. (1984). Impaired muscle function with aging. *Clin Orthop Rel Res*. 191, 193-210.

Bassey, E.J. and Ramsdale, S.J. (1994). Increase in femoral bone density in young women following high-impact exercise. *Osteoporosis Int*. 4, 72-75

Bassey, E.J., Fiatarone, M.J., Oneill, E.F, et al (1992). Leg extensor power and functional performance in very old men and women. *Clin Sci*. 82, 321-327.

Cavanaugh, D.J. and Cann, C.E. (1988). Brisk walking does not stop bone loss in postmenopausal women. *Bone*. 98, 201-204.

Chrischilles, E., Sherman, T., and Wallace, R.(1994). Cost and health effects of osteoporotic fractures *Bone*, 15, 377-386.

Donatelle, Snow-Harter, Wilcox (1995).*Wellness: Choices for Health and Fitness*, Brooks Cole Publishing Co.

Drinkwater, B.L. (1994). C.H McCloy Research Lecture: Does physical activity play a role in preventing osteoporosis? *Res Q Exerc and Sport*, 65, 197-206.

Drinkwater, B.L., Nilson, K., Chestnut, C.H., Bremner, W J., Shainholtz, S., et al. (1984). Bone mineral content of amenorrheic and eumenorrheic athletes *N Eng J Med*, 311, 277-281.

Forwood, M.R. and Burr, D.B. (1993). Physical activity and bone mass: Exercises in futility? *Bone Mineral*, 21, 89-112.

Granhad, H., Jonson, R., and Hansson, T. (1987). The loads on the lumbar spine during extreme weight lifting. *Spine*, 12, 146-149.

Greenspan, S.L., Meyers, E. R., Maitland, L. A., et al. (1994). Fall severity and bone mineral density as risk factors for hip fracture in ambulatory elderly *JAMA*, 271, 128-133.

Hayes, W.C., Meyers, E.R., Morris, J.N., et al. (1993) Impact near the hip dominates fracture risk in elderly nursing home residents who fall *Calc Tiss Int*, 52, 192-198.

Huddleston, A.L., Rockwell, D., Kulund, D.N., et al. (1980) Bone mass in lifetime tennis players *JAMA*, 244, 1107-1109.

Kannus, P., Haapasalo, H., Sievanen, H., et al. (1994).The site-specific effects of long-term unilateral activity on bone mineral density and content. *Bone*, 15, 279-284.

Mack, P.B., LaChance, P.A.,Vose, G.P., et al. (1967). Bone demineralization of foot and hand of Gemini-Titan IV, Vand VII astronauts during orbital flight. *Am J Roent: Rad Ther Nucl Med*, 100, 503-511.

Melton, L.J. (1993). Hip fractures: A worldwide problem today and tomorrow. *Bone*, 14, S1-S8.

Nishimura, H., Fukuoka, H., Kiriyama, M., et al. (1994). Bone turnover and calcium metabolism during 20 days bed rest in young healthy males and females. *Acta Physiol Scan*, 150, Suppl 616, 27-35.

Recker, R.R., Davies, K.M., Hinders, S.M., et al. (1992). Bone gain in young adult women *JAMA*, 268, 2403-2408.

Reid, I.R., Plank, L.D., and Evans, M.C. (1992). Fat mass is an important determinant of whole body bone density in premenopausal women but not in men. *J Clin Endocrinol Metab*. 75, 779-782.

Robinson, T.L., Snow-Harter, C ,Taaffe, D.R., et al. (1995). Gymnasts exhibit higher bone mass than runners despite similar prevalence of amenorrhea and oligomenorrhea. *J Bone Miner Res*. 10, 26-35.

Slemenda, C.W., Miller, J.Z., Hui, S.L., et al. (1991). Role of physical activity in the development of skeletal mass in children. *J Bone Miner Res*. 6, 1227-1233.

Snow-Harter, C., Bouxsein, M., Lewis, B., et al. (1990). Muscle strength as a predictor of bone mineral density in young women. *J Bone Miner Res*. 5, 589-595.

Snow-Harter, C., Robinson, T, Shaw, J., et al. (1993). Determinants of femoral neck mineral density in pre and postmenopausal women. *Med Sci Sports Exerc*. 25, Suppl S153.

Sowers, M.R., Kshirsagar, A., Crutchfield, M.M., and Updike, S. (1992). Joint influence of fat and lean body composition compartments on femoral bone mineral density in premenopausal women. *Am J Epidemiol*. 136, 257-265.

Taaffe, D.R., Snow-Harter, C., Connolly, D.A., et al. (1995). Differential effects of swimming versus weight bearing activity on bone mineral status of eumenorrheic athletes. *J Bone Miner Res*. 10, 588-593.

Vandervoort, A., Hill, K., Sandrin, M., et al. (1990). Mobility impairment and falling in the elderly. *Phys Ther Can*. 42, 99-107.

Chapter 43

Health Benefits Of Physical Activity During Childhood And Adolescence

Introduction

The beneficial effects to health of enhanced physical activity (PA) during adult years are numerous. There is mounting evidence that such benefits include a reduction in morbidity and mortality from diseases of several body systems (Bouchard et al., 1994). Much less evidence is available regarding the effects of an active lifestyle during childhood and adolescence on adult health.

The main reason for the paucity of information on the possible carry-over of benefits from childhood to adulthood is the lack of longitudinal studies that have followed the same individuals over many years. Ideally, one would need to randomly assign children into those who are given enhanced PA programs and those who remain sedentary over years and then observe the long-term effects of PA or of inactivity. On ethical grounds, such studies are hard to justify (it is unethical to demand that children not engage in PA for an extended period of time). In addition, they are extremely expensive and logistically most complicated. A second best alternative would be to conduct controlled intervention studies that last shorter periods and include several groups of subjects who span a wide age range (from childhood to middle age). Such "mixed longitudinal" studies are feasible, but have yet to be launched. Another approach is to identify

Physical Activity And Fitness Research Digest, Series 2, No. 4, December 1995.

adults with and without diseases and question them about their PA during earlier years. Such "retrospective" studies are easier to perform, but their outcome depends on the ability of people to correctly remember and report their PA behavior during earlier years. Conclusions derived from retrospective studies are less valid than those derived from longitudinal interventions.

The purpose of this article is to briefly examine the current evidence that enhanced PA during childhood and adolescence imparts immediate health benefits, or reduces risk for adult chronic disease. Emphasis will be given to the following conditions: obesity, hypertension, abnormal plasma lipoprotein profile and osteoporosis. The table on page 586 is a summary of the evidence attesting to such benefits.

Short-Term Benefits

Before analyzing the carry-over effects of childhood PA, one should identify the **immediate** effects of a training program (or an active lifestyle) on health-related risk factors. These are measured while the program is still in progress, or immediately upon its conclusion. Evidence for such benefits has been sought from intervention training programs that last a few weeks or several months at the most. An alternative approach has been cross-sectional studies which compare children (or youth) who habitually engage in athletic pursuit, with those who lead a sedentary lifestyle. The drawback of the latter approach is that differences in health-related risk between groups might not be a result of the physical activity per se. They may instead reflect heredity or events that took place before the child became physically active.

Body Fatness (see Bar-Or & Baranowski, 1994, for a review). Many, although not all, cross-sectional studies suggest that obese children and youth are less active than their leaner peers. There is only scant evidence, though, that inactivity **is a cause of** juvenile obesity (Roberts, 1993). Training studies with non-obese youth have shown little or no reduction in body adiposity (Wilmore, 1983). However, enhanced PA with or without a low-calorie diet, did reduce % body fat or excess body weight in obese children and youth.

Blood Pressure (see Alpert & Wilmore, 1994, for a review). Some cross-sectional studies show a slightly higher resting blood pressure among sedentary adolescents, compared with their active peers. Most studies, however, do not show such a difference, particularly if the groups have the same adiposity level. Training of healthy, previously inactive children or adolescents who have a normal blood pressure induces little (1-6 mmHg) or no drop in blood pressure. However, in adolescents with hypertension, training over several months does induce a reduction of both systolic and diastolic blood pressure. Even though such a reduction is modest (around 10 mmHg), it may be beneficial for some individuals with mild hypertension who otherwise may require medication to control their blood pressure. The training programs that induced a decline in blood pressure were comprised mostly of aerobic activities. In one study (Hagberg et al., 1984), the inclusion of a 5-month weight training regimen following a 6-month aerobic program further reduced the blood pressure of adolescents with hypertension. Such beneficial effects of exercise disappear within several months of termination of the program.

Blood Lipids (see Armstrong & Simons-Morton, 1994, for a review). Based on some cross-sectional studies, children and adolescents who are physically active, or whose aerobic fitness is high, have a more favorable blood lipid profile than their sedentary, or less fit, peers. This difference is particularly apparent in high-density lipoprotein cholesterol (HDL-C = the "good" cholesterol), which is higher in the active groups. Other cross-sectional comparisons, however, do not reveal such differences. In most of the cross-sectional studies it is impossible to separate a high activity level from a high fitness level.

Training studies of several weeks' duration have failed to show any beneficial effect on the blood lipid profile in healthy children or adolescents. More beneficial responses have been shown for groups who have a high coronary risk. These include children and adolescents with insulin-dependent diabetes mellitus, obesity, or with at least one parent who has three or more coronary risk factors.

Skeletal Health (see Bailey & Martin, 1994, for a review). The possible link between skeletal health and PA has received attention in recent years with the finding that physically active post-menopausal women, and elderly populations in general, have a higher bone mineral density (BMD) and less osteoporosis than less active controls. One of the determinants of bone health in old age is the "peak" BMD reached by young adulthood. Bone mass and BMD subsequently (and inevitably) decline with the years, until the bones become fragile.

This topic has an important pediatric relevance, because the great majority of bone build-up occurs during adolescence. A question of major public health relevance is whether enhanced PA during childhood and adolescence will result in a higher peak BMD.

Cross-sectional comparisons have shown that young athletes in weight-bearing sports such as gymnastics, soccer and volleyball (but not in non-weight-bearing sports such as swimming) have a higher BMD than do non-athletes. Likewise, bones of the dominant limb in "asymmetrical" sports, such as tennis or little-league pitching, have a higher BMD than the non-dominant limb. Conversely, bones of a limb immobilized for several weeks or months had a lower BMD than in the contralateral, non-immobilized limb.

Retrospective studies, in which adults were asked about their PA during childhood, suggest that women who had been physically active during childhood had a higher BMD in the 3rd and 4th decades of life than women who had been less active as children.

Longitudinal results of weight-bearing training programs are equivocal. Most controlled interventions yielded little or no increase in BMD or bone mass of exercising adolescents (e.g., Blimkie et al., 1993).

Carry-Over to Adult Life

There are several models that may explain a possible link between an adult person's health and her or his activity behavior in earlier years. As suggested by Blair et al. (1989) there are conceivably three avenues by which an enhanced PA level during childhood might improve adult health:

1. Childhood activity improves child health which, in turn, is beneficial to adult health.

2. An active lifestyle during childhood has a direct benefit to health in later years.

3. An active child becomes an active adult who, in turn has a lower risk for disease than an inactive adult.

Research provides no proof, or disproof. for any of these links. However, because a sedentary lifestyle in adults has been proven to entail a high risk for several chronic diseases (Bouchard et al., 1994), the most plausible link is that an active lifestyle during childhood and adolescence would be carried over through adulthood which, in turn, would reduce risk for disease. There are, however, no prospective studies that have tracked activity patterns from childhood to adulthood. Even though activity patterns and attitudes towards PA remain quite stable during late adolescence (but less so around age 10-12 years) (Malina. 1990), there is a low relationship between the two.

How Much Physical Activity?

There are practically no data as to the **optimal dose** of PA during childhood and adolescence, that might maintain and/or enhance health. However, a group of experts from various countries has recently generated a consensus statement (Sallis & Patrick, 1994), which includes the following guidelines for adolescents:

1. **All adolescents should be physically active daily, or nearly every day**, as part of play, games, sports, work, transportation, recreation, physical education, or planned exercise; in the context of family, school, and community activities.

2. Adolescents should engage in **three or more sessions per week** of activities that last 20 minutes or more at a time and that require **moderate to vigorous** levels of exertion.

There is no formal consensus statement for pre-adolescents although Corbin, Pangrazi, and Welk (1994) have made recommendations for physical activity levels for this group in a previous issue of the *President's Council on Physical Fitness and Sports Physical Activity and Fitness Research Digest* (see Chapter 39).

Summary and Conclusion

Based on current information, no long-term studies exist that support or reject the notion that physical activity during childhood and adolescence is beneficial to adult health There is, however, some evidence for short-term benefits of enhanced PA during the early years, particularly among children and youth who are at a high risk for chronic illness in later years. Much more research is needed to further study this important issue. In particular, it is essential to identify means of keeping young people motivated to maintain an active lifestyle as they reach young adulthood and middle age.

Possible Effects of Enhanced Physical Activity During Childhood and Adolescence on Risk for Chronic Disease

Observed Variable/Risk	Cross-Sectional Comparisons	Short-Term Effects of Intervention Programs	Carry-Over to Adult Life
Adiposity/ Obesity	Obesity is associated with hypoactivity	*General Population:* little or no reduction in % fat *Obese:* reduction in % fat pretraining levels in most patients	*General Population:* No information *Obese.* % fat returns to
Resting Blood Pressure/ Hypertension	Less active groups have similar or slightly higher BP compared with active groups	*General Population:* Little or no reduction in blood pressure *Hypertensives:* 5-12 mmHg reduction in SBP and less in DBP	*General Population:* No information *Hypertensives:* BP returns to pre-training values within weeks
Blood Lipid Profile	Young athletes sometimes have a better profile than sedentary controls (mostly in HDL-cholesterol)	*General Population:* No improvement in profile *High-risk Population:* Improved profile	*General Population:* No information *High-risk Population:* No information
Bone Mineral Density/ Osteoporosis	Athletes (weight bearing activities) have higher BMD than non-athletes.	Immobility induces loss of BMD. Training over several months induces no increase in BMD.	Retrospective data suggest a possible carryover.

BMD = bone mineral density; **BP** = blood pressure; **DBP** = diastolic blood pressure; **HDL** = high-density lipoprotein; **SBP** = systolic blood pressure.

The contrast between cross-sectional data and those generated through training studies is intriguing. The former suggest favorable health characteristics among active children and youth. compared with sedentary controls. Training studies, on the other hand, show little or no beneficial effect of training among healthy children and youth. This contrast may reflect a pre-selection of those who become active, and are healthier to start with, vs those who choose to pursue a sedentary lifestyle. It is possible, though, that interventions more vigorous than those commonly used in research would yield greater effects. It has been shown, for example, that army recruits who undergo an intense 8 hours per day training regimen for several months respond with an increase in bone mineral content (Margulies et al., 1986) and an improved lipid profile (Rubinstein et al., 1995). Likewise, it is possible that longer interventions (e.g., 1-2 years) than those used in most studies would yield more positive training-induced results.

References

Alpert, B.S., & Wilmore, J.H. (1994). Physical activity and blood pressure in adolescents. *Pediatric Exercise Science, 6,* 361-380.

Armstrong, N., & Simons-Morton, B. (1994). Physical activity and blood lipids in adolescents. *Pediatric Exercise Science, 6,* 381-405.

Bailey, D.A., & Martin, D.A. (1994). Physical activity and skeletal health in adolescents. *Pediatric Exercise Science, 6,* 330-347.

Bar-Or, O. (1994). Childhood and adolescent physical activity and fitness and adult risk profile. In C. Bouchard, R.J. Shephard, & T. Stephens (Eds.), *Physical Activity fitness, and Health. International Proceedings and Consensus Statement* (pp. 931-942) Champaign IL: Human Kinetics

Bar-Or, O., & Baranowski, T. (1994). Physical activity adiposity and obesity among adolescents. *Pediatric Exercise Science, 6* 348-360.

Bar-Or, O., & Malina, R.M. (1995). Exercise during childhood and adolescence. In L.W. Y. Cheung, & J.B. Richmond (Eds.), *Child Health, Nutrition, and Physical Activity* (pp. 79-123), Champaign, IL: Human Kinetics.

Blair, S.N., Clark D.B. & Cureton, K.J. (1989). Exercise and fitness in childhood: implications for a lifetime of health. In C.U.

Gisolfi, & D.L. Lamb (Eds.), *Perspectives in Exercise Science and Sports Medicine,* Vol 2 Youth Exercise and Sport (pp. 401-430), Indianapolis: Benchmark Press.

Blimkie, C., Rice, S., Webber, C., Martin, J., Levy, D., & Gordon, C. (1993). Effects of resistance training on bone mass and density in females. *Medicine & Science In Sports & Exercise,* 25, S48.

Bouchard C., Shephard R.J., & Stephens T. (Eds.) (1994). *Physical Activity, Fitness and Health. International Proceedings and Consensus Statement.* Champaign, IL: Human Kinetics.

Calfas, K.J., & Taylor, W. C. (1994). Effects of physical activity on psychological variables in adolescents. *Pediatric Exercise Science,* 6, 406-423.

Corbin, C.B., Pangnizi, R.P. & Welk, G.J. (1994). Toward an understanding of appropriate physical activity levels for youth. *President's Counsel on Physical Fitness and Sports Physical Activity and Fitness Research Digest.* 1 (8): 1 -8.

Hagberg, J.M., Ehsani, A.A., Goldring, D., Hernandez, A., Sinacore, D.R., & Holloszy, J.O. (1984). Effect of weight training on blood pressure and hemodynamics in hypertensive adolescents. *Journal of Pediatrics,* 104,147-151.

Malina, R.M. (1990). Growth, exercise, fitness and later outcomes. In C. Bouchard, R.J. Shephard, T. Stephens, J.R. Sutton, & B.D. McPherson (Eds.), *Exercise, Fitness and Health: A Consensus of Current Knowledge* (pp. 637-653, Champaign, IL: Human Kinetics.

Margulies, J.Y., Simkin, A., Leichter, I., Bivas, A., Steinberg, R., Giladi, M., Stein, M., Kashtan, H.,& Milgrom, C. (1986). Effect of intense physical activity on the bone-mineral content in the lower limbs of young adults. *Journal of Bone and Joint Surgery,* 68, 1090-1093.

Roberts, S.B. (1993). Energy expenditure and the development of early obesity. *Annals of the New York Academy of Medicine,* 699, 18-25.

Rubinstein, A., Burstein, R., Lubin, F, Chetrit, A., Dann, E.J., Levtov, O., Geter, R., Deuster, P.A., & Dolev, E. (1995). Lipoprotein profile changes during intense training of Israeli military recruits. *Medicine & Science in Sports & Exercise,* 27, 480-484.

Sallis, J.F. & Patrick, K. (1994). Physical activity guidelines for adolescents: consensus statement. *Pediatric Exercise Science*, 6, 302-314.

Wilmore, J.H. (1983). The 1983 C.H. McCloy Research Lecture. Appetite and body composition consequent to physical activity. *Research Quarterly of Exercise and Sport*, 54, 415-425.

Chapter 44

Physical Activity and Women's Health

A Note From The Editors

Many more women are active today compared to when the first studies of activity in America were conducted. However, as a group. girls and women are still less active than boys and men. Some of this difference in activity between males and females can be explained by the historical disparity in opportunities for females. Since 1972, when Title IX was implemented, more females have become involved in organized sport. We have yet to discover the effects of this increased participation on lifetime activity among females.

Much of the literature concerning health benefits of physical activity is based on studies done primarily with men. Only recently have large scale studies been initiated to investigate the effects of physical activity on women's health and wellness. Chris Wells, the author of this issue of the Digest, has been a pioneer in the study of physical activity for women. As you will see, much more research studying girls and women is necessary, but much has been accomplished in recent years. Diseases often thought to be "diseases of men" affect women as well as men. The evidence now suggests there are many health benefits for females who become regularly involved in physical activity.

This article clearly shows that women, especially women of color, are more likely to be sedentary. Sedentary living increases risk of

Physical Activity and Fitness Research Digest, Series 2, No. 5, March, 1996.

heart disease, various cancers, hypertension, stroke, and non insulin diabetes. Controlling body fatness, another factor that is related
to increased risk of chronic diseases, is also associated with inactivity. Continued efforts that focus on increasing physical activity among
girls and women will reduce the risk of chronic diseases and death.

Introduction

Healthy People 2000 sets forth the nation's health goals for the next
decade (Public Health Service, 1990). One of three primary goals is
to reduce health disparities among Americans. This goal addresses
reducing preventable disease and death from chronic diseases among
racial and ethnic minorities in the United States. Also of importance
is the disparity that exists among women as compared to men and
among women of different racial and ethnic groups. It is significant
that of 8 priorities for health promotion and disease prevention, increased physical activity and fitness leads the list. If we could increase
physical activity and decrease obesity, the reasoning goes, much of
the premature death, disease, and disability of high risk populations
could be virtually eliminated. But, what is the relationship between
physical activity and health in women? Can a strong case be made
for increasing physical activity in women as a primary preventive
measure for major chronic disease? Will increasing physical activity
reduce risk of disease and improve the health and wellness of women?
Is physical activity as beneficial for women as research has shown it
to be for men?

This *Digest* will address this issue by presenting the growing body
of evidence for the beneficial relationships between physical activity
(including exercise and physical fitness) and the major chronic diseases in women, with special reference to race and ethnicity. It will
be evident that American women need to make significant lifestyle
modifications to alter their health risks, and that health and educational professionals must mount new efforts to develop culturally
appropriate and sensitive health programs and educational materials.

But, first, how physically active are American women?

How Physically Active Are American Women?

The most current data on habitual physical activity are from the
Behavioral Risk Factor Surveillance System (BRFSS), a state-based,

random-digit-dialed telephone survey that collects self-reported information from a representative sample of people 18 years of age and older. In 1992, BRFSS data were available from 55,506 women from 48 states and the District of Columbia (Prevalence of recommended levels...1995). These women were asked about the frequency, duration, and intensity of their leisure-time physical activity (LTPA) during the preceding month. Respondents were categorized as having (1) no LTPA, (2) irregular activity that did not meet the recommended criteria for either vigorous physical activity (220 minutes per day of vigorous physical activity on 23 days per week) or the newer moderate activity recommendation (accumulation of >30 minutes per day of moderate activity on >5 days per week) (Summary Statement, CDC and ACSM, 1993). Only 27.1% of these women reported participation in recommended activity levels, and 30.2% reported no leisure-time physical activity whatsoever. The prevalence of no LTPA increased with age from 25.6% among women 18 to 34 years to 42.1 % among women over age 65. Racial/ethnic disparity was clearly evident. Black non-Hispanic women were less likely to be active (43.6%) than Hispanic women (40.2%) or white non-Hispanic women (27.6%). Physi-

---

Table 1.

Prevalence of Sedentary Lifestyle in U.S. Women, by Race, Ethnicity, and Education Level. Behavioral Risk Factor Surveillance System, United States, 1991-1992.

Women	White	Black	Hispanic	Native American/ Alaskan Native	Asian/ Pacific Islander
Sedentary Lifestyle	56.4	67.7	61.9	64.1	64.7
Education Level					
< 12 years	72.0	78.2	73.6	76.6	68.5
12 years	63.3	70.0	58.2	70.5	70.0
> 12 years	48.8	59.5	53.4	49.9	62.4

Adapted from: Prevalence of selected risk factors for chronic disease by education level in racial/ethnic populations—United States, 1991-1992. *Morbidity and Mortality Weekly Report*, 43 (48), pp. 895 & 897, December 9,. 1994.

cal inactivity was inversely related to income. Women with <$14,999 annual household income were most likely to have no LTPA (40.2%), and women with >$50,000 annual income were least likely to have no LTPA (21.2%).

BRFSS data from 1991 and 1992 were combined to increase precision of prevalence estimates for minority populations (Prevalence of selected..., 1994). Sedentary lifestyle was defined as reported participation in fewer than three 20-minute sessions of LTPA per week excluding usual job related physical activity. A sedentary lifestyle was reported most frequently among black women (68%) and least frequently among white women (56%). When racial/ethnic data were further stratified by level of education, the prevalence of sedentary lifestyle varied inversely with education within all five population groups. These data are shown in Table 1.

Other estimates of physical activity among American women have been equally low. Caspersen et al. (1986) estimated that 30.2% of American women were sedentary, 31.3% were irregularly active, 31.5% were regularly active at low levels of intensity, and that only 7% of women were sufficiently active to achieve the 1990 physical activity objectives for the nation. Ford et al. (1991) reported that women of higher socioeconomic status (SES) living in Pittsburgh spent significantly more time per week in LTPA, job-related physical activity, and household physical activity than did lower SES women. They estimated that only 7% of lower SES women expended 22,000 kcal/week, the energy expenditure linked to lower all-cause mortality in college alumni (Paffenbarger et al., 1986), compared to 16.8% of higher SES women.

Under the general assumption that low habitual energy expenditure results in obesity (excessive body fat), another way to estimate population specific physical activity is to assess body weight relative to height. BRFSS data on prevalence of overweight using body mass index (BMI = weight in kilograms divided by height in meters squared) 227.3 as the definition of overweight, indicates that black women have the highest prevalence of overweight (37.7%), followed by American Indian/Alaskan Native women (30.3%), Hispanic women (26.5%), white women (21.7%), and Asian/Pacific Islander women (10.1%) (Prevalence of selected...,1994). In addition, the prevalence of overweight varied inversely with level of education with all five population groups. Except for the low prevalence of overweight in Asian/Pacific Islander women, these values correspond to those of Table 1 for sedentary lifestyle.

Leading Causes of Mortality in American Women

In 1990, four of the ten leading causes of death in American women are chronic diseases directly associated with modifiable behavioral factors including physical inactivity or sedentary lifestyle. They are heart disease, certain forms of cancer (specifically, breast and colon cancers), cerebro-vascular disease (hypertension and stroke), and non-insulin-dependent diabetes mellitus (NIDDM) (National Center for Health Statistics, 1993). McGinnis and Foege (1993) summarized reports that attributed dietary factors and sedentary lifestyles with 22 to 30% of cardiovascular deaths, 20 to 60% of cancer deaths, and 30% of diabetes deaths. The only more prominent behavioral contributor to mortality than diet and physical inactivity was use of tobacco.

Table 2 presents age-adjusted mortality rates for chronic diseases associated with sedentary lifestyle in U.S. women by race and ethnicity. Coronary heart disease (CHD) and cerebrovascular disease (stroke) are the two leading causes of death in all five population groups. Diabetes ranks as the third leading cause of death from chronic disease in black, Hispanic, Native American/Alaskan Native and Asian/Pacific Islander women (exceeding death rates from lung cancer, breast cancer, chronic obstructive pulmonary disease, and colorectal cancer) (Centers for Disease Control . . . , 1994).

Table 2. Age-Adjusted Mortality Rates*, U.S. Women, 1990.

	White	Black	Hispanic	Native American/ Alaskan Native	Asian/ Pacific Islander
CHD	130.2	148.3	147.1	74.5	73.7
Stroke	45.8	68.7	45.4	314.0	43.7
Breast Cancer	29.1	33.4	25.0	12.1	11.9
Colorectal Cancer	17.0	22.9	15.0	9.7	9.9
Diabetes	14.8	37.1	27.6	31.0	11.8

Adapted from: Centers for Disease Control and Prevention (1994). *Chronic Disease in Minority Populations*, pp. C-3, C-4, Atlanta, GA: Centers for Disease Control and Prevention.

*Rate per 100,000 persons adjusted to the 1980 standard U.S. population.

Morbidity data correspond closely to mortality data. Table 3 provides age-adjusted prevalence of chronic disease in U.S. women between 1986-1990. Health disparities among racial/ethnic groups are evident with exceedingly high morbidity from chronic diseases that are major causes of death among black, Hispanic, and Native American/Alaskan Native women compared to white and Asian/Pacific Islander women.

Table 3. Age-Adjusted Prevalence* of Chronic Disease, U.S. Women, 1986-1990.

	White	Black	Hispanic	Native American/ Alaskan Native	Asian/ Pacific Islander
Hypertension	10.96	19.73	10.55	13.82	8.35
Diabetes	2.36	4.89	3.53	5.04	2.38
Coronary Heart Disease	1.83	1.42	3.53	n.a.	n.a.
Stroke	0.98	1.20	1.10	n.a.	n.a.

*Per 100,000.

Adapted from: Centers for Disease Control and Prevention (1994). *Chronic Disease in Minority Populations*, Atlanta, GA: Centers for Disease Control and Prevention.

The remainder of this *Digest* will describe evidence linking sedentary lifestyle/physical inactivity with diseases of the heart, hypertension and stroke, breast and colorectal cancer, and non-insulin-dependent diabetes mellitus.

Physical Inactivity and Diseases of the Heart in Women

According to the American Heart Association, in 1991, 51.8 to of all deaths from "total cardiovascular diseases" occurred in women (American Heart Association, 1994). The Nationals Heart, Lung, and Blood Institute (Public Health Service, 1992) reports that 1 in 10 women 45 to 64 years of age has some form of heart disease, and that this increases to 1 in 4 in women over age 65. Major modifiable risk factors include smoking, high blood cholesterol, high blood pressure, and physical inactivity. The following discussion will exclude smoking.

Physical Activity and Blood Cholesterol in Women

A blood lipid profile that places an individual at risk consists of elevated total cholesterol (TC), elevated low-density lipoprotein-cholesterol (LDL-C), and elevated triglycerides (TG). High levels of high-density lipoprotein-cholesterol (HDL-C) are considered protective from CHD. Women generally have higher HDL-C and lower LDL-C values than men prior to menopause. This is attributed to estrogen which interferes with the uptake of LDL-C in arterial walls. Following menopause, HDL-C values decline, LDL-C values increase, and TC values increase, sometimes well above those of age-matched men.

Following a meta-analysis to examine the effect of exercise training on serum lipids in women, Lokey and Tran (1989) concluded that training was associated with lower TC, TG, and TC/HDL-C, but no differences in HDL-C or LDL-C. The average age of the subjects was 29.5 years, and the women with the most atherogenic lipid profiles benefited the most. In 20 to 40 year old women, 24 weeks of walking yielded an increase in HDL-C independent of walking intensity (Duncan, et al., 1991). In the Healthy Women's Study, a longitudinal study that is following originally premenopausal women through menopause, women with higher physical activity had the least age-related weight gain and a decline in HDL-C (Owens et al., 1992). At the beginning of the study, only women reporting >2000 kcal/week energy expenditure had significantly better profiles for TC, TG, LDL-C and HDL_2-C (Owens, et al., 1 990).

In a recently published review, Shoenhair and Wells (1995) concluded that cross-sectional data strongly support an inverse relationship between current physical fitness and TC, TG, TC/HDL-C, and HDL-C/LDL-C. HDL-C values appear to be elevated in only the most highly fit women. Pre- and postmenopausal athletes have less atherogenic lipid profiles than sedentary or less active women matched for age and menopausal status (Rainville & Vaccaro, 1984; Harting et al., 1984; Stevenson et al., 1995).

Physical Activity and Blood Pressure in Women

In the Healthy Women's Study, systolic blood pressure was lower in women expending >500 kcal per week, and diastolic blood pressure was lower in those expending >1000 kcal/week compared to sedentary women (Owens et al., 1990). In the Stanford Community Health Survey, lower diastolic blood pressure was associated with both vigorous exercise (Sallis, et al., 1986a) and moderate-intensity exercise (Sallis et al., 1986b). In 1991, Reaven et al. reported a significant inverse relationship between physical activity and blood pressure in women. They reported that the most active women had systolic blood pressures 9-24 mmHg lower and diastolic blood pressures 3- 13 mmHg lower than the least active women after accounting for differences in body mass index.

A strong relationship also appears to exist between physical fitness and blood pressure in women. In the Aerobics Center Longitudinal Study, Gibbons et al. (1983) reported that cardiovascular fitness was independently associated with lower blood pressure. In Canadian women, blood pressure was significantly lower in subjects with the highest fitness classification (Jette et al., 1992).

Physical Inactivity and Cardiovascular Disease in Women

Very few studies have been completed on physical inactivity and CVD in American women (for an extensive review including international literature, see Schoenhair & Wells, 1995). In a homogeneous population of 17,000 Seventh-Day Adventist women, a population at relatively low risk for CVD, occupational and leisure-time activity was combined and subjects were grouped into three activity classifications. A strong inverse relationship was found between physical activity and CHD mortality. Relative risk ratios for the "high", "moderate", and "low" activity groups were .41, .61, and 1.0, respectively (Fraser et al., 1992). After 24 years of observation, an active lifestyle lowered the age-adjusted incidence of CHD and myocardial infarction in Framingham women by a factor of 2.5 (Kannel & Sorlie, 1979).

In a classic prospective study of all-cause mortality in the predominantly white, upper SES population of the Aerobics Center Longitudinal Study, Blair et al. (1989) reported a strong inverse relationship between cardiorespiratory fitness and death from cardiovascular disease. Women in the lowest quintile of physical fitness had an age-adjusted death rate from cardiovascular disease of 7.4 (per 10,000 person-years) compared to 2.9 and 0.8 for women in fitness groups 2-3 and 4-5. Women in the lowest fitness category had an age-adjusted relative risk of 8.0 when compared with women in fitness quintiles 4 and 5.

In summary, there is strong observational and experimental evidence that physical inactivity plays a significant role in the development of cardiovascular disease in women, and that habitual physical activity and at least a moderate level of cardiorespiratory fitness offers protection from these diseases in women as well as in men.

Physical Inactivity, Hypertension and Stroke in Women

Non-fatal stroke is the leading cause of disability in American women. Risk factors for stroke include hypertension, heart disease, and smoking. Approximately two-thirds of all stroke victims have hypertension (HT). Until age 64, HT is more prevalent in men, and thereafter, is more prevalent in women (Cowley et al., 1992). There is increasing prevalence of HT with age, and wide disparity among race/ethnic groups ranging from 2% in young white women to 83% in black women over 65 (Public Health Service, 1990, p. 392).

In the subjects originally studied by Gibbons et al. (1983), and followed for 1 to 12 years, Blair et al. (1984) reported that low physical fitness was an independent contributor to the risk of developing hypertension (RR=1.52) after controlling for sex, age, baseline blood pressure, baseline body mass index, and follow-up interval. In a related study, lower fitness was significantly related to the increased incidence of nonfatal stroke (Blair et al., 1989).

A strong inverse relationship between LTPA and death from stroke was observed in postmenopausal women (Paganini-Hill et al., 1988). Those who were physically active less than 30 minutes per day had twice the age-adjusted mortality from stroke as women who were active at least one hour per day.

Although there is less research available, it seems clear that habitual physical activity reduces the risk of hypertension in women, and consequently, is a primary preventive measure against stroke.

Physical Inactivity and Breast and Colorectal Cancers in Women

Data on cancer relative to physical activity have been inconsistent and difficult to interpret because cancer represents not one disease, but many distinct, site-specific diseases. To further complicate the situation, risk factors are specific to each disease. Nevertheless, over the past decade, increasing evidence indicates that physical activity is associated with decreased overall cancer mortality and decreased incidence of specific types of cancers (Sternfeld, 1992; Lee, 1995). The cancer site most frequently studied in relation to physical activity is colon cancer, and findings overwhelmingly support an inverse relationship. The two most likely potential mechanisms by which physical activity may be protective of colon cancer are (1) shortened intestinal transit time, and (2) decreased levels of body fat. Shortened intestinal transit time is thought to decrease the amount of contact between possible carcinogenic substances and intestinal mucosa, but evidence remains controversial on this matter. For several cancers (including colon and breast cancers), high levels of body fat are associated with increased risk.

Most research on physical activity and colon cancer has focused on occupational physical activity in men. Clearly, men with sedentary jobs have increased risk of colon cancer (Sternfeld, 1992). One of the most comprehensive studies that included women was a case-control study of Utah residents that took into account differences in dietary patterns and body weight, confounding factors not usually controlled (Slattery et al., 1988). Comparing both occupational and leisure-time activities, the sedentary individuals of both sexes were at nearly 2-fold increased risk for colon cancer.

The relationship between physical activity and breast cancer is less clear, but several studies in American women suggest that risk may be lowered in those who are habitually active. An extensive review of this subject is now available including international studies (Kramer & Wells, 1996). Only studies utilizing American subjects are reviewed here. In 1985, Frisch et al. assessed prevalence of breast cancer in 5398 former collegiate women athletes and nonathletes from 10 colleges and universities from classes spanning 56 years. A higher percentage of former athletes reported they were currently exercising than nonathletes. Comparing the prevalence of breast cancer between the two groups, the nonathletes had 1.85 times the risk of the former athletes, strong evidence for an inverse relationship between lifetime physical activity and breast cancer.

From the National Health and Nutrition Examination Survey database (NHANES I), Albanes et al. (1989) examined breast cancer incidence relative to baseline recreational and non-recreational physical activity levels. After 10 years of follow-up, pre-menopausal women with high levels of activity were associated with slightly increased risk of breast cancer. Among postmenopausal women, however, high physical activity conferred a protective effect.

More recently, Bernstein et al. (1994) studied the timing of physical activity relative to estrogen exposure in premenopausal women from Los Angeles County. Using a case-control study design, they report a strong dose response relationship between leisure-time exercise since menarche and decreased risk of breast cancer. Women reporting 3.8 or more hours per week of exercise since menarche had a 50% reduction in breast cancer risk. A 30% reduction was observed in women reporting 1-3 hours per week of exercise since menarche. A slightly weaker relationship was observed among nulliparous women. The observed benefit of exercise was attributed to reduced exposure to endogenous estrogen subsequent to shorter luteal phases and higher incidence of anovulatory menstrual cycles.

High to moderate levels of habitual physical activity may decrease lifetime exposure to endogenous sex hormones in two ways: (1) prior to menopause, high levels of physical activity may delay menarche, decrease the number of ovulatory cycles, and hence reduce exposure to endogenous estrogen (Frisch et al., 1980; Bernstein et al., 1987), and (2) following menopause, maintenance of low levels of adipose tissue may mediate the conversion of androgenic compounds to extraglandular estrogen (Siiteri, 1987; Hershcopf & Bradlow, 1987)

In summary, lifetime physical activity appears to reduce the risk of colon cancer and breast cancer in white women, but there is an obvious need to incorporate minority women into future research on these topics.

Physical Inactivity and Non-Insulin-Dependent Diabetes Mellitus in Women

About 14 million Americans have diabetes, with 95% having non-insulin-dependent diabetes mellitus (NIDDM). Tables 2 and 3 above indicate that certain minority women have exceedingly high mortality and prevalence rates from this adult-onset chronic disease. Diabetes is a leading cause of death in women and a leading cause of adult blindness, leg and foot amputations, circulatory disease, kidney failure, and birth defects. In NIDDM, the pancreas may secrete insulin, but cells and tissues of the body are insulin resistant, and consequently, patients are characterized by high levels of insulin (hyperinsulinemia) and blood glucose (hyperglycemia). Those at highest risk for NIDDM include the overweight or obese. and particularly, those over 40 years of age (American Diabetes Association, 1992).

According to the American Diabetes Association (1990), an appropriate exercise program should be an adjunct to diet and/or drug therapy to improve glycemic control, reduce cardiovascular risk factors, and increase psychological well-being in women with NIDDM. Individuals who are most likely to respond favorably are those with moderate glucose intolerance and hyperinsulinemia. Unfortunately, findings from the 1990 National Health Interview Survey (Ford & Herman, 1995) indicate that women with diabetes are less likely to report exercising regularly than women without diabetes. A comparison of the effects of exercise on insulin sensitivity in women with NIDDM recently revealed that low intensity exercise was as effective as high intensity exercise in enhancing insulin sensitivity (Braun et al., 1995). Duration of the two exercise regimes was adjusted so that energy expenditure was equal. This is important because obesity, diabetic complications, and general lack of physical fitness are common in women with glucose intolerance or NIDDM. Prescription of low intensity exercise is no doubt safer and more practicable, especially for older women with NIDDM. A recent community based study (San Luis Valley Diabetes Study) also demonstrated this. Higher levels of physical activity were associated with improved insulin action in individuals with impaired glucose tolerance (Regensteiner et al., 1995), further supporting the concept that habitual physical activity reduces incidence of impaired glucose tolerance and lowers morbidity from NIDDM.

Two studies directly indicate that habitual physical activity in women is a promising approach to the primary prevention of NIDDM. In one, Frisch and colleagues (1986) report a significantly lower prevalence of diabetes among every age group (20 to more than 70 years) in 5398 women who engaged in long-term athletic activity compared to their nonathletic classmates. In the other investigation, reduced incidence of NIDDM among women who exercised regularly was observed in a prospective cohort of 87,253 women 34 to 59 years (Manson et al., 1991).

In summary, regular physical activity has an important role in both treatment and prevention of NIDDM through its association with reduced body weight, and its independent effects on insulin sensitivity and glucose tolerance.

Obesity, Morbidity, and Mortality in Women

Data from nationally representative cross-sectional surveys reveals that prevalence of overweight in U.S. women has increased in all age groups since the sixties (Kuczmarski et al., 1994). These data also indicate that the prevalence of obesity is substantially higher in black, Hispanic, Pacific Islander, and Native American and Alaskan Native women than in white women (Kuczmarski et al., 1994; Kumanyika, 1993). Altogether, about 32 million American women are overweight or obese. In addition, the particularly high-risk upper body fat distribution (central adiposity) occurs to a greater extent in some minority populations than in whites (Kumanyika, 1993).

High body weight or weight gain since age 18 in women has been associated with coronary heart disease (Willett et al., 1995), all-cause mortality (Manson et al., 1995), and hyperinsulinemia (fasting insulin and insulin following glucose load) (Wing et al., 1992). Lowest mortality among U.S. women was observed in those who weighed at least 15% less than the U.S. average for women of similar age and whose weight had been stable since early adulthood (Manson et al., 1995).

Cleary, high body weight and body fat in women is related to increased incidence of coronary heart disease, hypertension, NIDDM, breast cancer, and all-cause mortality. Greater attention to prevention and treatment of obesity in minority populations may help to address critical health issues in American women (St. Jeor, 1993).

Conclusion

There is an obvious national shortfall in closing the gap in health disparities among Americans—especially, American women. We have failed—in physical education and sport, and in medicine—to clarify the importance of habitual physical activity, physical fitness, and maintenance of "normal" body weight to good health. One major reason is that we have attempted to use health messages, programs and approaches based on white, middle-class values and culture, and then wondered why they were not enthusiastically embraced. Research and educational efforts must focus on conceptually-based programs in schools and communities that are culturally-sensitive and ethnic-specific.

References

Albanes, D. Blair, A., and Taylor, P.R. (1989). Physical activity and risk of cancer in the NHANES I population. *American Journal of Public Health,* 79, 744-750.

American Diabetes Association. (1992). Alexandria, VA.

American Diabetes Association. (1990). Diabetes mellitus and exercise. Position Statement of the American Diabetes Association. *Diabetes Care,* 13, 804-805.

American Heart Association. (1994). *Heart and Stroke Facts: 1995 Statistical Supplement.* Dallas: TX. American Heart Association.

Bernstein, L., Henderson, B.E., Hanisch, R., Sullivan-Halley, J., and Ross, R.K. (1994). Physical exercise and risk of breast cancer in young women. *Journal of the National Cancer Institute,* 86, 1403-1408.

Bernstein, L., Ross, R.K., Lobo, R.A., Hanisch, R., Krailo, M.D., and Henderson, B.E. (1987). The effects of moderate physical activity on menstrual cycle patterns in adolescence: implications for breast cancer prevention. *British Journal of Cancer,* 55, 681-685.

Blair, S.N., Goodyear, N.N, Cooper, K.H., and Smith, M. (1984). Physical fitness and incidence of hypertension in healthy normotensive men and women. *Journal of the American Medical Association,* 252, 487-490.

Blair, S.N., Kohl, H.W., Paffenbarger, R.S., Clark, D.G., Cooper, K.H., and Gibbons, L.W., (1989). Physical fitness and all-cause mortality: A prospective study of healthy men and women. *Journal of the American Medical Association,* 262, 2395-2401.

Braun, B., Zimmermann, M.B., and Kretchmer, N. (1995). Effects of exercise intensity on insulin sensitivity in women with non-insulin-dependent diabetes mellitus. *Journal of Applied Physiology,* 78, 3000-3036.

Caspersen, C.J., Christenson, G.M., and Pollard, R.A. (1986). Status of the 1990 physical fitness and exercise objectives—evidence from NHIS 1995, *Public Health Reports,* 101, 587-592.

Centers for Disease Control and Prevention. (1994). *Chronic disease in Minority Populations*. Atlanta: Centers for Disease Control and Prevention.

Cowley, A.W. Jr., Dzau, V. Buttrick, P., Cooke, J., Devereux, R.B., Grines, C.L., Haidet, G.C., and Thames, M.C. (1992). Working group on noncoronary cardiovascular disease and exercise in women. *Medicine and Science in Sports and Exercise*, 24, S277-S287.

Duncan, J.J., Gordon, N.F., and Scott, C.B. (1991). Women walking for health and fitness: how much is enough? *Journal of the American Medical Association*, 266, 3295-3299.

Ford, E.S. and Herman, W.H. (1995). Leisure-time physical activity patterns in the U.S. diabetic population. *Diabetes Care*, 18, 27-33.

Ford, E.S., Merritt, R.K., Heath, G.W., Rowell, K.E., Washburn, R.A., Kriska, A., and Heile, G. (1991). Physical activity behaviors in lower and higher socioeconomic status populations. *American Journal of Epidemiology*, 133, 1246-1256.

Fraser, G.E., Strahan, T.M., Sabate, J., Beeson, W.L., and Kissinger, D. (1992). Effects of traditional coronary risk factors on rates of incident coronary events in a low-risk population: The Adventist Health Study. *Circulation,* 86, 406-413.

Frisch, R.E., Wyshak, G., Albright, T.E., Albright, N.L., and Schiff, I. (1986). Lower prevalence of diabetes in female former college athletes compared with nonathletes. *Diabetes,* 35, 1101-1105.

Frisch, R.E., Wyshak, G., Albright, N.L., Albright, T.E., Schiff, L., Jones, K.P., Witschi, J., Shiang, E., Koff, E., and Marguglio, M. (1985). Lower prevalence of breast cancer and cancers of the reproductive system among former college athletes compared to non-athletes. *British Journal of Cancer,* 52, 885-891.

Frisch, R.E., Wyshak, G., and Vincent, L. (1980). Delayed menarche and amenorrhea in ballet dancers. *New England Journal of Medicine,* 303, 17-19.

Gibbons, L.W., Blair, S.N., Cooper, K.H., and Smith, M. (1983). Association between coronary heart disease risk factors and physical fitness in healthy adult women. *Circulation,* 67, 977-983.

Harting, G.H., Moore, C.E., Mitchell, R., and Kappus, C.M. (1984). Relationship of menopausal status and exercise level to HDL cholesterol in women. *Experimental and Aging Research,* 10, 13-18.

Hershcopf, R.J. and Bradlow, H.L. (1987). Obesity, diet, endogenous estrogens and the risk of hormone-sensitive cancer. *American Journal of Clinical Nutrition,* 45, 283-289.

Jette, M., Sidney, K., Quenneville, J., and Landry, F. (1992). Relation between cardiorespiratory fitness and selected risk factors for coronary heart disease in a population of Canadian men and women. *Canadian Medical Association Journal,* 146, 1353-1360.

Kannel, W.B. and Sorlie, P. (1979). Some health benefits of physical activity: The Framingham study. *Archives of Internal Medicine,* 139, 857-861.

Kramer, M.M. and Wells, C.L. (1996). Does physical activity reduce risk of estrogen-dependent cancer in women? A review. *Medicine and Science in Sports and Exercise,* (in press).

Kuczmarski, R.J., Flegal, K.M., Campbell, S.M., and Johnson, C.L. (1994). Increasing prevalence of overweight among U.S. adults: The National Health Examination Surveys, 1960 to 1991. *Journal of the American Medical Association,* 272, 205-211.

Kumanyika, S.K. (1993). Special issues regarding obesity in minority populations. *Annals of Internal Medicine,* 119, 650-654.

Lee, I. (1995). Physical activity and cancer. *PCPFS Physical Activity and Fitness Research Digest.* 2 (2). Washington, D.C.: PCPFS.

Lokey, E.A. and Tran, Z.V. (1989). Effects of exercise training on serum lipid and lipoprotein concentrations in women: A meta-analysis. *International Journal of Sports Medicine,* 10, 424-429.

Manson, J.E., Rimm, E.B., Stampfer, M.J., Colditz, G.A., Willett, W.C., Krolewski, A.S., Rosner, B., Hennekens, C.H., and Speizer, F.E. (1991). Physical activity and incidence of non-insulin-dependent diabetes mellitus in women. *The Lancet,* 338, 774-778.

Manson, J.E., Willett, W.C., Stampfer, M.J., Colditz, G.A., Hunter, D.J., Hankinson, S.E., Hennekens, C.H., and Speizer, F.E. (1995). Body weight and mortality among women. *New England Journal of Medicine,* 333, 677-685.

McGinnis, J.M. and Foege, W.H. (1993). Actual causes of death in the United States. Journal of the American Medical Association, 270, 2207-2212.

National Center for Health Statistics. Advance Report of Final Mortality Statistics, 1990. Hyattsville, MD: Department of Health and Human Services, 1993. *Monthly Vital Statistics Report,* 41 (7).

Owens, J.F., Matthews, K.A., Wing, R.R., and Kuller, L.H. (1992). Can physical activity mitigate the effects of aging in middle-age women? *Circulation,* 85, 1265-1270.

Owens, J.F., Matthews, K.A., Wing, R.R., and Kuller, L.H. (1990). Physical activity and cardiovascular risk: A cross-sectional study of middle-aged premenopausal women. *Preventive Medicine,* 19, 147-1457.

Paffenbarger, R.S., Jr., Hyde, R.T., Wing, A.K., and Hsieh, C.C. (1986). Physical activity, all-cause mortality and longevity of college alumni. *New England Journal of Medicine,* 314, 605-613.

Paganini-Hill, A., Ross, R.K., and Henderson, B.E. (1988). Post-menopausal estrogen treatment and stroke: A prospective study. *British Medical Journal,* 297, 519-522.

Prevalence of recommended levels of physical activity among women—Behavioral Risk Factor Surveillance System, 1992. (1995). *Morbidity and Mortality Weekly Report,* 44 (6), 105-108.

Prevalence of selected risk factors for chronic disease by education level in racial/ethnic populations—United States, 1991-1992. (1994). *Morbidity and Mortality Weekly Report,* 43 (48), 894-899.

Public Health Service. (1990). *Healthy People 2000: National Health Promotion and Disease Prevention Objectives.* Washington D.C.: Department of Health and Human Services. Publication PHS 91-50212.

Public Health Service. (1992). *The Healthy Heart Handbook for Women.* National Heart, Lung and Blood Institute. National Institutes of Health, Washington D.C.: NIH publication no. 92-2720.

Rainville, S. and Vaccaro, P. (1984). The effects of menopause and training on serum lipids. *International Journal of Sports Medicine,* 5, 137-141.

Reaven, P.D., Barrett-Connor, E., and Edelstein, S. (1991). Relation between leisure-time physical activity and blood pressure in older women. *Circulation*, 83, 559-565.

Regensteiner, J.G., Shetterly, S.M., Mayer, E.J., Eckel, R.H., Haskell, W.L., Baxter, J., and Hamman, R.F.(1995). Relationship between habitual physical activity and insulin area among individuals with impaired glucose tolerance. The San Luis Valley Diabetes Study. *Diabetes Care*, 18, 490-497.

Sallis, J.F., Haskell, W.L., Wood, P.D., Fortman, S.P., and Vranizan, K.M. (1986a). Vigorous physical activity and cardiovascular risk factors in young adults. *Journal of Chronic Diseases*, 39, 115-120.

Sallis, J.F., Heskell, W.L., Fortman, S.P., Wood, P.D., and Vranizan, K. (1986b). Moderate-intensity physical activity and cardiovascular risk factors: The Stanford Five-City Project. *Preventive Medicine*, 15, 561-568.

Shoenhair, C.L. and Wells, C.L. (1995). Women, physical activity, and coronary heart disease: A review. *Medicine, Exercise, Nutrition, Health*, 4 (4), 200.

Siiteri, P.K. (1987). Adipose tissue as a source of hormones. *American Journal of Clinical Nutrition*, 45, 277-282.

Slattery, M.L., Schumacher, M.C., Smith, K.R., West, D.W., and Abd-Elghany, N. (1988). Physical activity, diet, and risk of colon cancer in Utah. *American Journal of Epidemiology*, 128, 989-999.

St. Jeor, S.T. (1993). The role of weight management in the health of women. *Journal of the American Diabetic Association*, 93, 1007-1012.

Sternfeld, B. (1992). Cancer and the protective effect of physical activity: The epidemiological evidence. *Medicine and Science in Sports and Exercise*, 24, 1195-1209.

Stevenson, E.T., Davy, K.P., and Seals, D.R. (1995). Hemostatic, metabolic, and androgenic risk factors for coronary heart disease in physically active and less active postmenopausal women. *Arteriosclerosis, Thrombosis, and Vascular Biology*, 15, 23-31.

Summary Statement Workshop on Physical Activity and Public Health. (1993). Centers for Disease Control and Prevention and

American College of Sports Medicine. *Sports Medicine Bulletin*, 24 (4), 7.

Willett, W.C., Manson, J.E., Stampfer, M.J., Colditz, G.A., Rosner, B., Speizer, F.E., and Hennekens, C.H. (1995). Weight, weight change, and coronary heart disease in women: Risk within the "normal" weight range. *Journal of the American Medical Association*, 273, 461-465.

Wing, R.R., Matthews, K.A., Kuller, L.H., Smith, D., Becker, D., Plantinga, P.L., and Meilahn, E.N. (1992). Environmental and familial contributions to insulin levels and change in insulin levels in middle-aged women. *Journal of the American Medical Association*, 268, 1890-1985.

Chapter 45

Exercise, Obesity, and Weight Control

It is ironic that while millions of people are dying of starvation each year in most parts of the world, many Americans are dying as an indirect result of an overabundance of food. Further, billions of dollars are spent each year overfeeding the American public, which then leads to the spending of billions of dollars more each year on various weight loss methods. This review will investigate various aspects of overweight and obesity, and show how they are affected by physical activity. But first, we must define and differentiate between the terms overweight and obesity.

Overweight, Obesity and Their Assessment

The terms overweight and obesity are often used interchangeably, but this is technically incorrect as they have different meanings. Overweight is defined as a body weight that exceeds the normal or standard weight for a particular person, based on his or her height and frame size. These standards are established solely on the basis of population averages. It is quite possible to be overweight according to these standard tables and yet have a body fat content which is average or even below average. For example, almost all college and pro-

*Parts of this review were adapted with permission from: Wilmore, J.H., & Costill, D.L. (1994) *Physiology of Sport and Exercise*. Champaign, IL: Human Kinetics Publishers.

Physical Activity And Fitness Research Digest, Series 1, No. 6, May 1994.

fessional football players are overweight by these tables, but few are overfat. There are also people who are within the normal range of body weights for their height and frame size by the standard tables, but who have, in fact, excessive body fat.

Obesity is the condition where the individual has an excessive amount of body fat. This means that the actual amount of body fat, or its percentage of a person's total weight, must be assessed or estimated. A number of laboratory and field assessment techniques can provide reasonably accurate estimates of a person's body composition. Exact standards for allowable fat percentages, however, have not been established. But there is general agreement among clinicians and scientists that men over 25% body fat and women over 35% should be considered obese, and that relative fat values of 20% to 25% in men and 30% to 35% in women should be considered borderline obese.

Prevalence of Obesity and Overweight

The prevalence of obesity and overweight in the United States has increased dramatically over the past 30 years. On the basis of data from a large study conducted between 1976 and 1980 by the National Center for Health Statistics (National Center for Health Statistics, 1986), 28.4% of American adults aged 25 to 74 years are overweight. Between 13% and 26% of the U.S. adolescent population, 12 to 17 years of age, are obese, depending on gender and race, and an additional 4% to 12% are superobese. This represents a 39% increase in the prevalence of obesity when compared with data collected between 1966 and 1970. Equally alarming, there has been a 54% increase in the prevalence of obesity among children 6 to 11 years of age (Gortmaker, et al., 1987).

It has also been demonstrated that the average individual in this country will gain approximately one pound of additional weight each year after the age of 25 years. Such a seemingly small gain, however, results in 30 pounds of excess weight by the age of 55 years. Since the bone and muscle mass decreases by approximately one half pound per year due to reduced physical activity, fat is actually increasing by 1.5 pounds each year. This means a 45 pound gain in fat over this 30-year period! It is no wonder that weight loss is a national obsession.

The Control of Body Weight

It is important to have a basic understanding of how body weight is controlled or regulated, in order to better understand how one becomes obese. The issue of how body weight is regulated has puzzled scientists for years. It is rather remarkable that the body takes in an average of about 2,500 kcal per day, or nearly one million kcal per year. The average gain of 1.5 pounds of fat each year, which we just discussed, represents an imbalance between energy intake and expenditure of only 5,250 kcal per year (using 3,500 kcal to represent the energy equivalent of a pound of adipose tissue), or less than 15 kcal per day. Even with a weight gain of 1.5 pounds of fat, the body is able to balance the food intake to within 1 potato chip per day of what is expended! That is truly remarkable.

The ability of the body to balance its intake and expenditure has led scientists to propose that body weight is regulated within a narrow range similar to the way in which body temperature is regulated. There is excellent evidence for this in the animal research literature (Keesey, 1986). When animals are force-fed, or starved, for various periods of time, their weight will increase, or decrease, markedly, but they will always return to their original weight, or to the weight of the control animals (for those animals that naturally continue to increase weight throughout their life span), when allowed to go back to their normal eating patterns.

Similar results have been found in humans, although the number of studies has been limited. Subjects placed on semi-starvation diets have lost up to 25% of their body weight, but regained that weight within months of returning to a normal diet (Keys, et al., 1950). In overfeeding studies of Vermont prisoners, overfeeding resulted in weight gains of 15 to 25%, yet weight returned to its original level shortly after the completion of the experiment (Sims, 1976).

How is the body able to do this? The total amount of energy expended each day can be expressed in three categories: resting metabolic rate (RMR), the thermic effect of feeding (TEF), and the thermic effect of activity (TEA). RMR is your body's metabolic rate early in the morning following an overnight fast and 8 hours of sleep. The term basal metabolic rate (BMR) is also used, but generally implies that the person sleeps over in the clinical facility where the metabolic rate measurement will be made. Most research today uses resting metabolic rate. It accounts for 60 to 75% of the total energy expended each day.

The TEF, which represents the increase in metabolic rate that is associated with the digestion, absorption, transport, metabolism, and storage of the ingested food, accounts for approximately 10% of the total energy expended each day. There is probably also a wastage component included in the thermic effect of a meal, where the body is able to increase its metabolic rate above that necessary for the processing and storage of the ingested food. This component may be defective in obese individuals. The TEA, which is simply the energy expended above resting metabolic rate levels necessary to accomplish a given task or activity, whether it be washing your face or a brisk 3 mile walk, accounts for the remainder.

The body makes very important adaptations in each of these three components of total energy expenditure when there are major increases or decreases in the energy intake. With very low calorie diets, there are decreases in the RMR, TEF, and TEA. The body appears to be attempting to conserve its energy stores. This is dramatically illustrated by the decreases reported in resting metabolic rate of 20 to 30% or more within several weeks after patients begin a very low calorie diet. Conversely, with overeating RMR, TEF, and TEA all increase to prevent the unnecessary storage of a large number of calories. It is quite possible that all of these adaptations are under the control of the sympathetic nervous system, and play a major, if not the primary role in controlling weight around a given set-point.

Etiology of Obesity

The results of recent medical and physiological research show that obesity can be the result of any one, or a combination of many, factors. Its etiology is not as simple or straight-forward as was once believed. A number of experimental studies on animals have linked obesity to hereditary or genetic factors. Recent studies by Dr. Albert Stunkard at the University of Pennsylvania have shown a direct genetic influence on height, weight, and BMI (Stunkard, et al., 1986a, 1986b, 1990).

A study from Laval University in Quebec, Canada has provided possibly the strongest evidence of a significant genetic component in the establishment of obesity (Bouchard, et al., 1990). With periods of overfeeding of identical monozygotic twins (1,000 kcal above maintenance levels, six out of every seven days), there was a three-fold variation in the weight gained over 100 days between twin pairs, while there were relatively small differences within twin pairs. This is illustrated in Figure 1. Similar results were found for gains in fat mass, percentage body fat, and subcutaneous fat.

Obesity has also been experimentally and clinically linked with both physiological and psychological trauma. Hormonal imbalances, emotional trauma, and alterations in basic homeostatic mechanisms have all been shown to be either directly or indirectly related to the onset of obesity. Environmental factors, such as cultural habits, inadequate physical activity, and improper diets, also make major contributions to excessive fat gain. Thus, obesity is of complex origin, and the specific causes undoubtedly differ from one person to the next. Recognizing this fact is important both in the treatment of existing obesity and in the application of measures to prevent its onset.

Figure 1. Similarity within twin pairs of weight gain in response to a 1,000 kcal increase in dietary intake for 84 days of a 100 day period of study. Reprinted with permission from: Bouchard, C., Tremblay, A., Després, J.-P., Nadeau, A., Lupien, P.J., Thériault, G., Dussault, J., Moorjani, S., Pinault, S., & Fournier, G. (1990). The response to long-term overfeeding in identical twins. New England Journal of Medicine, *322,1477-1482. Each point represents one pair of twins (A and B). The closer the points are to the diagonal line, the more similar the twins are to each other.*

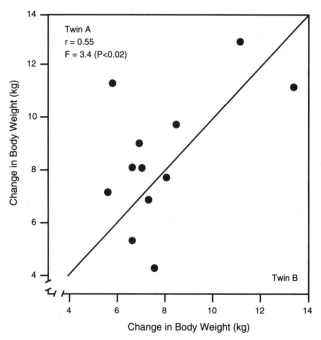

Health Implications of Overweight and Obesity

There is an increased risk for general excess mortality associated with overweight and obesity. This relationship is curvilinear as is illustrated in Figure 2. A large jump in risk occurs when the Body Mass Index (BMI) exceeds a value of 30 kg/m2. The BMI is a simple ratio of body weight divided by height squared, and provides an estimate of obesity. The causes of the excess mortality associated with obesity and overweight include heart disease, hypertension, and diabetes.

It has been recognized since the 1940s that there are major gender differences in the way in which fat is stored or patterned in the body. Males tend to pattern fat in the upper regions of the body, particularly in the abdominal area, while females tend to pattern fat in the lower regions of the body, particularly in the hips, buttocks and thighs. When obese, the male pattern is referred to as upper body, "apple-shaped," or android obesity, and the female pattern is referred to as lower body, "pear-shaped," or gynoid obesity. Research beginning in the late 1970s and early 1980s clearly established upper body obesity as a risk factor for heart disease, hypertension, stroke, elevated blood lipids, and diabetes (Björtorp, et al., 1988). Further, upper body obesity appears to be more important as a risk factor for these diseases than total body fatness. With upper body obesity, the increased risk may be the result of the location of these depots in close proximity to the portal circulatory system.

General Treatment of Obesity

In theory, weight control seems to be a very simple matter. The energy consumed by the body in the form of food must equal the total energy expended, which is the sum of the RMR, TEF, and TEA. The body normally maintains a balance between caloric intake and caloric expenditure. However, when this balance is upset, a loss or gain in weight will result. It would appear that both weight losses and weight gains are largely dependent on just two factors—dietary intake and habitual physical activity. This now appears to be an oversimplification considering the results of the overfeeding study of monozygotic twins discussed earlier in this review, where there was considerable variation in the weight gained for the same amount of overfeeding (Bouchard, et al., 1990). Thus, not everyone will respond the same to the same intervention. This must be considered when designing treatment programs for individuals attempting to lose

Figure 2. Relation of body mass index to excess mortality. From: Bray, G.A. (1985). Obesity: definition, diagnosis and disadvantages. Medical Journal of Australia, *142: S2-S8.*

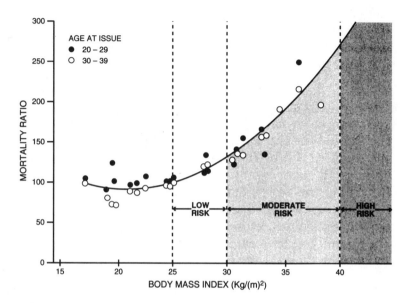

weight. Also, it is important for the individual trying to lose weight to understand this fact, so that he or she will not get discouraged.

Many special diets have achieved popularity over the years, including the Drinking Man's Diet, the Beverly Hills Diet, the Cambridge Diet, the California Diet, Dr. Stillman's Diet, and Dr. Adkin's Diet. Each claims to be the ultimate in terms of effectiveness and comfort in weight loss. Some of the more recent diets have been developed for use either in the hospital or at home under the supervision of a physician. These are referred to as very low calorie diets, as they allow only 350 to 500 kcal of food per day. Most of these have been formulated with a certain amount of protein and carbohydrate in order to minimize the loss of fat-free tissue. Research has shown that many of these diets are effective, but no one single diet has been shown to be any more effective than any other. Again, the important factor is the development of a caloric deficit, while maintaining a balanced diet that is complete in all respects with regard to vitamin and mineral requirements. The diet that meets these criteria and is best suited to the comfort and personality of each individual is the best diet.

Generally, improper eating habits are at least partially responsible for most weight problems, so any given diet should not be looked on as a "quick fix." The individual should be instructed to make permanent changes in his or her dietary habits, particularly reducing the intake of fat and simple sugars. Just eating a low fat diet will gradually bring weight down to desirable levels for most individuals without restricting the quantity of food eaten. For most individuals, reducing the total caloric intake by not more than 250 to 500 kcal per day would be sufficient to accomplish the desired weight loss goals.

Behavior modification has been proposed as one of the most effective techniques for dealing with weight problems. By changing basic behavior patterns, many associated with eating, major weight losses have been achieved. Further, these weight losses appear to be much more permanent, in that the weight is less likely to be regained. This approach appeals to most people since the techniques seem to make sense. For example, individuals might not have to reduce the amount of food they eat, but simply agree that all eating will be done in one location. Or, the individual will be allowed to eat as much as he or she wants, but it must be eaten with the first helping—no second helpings! There are a number of very simple things that can be done to regulate the individual's eating behavior which can result in substantial weight loss.

Hormones and drugs have also been used to assist patients in weight loss, mainly through increasing their RMR. Surgical techniques are also used in the treatment of extreme obesity, but only as a last resort where other treatment procedures have failed and the obesity constitutes a life-threatening situation.

The Role of Physical Activity in Weight Reduction and Control

Inactivity is a major cause of obesity in the United States. In fact, inactivity might be a far more significant factor in the development of obesity than overeating! Thus, exercise must be recognized as an essential component in any program of weight reduction or control.

The Excess Post-Exercise Oxygen Consumption (EPOC)

It has often been stated that physical activity has only a limited influence on changing body composition, and that even exercise of a vigorous nature results in the expenditure of too few calories to lead to substantial reductions in body fat. Yet, research has conclusively demonstrated the effectiveness of exercise training in promoting major alterations in body composition. How do we account for this apparent conflict?

When estimating the energy cost of an activity, it is typical to multiply the average or steady-state rate of energy expenditure for a specific activity times the minutes engaged in that activity. However, the metabolism remains elevated following exercise. This was, at one time, referred to as the oxygen debt, but is now referred to as the excess post-exercise oxygen consumption (EPOC). The recovery of the metabolic rate back to pre-exercise levels can require several minutes for light exercise, several hours for very heavy exercise, and up to 12 to 24 hours or even longer for prolonged, exhaustive exercise.

The EPOC can add up to a substantial energy expenditure when totaled over the entire period of recovery. If the oxygen consumption following exercise remains elevated by an average of only 50 ml/min or 0.05 liter/min, this will amount to approximately 0.25 kcal/min or 15 kcal/hr. If the metabolism remains elevated for five hours, this would amount to an additional expenditure of 75 kcal that would not normally be included in the calculated total energy expenditure for that particular activity. This major source of energy expenditure, which occurs during recovery, but is directly the result of the exercise bout, is frequently ignored in most calculations of the energy cost of various activities. If the individual in this example exercised five days per week, he or she would have expended 375 kcal, or lost the equivalent of approximately 0.1 pounds of fat in one week, or 1.0 pounds in 10 weeks, just from the additional caloric expenditure during the recovery period alone.

Changes in Weight and Body Composition with Exercise Training

A number of studies have shown major changes in both weight and body composition with exercise training. In one study, the investigators investigated the changes in body composition with diet, exercise, and a combination of diet and exercise (Zuti and Golding, 1976). A caloric deficit of 500 kcal per day was maintained by each of three groups of adult women during a 16-week period of weight loss. The diet-only group reduced their normal daily intake by 500 kcal per day, but did not alter their activity levels. The exercise-only group increased their activity by 500 kcal per day, but did not alter their diet. The combination group reduced their caloric intake by 250 kcal and increased their activity by 250 kcal. While there were similar decreases in body weight, the two groups that exercised lost substantially more body fat. A major difference between the two exercise groups and the diet-only group was the gain in fat-free body mass with exercise and its loss with diet-only.

In a second study, 72 mildly obese male subjects were assigned to one of several treatment programs, which included either exercise or non-exercise in combination with different dietary treatments. While the exercise and non-exercise groups lost similar amounts of weight, the exercise group lost significantly more fat weight and did not lose fat-free mass. The non-exercising group lost a significant amount of fat-free mass (Pavlou, et al., 1985).

Not all studies have been able to demonstrate such dramatic changes in weight and body composition with exercise training. However, most studies have found similar trends, in that total weight decreases, fat weight and relative body fat decrease, and fat-free mass is either maintained or increases (Ballor and Keesey, 1991; Stefanick, 1993; Wilmore, 1983). While most of these studies have used aerobic training, several studies have shown impressive decreases in body fat and increases in fat-free mass with resistance training. The evidence is clear that exercise is an important part of any weight loss program. However, it is also clear that to maximize decreases in body weight and body fat, it is necessary to combine exercise with decreases in caloric intake.

Mechanisms for Change in Body Weight and Composition

In looking for ways to explain the above changes in body weight and composition with exercise, it is important to consider both sides of the energy balance equation. When evaluating energy expenditure, it is useful to consider each of the three components of energy expenditure: RMR, TEF, and TEA. When evaluating energy intake, it is also important to consider the energy that is lost in the feces (energy excreted), which is generally less than 5% of the total calories ingested.

The Energy Balance Equation
Energy Intake - Energy Excreted = RMR + TEF + TEA

It has been contended that exercise will stimulate the appetite to such an extent that food intake will be unconsciously increased to at least equal that expended during exercise. Jean Mayer, world-famous nutritionist, reported a number of years ago that animals exercising for periods of from 20 minutes up to one hour per day had a lower food intake than non-exercising control animals (Mayer, et al., 1954). He concluded from this and other studies that when activity is reduced to below a certain minimum level, a corresponding decrease in food intake does not occur and the animal or human begins to accumulate body fat. This has led to the theory that a certain minimum level of physical activity is necessary before the body can precisely regulate, or fine tune food intake to balance energy expenditure. A sedentary lifestyle might reduce the ability of the fine tuning device to control food intake precisely, resulting in a positive energy balance and a weight gain.

Exercise does, in fact, appear to be a mild appetite suppressant, at least for the first few hours following intense exercise training. Further, studies have shown that the total number of calories consumed per day does not change when one begins a training program, even with a greatly increased caloric expenditure. While some have interpreted this as evidence that exercise does not affect appetite, it might be more accurate to conclude that appetite was affected in that caloric intake did not increase in proportion to the additional caloric expenditure resulting from the exercise program. In studies conducted on rats, the food intake of male rats appears to be reduced with exercise training, while female rats tend to eat the same or even more than non-exercising control rats (Oscai, 1973). There is no obvious explanation for this gender difference, and so far similar results have not been reported in humans.

It is possible that the decrease in appetite occurs only with intense levels of exercise in which the increased catecholamine levels might suppress the appetite. It is also possible that the increased body temperature that accompanies high intensity activity, or almost any activity performed under hot and humid conditions, leads to a decreased appetite. When the weather is hot, or when there is an elevated body temperature as a result of illness, there is a loss in the desire for food. This might also explain why there is little or no desire to eat after a hard running workout, but a relatively strong craving for food following a hard swimming workout. In the pool, providing the water temperature is well below core temperature, the heat generated by

621

exercise is lost very effectively making it possible to better regulate core temperature.

The effect of exercise on the components of energy expenditure became a major topic of interest among researchers in the late 1980s and early 1990s. Of obvious interest is how exercise training might affect the RMR, since it represents 60% to 75% of the total number of calories expended each day. If a 25-year-old male's total caloric intake was 2,700 kcal per day, and his RMR accounted for just 60% of that total (0.60 x 2700 = 1620 kcal RMR), just a one percent increase in his RMR would be an extra 16 kcal expended each day, or 5,913 kcal per year. This small increase in RMR alone would account for the equivalent of a 1.7 pound fat loss per year!

The role of physical training in increasing RMR has not been totally resolved. Several cross-sectional studies have found that highly trained runners have higher RMRs than individuals of similar age and size who are untrained. However, other studies have not been able to confirm this (Poehlman, 1989). Few longitudinal studies have been conducted where untrained individuals are trained for a period of time and their changes in RMR are determined. Those longitudinal studies that have been conducted suggest that there might be an increase in RMR following training, but the data are not conclusive (Broeder, et al., 1992). Since RMR is closely related to the fat-free mass of the body, there is now interest in the possible use of resistance training to increase the fat-free mass in an attempt to increase RMR.

A number of studies have been conducted on the role of individual bouts of exercise and exercise training in increasing the TEF It is reasonably clear that a single bout of exercise, either before or after a meal, increases the thermic effect of that meal. Less clear is the role of exercise training on the TEF Studies have shown increases, others have shown decreases, and still others have shown no effect of exercise training on the TEF.

With respect to the specific loss of body fat with exercise, several research studies have pointed to the possible role of human growth hormone as being responsible for the increased fatty acid mobilization during exercise. Growth hormone levels do increase sharply with exercise and remain elevated for up to several hours in the recovery period. Other research has suggested that with exercise the adipose tissue is more sensitive to the sympathetic nervous system, or to the levels of circulating catecholamines, which would result in increased lipid mobilization. More recent research suggests that a specific fat-mobilizing substance, which is highly responsive to elevated levels of activity, is responsible. Thus, it is impossible to state with certainty which factors are of greatest importance in mediating this response.

Spot Reduction, Other Myths, and Exercise Devices

Many individuals, including athletes, believe that by exercising a specific area of the body, the fat in that localized area will be utilized, thus reducing the locally stored fat. Several early research studies reported results that tended to support the concept of spot reduction. However, later research suggested that spot reduction is a myth and that exercise, even when localized, draws from all of the fat stores of the body, not just from the local depots.

One study utilized outstanding tennis players to investigate the phenomenon of spot reduction, theorizing that they would be ideal subjects for studying spot reduction since they could act as their own controls, in that the dominant arm exercises vigorously every day for several hours, while the nondominant arm is relatively sedentary (Gwinup, et al., 1971). They postulated that if spot reduction was a reality, the nondominant (inactive) arm should have substantially more fat than the dominant (active) arm. In fact, while the arm girths were substantially greater in the dominant arm due to exercise-induced muscle hypertrophy, there were absolutely no differences between the arms in subcutaneous skinfold fat thicknesses. Another study reported no difference in the rate of change in fat cell diameters at the abdomen, subscapular and gluteal fat biopsy sites following a 27-day intense sit-up training program, indicating a lack of specific adaptation at the site of exercise training (Katch, et al., 1984). Researchers now theorize that fat is mobilized from either those areas of highest concentration or equally from all areas, thus negating the spot reduction theory. Changes in girth, such as the abdominal girth, can occur with exercise training, but these changes are the result of increased muscle tone, not fat loss.

During the latter part of the 1980s and early 1990s, various professional exercise groups promoted low intensity aerobic exercise to increase the loss of body fat. It has been clearly established that the higher the exercise intensity, the greater the body's reliance on carbohydrate as an energy source. With high intensity aerobic exercise, carbohydrate might supply 65% or more of the body's energy needs. These groups theorized that low intensity aerobic training would allow the body to use more fat as the energy source, thus more effectively reducing the body's fat stores. While it is true that the body uses a higher percentage of fat for energy at lower intensities of exercise, the total number of calories expended from the use of fat is not different. Furthermore, there are substantially more calories expended during the higher intensity workout for the same period of time.

With the popularity of exercise increasing, there are many gimmicks and gadgets on the market. While some of these are legitimate and effective, many are of no practical value for either exercise conditioning or weight loss. Three such devices were evaluated to determine the legitimacy of their claims: the Mark II bust developer; the Astro-Trimmer exercise belt; and the Slim-Skins vacuum pants. The last two devices claimed to take inches off of the abdomen, hips, buttocks and thighs in a matter of minutes, while the first device claimed to add 2 to 3 inches to the bust within 3 to 7 days. All three failed to produce any changes whatsoever when evaluated in tightly controlled scientific studies (Wilmore, et al., 1985a, 1985b). To gain the benefits from exercise it is necessary to actually do the work!

References

Ballor, D.L., & Keesey, R.E. (1991). A meta-analysis of the factors affecting exercise-induced changes in body mass, fat mass and fat-free mass in males and females. *International Journal of Obesity*, 15: 717-726.

Björntorp, P., Smith, U., & Lönnroth, P. (1988). Health Implications of Regional Obesity. *Acta Medica Scandinavica Symposium Series* No. 4, Stockholm: Almqvist & Wiksell International.

Bouchard, C., Tremblay, A., Després, J.-P., Nadeau, A., Lupien, P.J., Thériault, G., Dussault, J., Moorjani, S., Pinault, S., & Fournier, G. (1990). The response to long-term overfeeding in identical twins. *New England Journal of Medicine*, 322, 1477-1482.

Bray, G.A. (1985). Obesity: definition, diagnosis and disadvantages. *Medical Journal of Australia*, 142, S2-S8.

Broeder, C.E., Burrhus, K.A., Svanevik, L.S., & Wilmore, J.H. (1992). The effects of either high intensity resistance or endurance training on resting metabolic rate. *American Journal of Clinical Nutrition*, 55, 802-810.

Gortmaker, S.L., Dietz, W.H. Jr., Sobol, A.M., & Wehler, C.A. (1987). Increasing pediatric obesity in the United States. *American Journal of Diseases of Children*, 141, 535-540.

Gwinup, G., Chelvam, R. & Steinberg, T. (1971). Thickness of subcutaneous fat and activity of underlying muscles. *Annals of Internal Medicine*, 74, 408-411.

Katch, F.I., Clarkson, P.M., Kroll, W., McBride, T., & Wilcox, A. (1984). Effects of sit up exercise training on adipose cell size and adiposity. *Research Quarterly for Exercise and Sport*, 55, 242-247.

Keesey, R.E. (1986). A set-point theory of obesity. In, Brownell, K.D., & Foreyt, J.P. (eds). *Handbook of Eating Disorders: Physiology, Psychology and Treatment of Obesity, Anorexia, and Bulimia*. New York: Basic Books, Inc., pp. 63-87.

Keys, A., Brozek, J., Henschel, A., Mickelsen, O., & Taylor, H.L. (1950). *The Biology of Human Starvation*. Minneapolis: University of Minnesota Press.

Mayer, J., Marshall, N.B., Vitale, J.J., Christensen, J.H., Mashayekhi, M.B., & Stare, F.J. (1954). Exercise, food intake, and body weight in normal rats and genetically obese adult mice. *American Journal of Physiology*, 177, 544-548.

National Center for Health Statistics. (1986). *Health, United States, 1986*. DHHS Publ. No. (PHS) 87-1232. Public Health Service, Washington D.C.: U.S. Government Printing Office, December, 1986.

National Institutes of Health. (1985). Health implications of obesity: National Institutes of Health Consensus Development Conference Statement. *Annals of Internal Medicine*, 103, 1073-1077.

Oscai, L. B. (1973). The role of exercise in weight control. *Exercise and Sport Sciences Reviews*, 1, 103-123.

Pavlou, K.N., Steffee, W.P., Lerman, R.H. & Burrows, V. (1985). Effects of dieting and exercise on lean body mass, oxygen uptake, and strength. *Medicine and Science in Sports and Exercise*, 17, 466-471.

Poehlman, E.T. (1989). A review: exercise and its influence on resting energy metabolism in man. *Medicine and Science in Sports and Exercise*, 21, 515-525.

Sims, E.A.H. (1976). Experimental obesity, dietary-induced thermogenesis and their clinical implications. *Clinics in Endocrinology and Metabolism.* 5. 377-395.

Stefanick, M.L. (1993). Exercise and weight control. *Exercise and Sport Sciences Reviews,* 21, 363-396.

Stunkard, A.J., Foch, T.T., & Hrubec, Z. (1986a). A twin study of human obesity. *Journal of the American Medical Association,* 256, 51 -54.

Stunkard, A.J., Harris, J.R., Pedersen, N.L., & McClearn, G.E. (1990). The body-mass index of twins who have been reared apart. *New England Journal of Medicine,* 322, 1483-1487.

Stunkard, A.J., Sorensen, T.I.A., Hanis, C., Teasdale, T.W., Chakraborty, R., Schull, W.J., & Schulsinger, F. (1986b). An adoption study of human obesity. *New England Journal of Medicine,* 314, 193-198.

Wilmore, J.H. (1983). Body composition in sport and exercise: directions for future research. *Medicine and Science in Sports and Exercise,* 15: 21 -31.

Wilmore, J.H., Atwater, A.E., Maxwell, B.D., Wilmore, D.L., Constable, S.H., & Buono, M.J. (1985a). Alterations in body size and composition consequent to Astro-Trimmer and Slim-Skins training programs. *Research Quarterly for Exercise and Sport,* 56, 90-92.

Wilmore, J.H., Atwater, A.E., Maxwell, B.D., Wilmore, D.L., Constable, S.H., & Buono, M.J. (1985b). Alterations in breast morphology consequent to a 21-day bust developer program. *Medicine and Science in Sports and Exercise,* 17, 106-112.

Zuti, W.B., & Golding, L.A. (1976). Comparing diet and exercise as weight reduction tools. *Physician and Sportsmedicine,* 4, 49-53.

Index